IN WHOSE INTEREST?

IN WHOSE INTEREST?

The privatisation of child protection and social work

Ray Jones

First published in Great Britain in 2019 by

Policy Press
University of Bristol
1-9 Old Park Hill
Bristol
BS2 8BB
UK
t: +44 (0)117 954 5940
pp-info@bristol.ac.uk
www.policypress.co.uk

North America office:
Policy Press
c/o The University of Chicago Press
1427 East 60th Street
Chicago, IL 60637, USA
t: +1 773 702 7700
f: +1 773 702 9756
sales@press.uchicago.edu
www.press.uchicago.edu

© Policy Press 2019

British Library Cataloguing in Publication Data
A catalogue record for this book is available from the British Library.

Library of Congress Cataloging-in-Publication Data
A catalog record for this book has been requested.

ISBN 978-1-4473-5128-3 paperback
ISBN 978-1-4473-5129-0 Pub
ISBN 978-1-4473-5183-2 Mobi
ISBN 978-1-4473-5127-6 ePdf

Cover design by Liron Gilenberg
Printed and bound in Great Britain by TJ International, Padstow
Policy Press uses environmentally responsible print partners

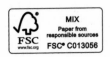

Contents

Foreword by Patrick Butler   vii

About the author   x

Introduction   1

Part 1: The recent history

one   How did we get here? The recent moves to privatise   7
children's social services and social work

two   Creeping political control: the Children and Social Work Bill 52
and anti-professionalism

three   The key players and their networks   91

Part 2: The long haul

four   The formation of the welfare state and its 1980s rejection 109
by Thatcher

five   Thatcher's levers and mechanisms to promote   117
marketisation and privatisation

six   Blair and New Labour's continuation of the journey   137
towards privatisation

seven   Cameron, the coalition and the Conservatives: 154
'Cambornism' and enhanced Thatcherism

Part 3: The impact of privatisation

eight   Privatisation of public services and the undermining 167
of the welfare state

nine   The experience and outcomes of privatising public services 177

ten   The impact to date of the privatisation of social care, 231
social services and social work

Part 4: Changing course

eleven No to TINA: an alternative journey for social work   263
and children's social services

Notes and references   307

Index   377

Foreword

A few years ago I attended a civil service briefing for journalists and stakeholders in a government department in Whitehall. The laptop computer driving the projector – which was to illustrate the theme of the briefing with a series of persuasive graphs and charts – was faulty. After 15 minutes of ineffective tinkering, the officials suggested we could go ahead without the slides. "Why not call IT, and get them to come and fix it?", I asked. Alas, that was impossible, I was sheepishly told. Under the terms of the department's outsourced IT maintenance contract, staff were allowed 30 repair calls a month. Any calls fulfilled by the private IT firm after that would be charged for at a massive premium. The department could not countenance that extra cost in an era of shrinking budgets. So laptops didn't always get fixed. A minor irritation in the great scheme of things, but a useful illustration in miniature of the pitfalls and paradoxes of the phenomenon of outsourced public services: cheaper doesn't always mean more efficient; leaner doesn't automatically mean more effective; and the contract is king.

'What matters is what works' was for some years a voguish rallying cry for those arguing for the privatisation of public services. It's an oddly disinterested phrase, one that suggests that the speaker doesn't care either way who provides the service, although in practice it almost invariably justifies a decision to introduce market disciplines into the welfare state, be it the NHS, older people's care, social security benefits assessments, probation services or even child protection. Privatisation, the enthusiasts proposed, was a matter of managerial common sense and organisational logic, rather than ideological preference. They bought wholesale the great claim of the silver-tongued outsourcers that 'contracting out' to private firms would be intrinsically more dynamic and efficient than leaving services with entrenched and hidebound state-run providers. Private firms would be more nimble, dynamic, and more innovative. A wave of the magic wand of market discipline would transform these moribund services, make them cheaper, better, more efficient.

Of course, state-run services need regular renewal. Without challenge and change they can be monolithic and ponderous, hiding unresponsive and unsafe services behind a flag of public sector virtue. All organisations can become complacent, and ineffective, stifling staff ingenuity and crucially losing focus on the needs of service users. What was curious was how privatisation was seen by some as the only way to re-energise public services. The privatisation hard-sell could be superficially impressive, especially when private firms submitted lower-cost contract bids. But when outsourcing did happen, it was often hard to see any sign of service innovation beyond holding down staff wage bills and slashing backroom costs. Moving in a big private firm often killed off local expertise and disrupted effective working relationships and networks. That brought with it unaccounted-for on-costs. And when public funding began to dry up post-2010 the outsourcers' claims became increasingly hollow. What was now apparent was that hived-off, arm's-length services weren't all that efficient: they were often too distant, too difficult to control (when close control was needed more than ever before); and on too many occasions negligent and incompetent. The likes of G4S, Atos and Carillion – recipients of billions of pounds of public contracts over the past decades – became bywords for greed, cruelty and scandalous mediocrity. If what mattered was what worked, it was clear that privatisation far too often wasn't working.

All this is brilliantly illuminated by Ray Jones in this compelling book. He traces the evolution of the ideology of public service privatisation and outsourcing in the UK from the Thatcherite 1980s onwards, from a relatively niche tool for hiving-off behind-the-scenes departments like payroll, up to and beyond the reckless and unprecedented attempts under the coalition government in 2014 to extend the privatisation boundaries by outsourcing frontline local authority child protection functions to private firms. The outraged public response to this proposal was striking: they saw clearly and immediately the blatant and horrifying conflicts of interests such a move entailed. You don't have to be a social worker to see that a decision as momentous as taking a child from its family could be hopelessly compromised if those in charge of putting the child into care have a potential financial interest in doing so. Or equally, that a decision not to safeguard an at-risk child could be prejudicially influenced if, say, a firm's contractual performance payments are predicated on limiting the numbers of children moving into care. Such matters, the public saw, are complex judgements in which the interests and safety of the child are paramount; not business decisions dictated by contractual requirements and profit margins.

The currently waning appetite for outsourcing is no surprise. As Ray rightly concludes: 'Markets [in public services] have not delivered what was promised on the tin. They have been no guarantee of economy, efficiency or effectiveness, and they have certainly not created equity and fairness. What they have generated is greater inequality and greater vulnerability as they have been exploited for personal gain and profit-taking.' In nearly two decades of reporting on social policy and public services, I have frequently drawn on Ray's wisdom, knowledge and explanatory flair for advice and commentary. He understands social justice, the history of social care and children's services, the political dynamics of government, both in Whitehall and town hall, and the real-life impact of policy decisions on very vulnerable children and families. All this he brings impressively to bear in this terrific book.

Patrick Butler
Social Policy Editor, The Guardian
November 2018

About the author

Dr Ray Jones is emeritus professor of social work at Kingston University and St George's, University of London. He has more than 40 years' experience as a social worker and has been a director of social services, chief executive of the Social Care Institute for Excellence and chair of the British Association of Social Workers. He is a frequent media columnist and commentator, and the author of six books, including the best-selling *The Story of Baby P: Setting the Record Straight* (Policy Press, 2014). In 2017 he received the Social Worker of the Year Award for Outstanding Contribution to Social Work.

Introduction

This book is intended as a contribution to the debate that needs to be further promoted about the government's policies for children's services and social care in England. This is a debate which has urgency, as the government has been moving at pace to pursue its intentions of rapidly increasing the privatisation of social work and developing an even greater marketplace in children's social services and child protection.

It is a book which focuses on England, as what is happening in England is quite different from the other administrations within the United Kingdom. Indeed, the privatisation policies being promoted in England go beyond what is happening anywhere else in the world. They now allow the assessment of children and families, the drafting of children in need and child protection plans, the initiation of court proceedings to remove children from families, and the subsequent decisions as to where children should live and with whom – all integral and crucial activities and responsibilities within statutory children's social work and local authority children's social services – to be contracted out to other organisations including commercial companies, and the big outsourcing companies have already been exploring the opportunities in the marketplace which is being created.

Although the focus of the book is social work, children's social services and child protection in England, it provides an alarm call to other countries and administrations where neoliberal ideology has since the 1980s become ingrained and where competitive marketisation and privatisation is now embedded, distorting the role and remit of what were public services.

In a series of moves fuelled by political ideology and dogma, although now more quietly expressed than previously, social work and social care in England, for children and for adults, are being taken beyond the boundaries of what had previously been

1

seen as sensible and acceptable. Recent Prime Ministers such as Tony Blair, and then David Cameron, and ministers such as Michael Gove and Andrew Lansley, have pushed ahead with the privatisation of public welfare services. When Mr Cameron led the Conservative–Liberal Democrat coalition government, his enthusiasm for the market and private sector and his rhetoric outstripped the aspirations and actions of Margaret Thatcher in the 1980s. Mrs May, his successor as Prime Minister, has shown no sign of changing script or course.

It is the combination of the continuing impact of the bankers' greed-created financial crisis of 2008[1,2] and the subsequent and related politically chosen policies of austerity targeted at poor people and communities, and at public services, that is immersing and overwhelming social work and social care. This is then used to create a narrative that social work and social care are failing, and the prescribed remedy is even more competition and commercialisation.

The journey leading to the current position, however, is a long one, going back 40 years to the mid-1970s. It is a journey now being directed for social work by a surprisingly small number of frequently networked players. The same names keep cropping up, especially among those working with the government to introduce the radical changes it intends for social work, and in particular social work with children and families, and child protection.

I have been taken on this journey myself through my professional career as a social worker and social services manager and director. I started to work in mental health services in 1967, qualified as a social worker in 1972, and now have had 50 years of working life within social work and social services. I have been carried along – and sometimes immersed – by the tidal flow of the waves of increasing marketisation of social care and social services and have been a bit player in some of the policy and practice action. Increasingly less willingly in the 1990s and 2000s I have had to respond to and to accommodate within the services in which I had a leadership role political ideologies and intentions with which I have felt less and less comfortable. But it is the most recent actions of government which have caused me greatest concern and which, if unchecked, will soon have undermined social work and removed social care from the public sector and the values of public and professional service.

This book recounts how powerful forces have across outsourced public services generally pursued profit at the expense of a public service ethos. The journey which is tracked in the book tells of services being taken to cliff edges and up cul-de-sacs, with the public left stranded and sometimes abandoned. And it has then been the remnants of those public services which have been called to the rescue to repair the damage created. It is a journey characterised by greed and exploitation that ranges from the awful Grenfell Tower fire tragedy to children and adults in care homes being left vulnerable by commercial interests trumping care and responsibility.

My 2014 book *The Story of Baby P: Setting the Record Straight*[3] gave an account of how the powerful forces of the press, politicians and the police worked together to target those who spent their working lives seeking to help and protect children for vilification and vengeance following the terrible death of a little boy. This book is also about powerful forces – the press and politicians again, but this time along with a profit-prioritised private sector – who have, through the narrative they have created and through their actions, undermined public services. Their actions too – as with those of *The Sun* tabloid newspaper and others involved in shaping 'the story of Baby P' – will have made the position of those who are vulnerable and who may need protection and assistance less safe.

The book is intended as a clarion call and warning shot about how the current political agenda, if not successfully resisted, will soon have reached the conclusion of making care and social work commercial commodities to be traded with the goal of generating a profit rather than providing a service. Rather like the much bigger, catastrophic issue of global warming, there is the possibility that we have already travelled too far and too fast to now be able to restrain and reverse an inevitable impetus and outcome. This, however, is not certain, so now is the time to be mounting a rearguard action and looking to change course.

Simon Cardy[4] and Paul Michael Garrett[5,6] have already written about the privatisation of children's social services; Kathy

Evans,[7] the chief executive of Children England, and others, have raised the alarm about opening up child protection to the marketplace and commercial companies;[8] Steve Rogowski has written about the increasing political control of social work;[9] and Carolyne Willow of Article 39 and the 'Together for Children' campaigning alliance have opposed the removal of children's rights.[10] These are all, however, still continuing contemporary concerns.

This book starts in Chapter One by charting the very recent developments for social work, children's services and child protection in England which have moved to open them up to a commercialised marketplace. Chapter Two gives particular attention to the very recent social work and children's services legislation which has increased political control of the profession of social work. Chapter Three focuses on the small number of key networked players who have been central to the recent developments. Chapters Four to Seven recount the longer journey, going back to the 1970s, which has provided the platform for the more recent changes. And Chapters Eight to Ten note how what is being put in place for children's social work and child protection replicates what has already happened to much of what were public services but with awful outcomes. But it does not have to be this way, and an alternative is sketched out in the final chapter.

The hope is that the fears described in this book will never come to fruition and that the ultimate result will not be privatised social work services for children and families where profit-focused commercial companies will have the powers to intrude into families and to take crucial decisions about the safety and welfare of children. But looking at what has already happened across the public sector, and at the rhetoric from recent governments in England, the signs are ominous. There is a need to be alert and active in challenging what has already been set in motion.

Part 1
The recent history

ONE

How did we get here? The recent moves to privatise children's social services and social work

For social work and social care it has been a time of crisis. Since 2010 there has been a 40% reduction in central government grant to local authorities,[1] and councils have also been restrained from increasing council tax to replace the government's shrinking funding. And despite the change of prime minister and chancellor in 2016, and Theresa May's rhetoric about helping the 'just managing',[2] those who are 'just managing' and those falling into, or entrenched in, poverty and not managing are promised more austerity, cuts and pain. What funding is available from the government is also being redirected away from areas of high deprivation to more affluent areas[3] – the areas which have been the source of the Conservative government's voting base.

In 2010 the 'New Labour' government's 13 years in power since 1997 came to an end. Although the government, and Gordon Brown as prime minister, were seen to have generally handled well the international banking crisis of 2008 – a crisis for which, however, it carried some responsibility with its previous policies of banking deregulation which let loose unrestrained banker greed and self-centred stupidity across much of the financial sector – it found the popular right-wing press had turned against it, which, in part, created the consequence that the public also looked for a political change.

Even then the Conservative party, with David Cameron as its relatively new leader, did not get a parliamentary majority. To the surprise of many, and especially many who had tactically voted Liberal Democrat in constituencies to defeat Conservative candidates, the Liberal Democrats led by Nick Clegg entered a partnership with the Conservatives to form a coalition government. With Mr Cameron as Prime Minister, George Osborne as Chancellor of the Exchequer, Michael Gove as Secretary of State for Education, and Andrew Lansley as Health Secretary, the die was cast for a future of politically chosen rapid and radical austerity, with the alternative of Keynesian economics of investment to generate employment and growth rejected. But not only was the policy of austerity and cuts rapid and radical, it has also been recidivist, repeated and reinforced year after year, returning public expenditure to the levels of the 1930s.[3] Public services have had their funding dramatically reduced.

At the same time those who especially use public services, such as the poor and those living in areas of high social need, have been made poorer, with some children and families and disabled adults moving from deprivation to destitution. Food and clothing banks (including clothing banks for babies) are the symbol which should now be seen as the trade mark of the coalition and the Conservative governments since 2010. There are now over four million children living in poverty in the UK, and this is projected to increase to over five million by 2021.[4]

This is the context in which social work, in England, is immersed. It is pulled away by the government from social work in the three other UK administrations which have quite a different view of social work and what it offers, with their focus on community, partnership working and public service rather than competition, fragmentation and commercialisation. In England social work is in the midst of creeping privatisation and creeping control by whoever forms the government of the day. And this insidious but coherent thrust towards privatisation and political control is gaining pace.

How to privatise child protection in six easy stages

In November 2013 I wrote a piece published by *The Guardian* which was headed 'How to privatise child protection in six easy stages'.[5] The six stages were, first: rubbish social workers through targeting them in serious case reviews while, secondly, other agencies and professions are placed at the margins of scrutiny and drift out of view. Thirdly, make statements about social workers being politically correct and naïve and then, fourthly, introduce a fast-track education programme which separates, divides and fragments the social work profession into too early specialisation and favours a small cohort of graduates over the majority of social work students. Fifthly, create children's social work and child protection systems which are overwhelmed by service cuts at the same time as more families are struggling because of changes in welfare benefits and the dysfunctional administration of benefits. Lastly, amidst all of these pressures have the national inspectorate make its standards harder to achieve and its gradings more undermining, with 'adequate' now badged as 'requires improvement'.

The Guardian article concluded by noting that:

> the way has been paved for Serco, G4S and venture capitalists to make money from child protection. It will not only lead to increasing costs, but will undermine one of the safest and strongest child protection systems in the world. It's frightening that Gove's government dogma is likely to lead to so much damage and disintegration leaving children less protected. This has been a government journey for some time, but now the destination has become much clearer.

Written in November 2013, the 'six steps to privatisation' turned out to be a considerable underestimate of the much bigger strides, and much greater pace, with which the government would push ahead during 2014. It also did not anticipate how the rhetoric would be ratcheted up several notches by Mr Cameron, the Prime Minister, over the next two years, as noted in the time-line below, and each of the developments noted on the timeline are covered in this chapter.

A timeline of government activity on children's social services, 2013–15

In whose interest?

DECEMBER 2015

CAMERON'S SPEECH ON SIX MONTH DEADLINE ON IMPROVEMENT OR REMOVAL OF SERVICES

CAMERON'S MARKET INSURGENTS SPEECH

CAMERON'S SPEECH ON SOCIAL WORKERS NOT USING COMMON SENSE

DECEMBER 2014

DfE IMPROVEMENT PARTNERS MEETING

DEREGULATION STATUTORY CHANGE

NEW STATUTORY REGULATIONS PUBLISHED ALLOWING CONTRACTING OUT TO PRIVATE AND NOT-FOR-PROFIT PROVIDERS

DfE MARKET-MAKING MEETING

LAINGBUISSON MARKET REVIEW COMMISSIONED

DECEMBER 2013

DRAFT STATUTORY OUTSOURCING REGULATIONS PUBLISHED

GOVE'S SPEECH ON SOCIAL WORKERS TOO CONCERNED WITH POVERTY

10

The two 2014 changes in statutory regulations

The greatest leap forward on the privatisation journey was in April 2014. The government on the day before Good Friday and the Easter bank holiday weekend launched, with no fanfare or publicity, a consultation about changing regulations so that any organisation could be contracted to provide statutory children's social work and child protection services.[7] Not only was this consultation initiated quietly and originally received no attention or profile, but it was also set up as a six-week internet-based consultation on the government's website, with the six weeks including not just the Easter holiday period but also the two May bank holidays.[*]

When the consultation was spotted, I contacted Patrick Butler at *The Guardian* and asked how it might be given publicity and profile. The concern was that the proposals would allow statutory children's social work and child protection to be contracted outside of local authorities, including to private commercial businesses. I was advised that if a significant number of people with credibility and expertise were to send a letter to *The Guardian* expressing concern it might be published on the Letters page, with the possibility of it also getting coverage in the news pages.

A letter was drafted and by the end of the day, and using the Association of Professors of Social Work group email address list, 37 professors of social work had signed and the letter was submitted. The following day not only was the letter published,[8] but *The Guardian* covered it as the front-page story, with Butler writing:

> The power to take children away from their families could be privatised along with other child protection

---

[*] If six weeks seems a short time for a government national consultation, it is three times the time allowed, only two weeks, in 2017 for a national 'Consultation on the Revised Statutory Guidance for Local Authorities on the Care of Unaccompanied Asylum Seeking and Trafficked Children', which was to run from 3 March until 17 March 2017 (https://consult.education.gov.uk/children-in-care/care-of-unaccompanied-and-traffickedchildren/supporting_documents/Consultation%20 Document.pdf) and was criticised by the British Association of Social Workers (https://outlook.live.com/owa/?path=/attachmentlightbox).

services under controversial plans the government has quietly announced. The proposal from Michael Gove's Department for Education (DfE) to permit the outsourcing of children's social services in England to companies such as G4S and Serco has alarmed experts. They say profit-making companies should not be in charge of such sensitive family matters, and warn that the introduction of the profit motive into child protection may distort the decision-making process. A DfE consultation paper published last month argues that enabling local authorities to outsource children's social services will encourage innovation and improve outcomes for at-risk youngsters. Private providers will allow authorities to 'harness third-party expertise' and 'stimulate new approaches to securing improvements' for safeguarding services outside 'traditional hierarchies', the document says.[9]

It was clear the proposed change in regulation would have allowed private, for-profit, companies, among what the DfE called 'third party providers', to be contracted to provide children's social work and child protection services:

The DfE said it was responding to demand from councils and there was no requirement for any council to outsource to a private company. 'There will be no obligation for councils to take up these freedoms and any that do will still be held accountable by Ofsted. We will take into account all responses to the consultation before setting out next steps'.[10]

'No requirement', but private companies were to be allowed to be awarded these contracts.

Following the coverage in *The Guardian* and other media, including the BBC,[11] three public petitions were launched opposing the government's proposals. By the end of the brief consultation period, 71,797 people had signed the petitions and the government had also had 1,315 responses to the consultation, 94% of whom disagreed with the government's proposals.[12]

The government published at the end of June 2014 its comments on the feedback received from the consultation. It noted that:

> By far the most common theme [within the responses to the government's consultation paper] was the prospect of 'privatising children's services' and the introduction of a potentially contradictory profit making imperative to work with vulnerable children ... A related point was that local authorities would be motivated in their choice of provision by questions of cost rather than quality ... [There were also concerns about] the dilution of local authority accountability [and about] the break up or fragmentation of services that would result from delegation of functions.[13]

The message to the government was clear – there should be no contracting of statutory children's social work services to private profit-making companies. And the reasons for the message were also clear – there should be no distortion introduced by companies seeking profits, no overwhelming focus on cost rather than quality, no confused accountability and no fragmentation.

Did the government hear and take on board the overwhelming and consistent consultation response? Apparently, it did, stating that:

> The Government recognises the scale of concern in relation to the inclusion of a profitmaking motive in the proposed range of additional delegable functions – in particular child protection. The government's intentions in bringing forward these proposals was to allow local authorities to consider a broader range of delivery and reporting structures, enabling greater structural innovation and the harnessing of external expertise in pursuit of improved social work practice and better outcomes for children. The proposals were concerned with improving the quality of children's services, rather than savings, 'privatisation' or profitmaking. Indeed the local authorities currently

exploring possibilities are considering mutualised and community-interest structures. In this context, the Government is happy to respond directly to the primary concern raised in the consultation and is making an amendment to the draft regulations which would prevent profit-making bodies from carrying out additional delegable functions on behalf of local authorities ... Whatever arrangements a local authority chooses to pursue, Ofsted will continue to inspect all children's services, will look at arrangements with commissioned providers, and issue judgments on the local authority's performance in meeting its duties.[14]

A few reflections on the above statement from the government. First, the government acknowledged the high level of concern and opposition to its Spring 2014 proposals. Secondly, why it singled out 'privatisation' as a concern to be placed in inverted commas is a mystery, suggesting that there was no such process as 'privatisation'. Thirdly, having acknowledged the concerns, and presumably accepting their validity, the government stated it would change its intentions and make it explicit that for-profit bodies would not be allowed to receive contracts from local authorities giving them delegated responsibility for statutory social work and child protection services. And, fourthly, all of these services, whether provided directly by a local authority or contracted to a not-for-profit organisation, would still continue to be inspected in their own right by Ofsted.

However, even without the possibility of private commercial companies being contracted to provide statutory children's social services, this was still a fundamental change of principle and practice being taken forward by the coalition government. It meant that no longer would children in need and child protection assessments have to be undertaken by local authorities. No longer would local councils have to take decisions themselves about seeking court orders to remove children from their families. And councils would not be the only bodies that could initiate care proceedings and, if care orders were made by the courts, decide where and with whom children would live away from their families.

All of these statutory responsibilities, and more, could be contracted outside of local authorities to charities, trusts, and community interest companies. In the past, only local authorities could hold these crucial responsibilities, and take these major decisions, about the welfare and safety of children. The National Society for the Prevention of Cruelty to Children (NSPCC) had historically had the power to investigate child abuse concerns and to make applications for care proceedings to remove children from families, but it stopped using these powers in the 1980s and no longer is a front-line child protection agency undertaking child abuse investigations.

Now local authorities were to be able, if they chose, to delegate these major state responsibilities to others, albeit with the local authority still accountable as the body contracting out these services. But the government was clear – the responsibilities must not and could not be contracted to profit-making bodies.

On a Friday at about 1 pm, I had a phone call from a senior civil servant in the Department for Education. He told me that in response to the concerns raised through the consultation the government was announcing that afternoon that it was changing the draft statutory regulation. It would be made clear that profit-making companies would not be allowed to receive contracts to provide statutory children's social work and child protection services. I commented that this was a positive reaction by the government. But I also noted that what was still being proposed and intended was a fundamental change, and there should still be concerns that crucial roles in safeguarding and protecting children would be able to be contracted outside of local authority direct provision and that public accountability for these services would only be through the management of a contract.

I was intrigued why I had received the phone call. I had never received such a call from a senior civil servant before or since. Was it just a courtesy call as I had had a role in making public an issue which the government had seemed to me to be quietly slipping under the radar? If so, presumably others who had contributed to making the issue and the concerns public would also have had phone calls. As far as I know, no one else received such a phone call. Or was it that – unlike the lack of profile and publicity for the government's intended changes when the initial consultation was very quietly launched only eight weeks before – this time the government wanted to ensure as much media coverage as possible, and maybe it was anticipated I would that afternoon be alerting my media contacts to the government's change of policy?

Whatever was intended, I did nothing, in part because I realised on reflection that I had not clearly understood the nature of the call, and whether the information I had been given was embargoed until the Department for Education issued its public and press statement. However, at about 4 pm I had a call from Patrick Butler at *The Guardian* asking if I had seen the then recently issued Government statement. *The Guardian's* coverage the following day was headed 'Government U-turn over privatising child protection services' and went on to note that:

> Proposals to allow local authorities in England to privatise child protection services have been abandoned. The Department for Education said on Friday that profit-making organisations would be barred from carrying out core child safeguarding duties, although councils would still be able to bring in charities and not-for-profit firms if they wished. The decision follows criticism from experts – including social work academics, professionals and charities – that opening up child protection to the market would distort decision-making and dilute local accountability over sensitive matters such as taking a child into care … Ministers had argued that allowing the outsourcing of child protection would enable more innovative approaches and improve services for youngsters at risk, but the strength of opposition forced them into a swift climb down.[15]

The Guardian report further noted that:

> Ray Jones, professor of social work at Kingston University, who organised a letter condemning the

move signed by 37 leading social work academics, also applauded the U-turn. Local authorities can still contract out these responsibilities to not-for-profit organisations, but there is no route in here for the likes of G4S, Serco, Virgin Healthcare and Atos.

(However, I was wrong, and the government was shortly to be found to be somewhat ingenuous.)

The article continued:

The children's minister, Edward Timpson, said: "We want to offer local authorities the freedom to deliver services differently in order to achieve better outcomes for vulnerable children – to make the adequate good and the good outstanding. If we are going to achieve the very best for our most vulnerable children, we must harness the expertise, passion and drive of all those who want to serve children's needs."

Edward Timpson was the Children's Minister leading for the government on the proposed changes to the children's services statutory regulations in 2014. He had been a long-serving children's minister in the Department for Education, and was still in post in 2017 leading for the government on the Children and Social Work Bill. It was the recollection of the government's less than straightforward actions and statements in 2014 which led some to be less trusting of the government's intentions in 2017.

What happened in 2014 was that when the government did issue its revised draft statutory regulation it did not do what it had been understood to have promised. It did not exclude private, for-profit, organisations from receiving contracts to provide statutory children's social work and child protection services. This is what it said instead in the 'Explanatory Memorandum' to the new statutory regulations:

The regulations will not prevent an otherwise profit-making company from setting up a separate non-profit making subsidiary to enable them to undertake such functions.[16]

It also stated that:

> Local authorities will remain ultimately accountable
> for decisions taken by the third party to which they
> delegate functions. As with the present arrangements,
> it will be entirely for local authorities to decide
> whether or not to delegate functions.[17]

Despite the previous undertaking that commercial, for-profit, companies would not be allowed to be contracted to provide statutory children's social work and child protection services, the regulation which was introduced in September 2014 explicitly noted that they could now do so, albeit that they would have to set up a not-for-profit subsidiary (from which, as will be noted below, they could then make a profit).

So what had been said by the government in the summer of 2014 was found to be misleading. It was soon to be found that the statement that it would be 'entirely for local authorities to decide whether or not to delegate functions' was also misleading, as the government had the power, which it has since used, to move statutory children's social services outside of some local authorities.

It proved impossible to get much media coverage or traction on the story of how the government had made misleading statements in the summer and that for-profit companies would now be able to provide child protection and statutory children's social work services and to have delegated to them the powers to intrude and intervene within families. The story was no longer 'news'. It had been covered in May and in June and had moved past its sell-by-date.

In September 2014 when the revised draft statutory regulation was considered and debated in Parliament, what was presented by Mr Timpson on behalf of the Conservative and Liberal Democrat coalition government went unopposed by the Labour opposition.

There were informed Labour members of Parliament who wanted the opposition to vote against the revised draft regulation, but they were not, despite their requests, appointed by Labour to the committee considering the regulatory proposal. Three Labour MPs, in particular, were active in the discussions in the Committee considering the draft regulation, but two were present as voluntary attendees rather than appointed committee members. Each had a professional background as a social worker within local authority children's services.

The first was Steve McCabe. At the time he was the shadow Children's Minister. A Birmingham MP since 1997, elected at the same time as Tony Blair became Prime Minister and 'New Labour' came into government, McCabe had previously qualified and worked as a social worker, manager of a hostel for adolescent boys, social work lecturer and social work education advisor within the Central Council for the Education and Training of Social Workers (CCETSW). He led for Labour in the House of Commons consideration of the revised draft regulation. Here is what he said in the committee discussion:

> If people's worse fears are realised and these measures prove to be the route to fragmentation, unaccountable, unregulated provision, riddled with conflicts of interest and dubious financial incentives, a future Government will have to repeal them. By that time, however, thousands of children might have suffered needlessly.[18]

As the shadow Children's Minister, it is surprising, having had the very serious concerns expressed above, that he and the Labour opposition did not seek to have a vote on the draft regulation but allowed it to be progressed without formal opposition.

Meg Munn became an MP in 2001. Within the Labour government she had been a Minister for Women and Equalities, and a minister in the Foreign Office. In 2015 she did not seek re-election as an MP. Prior to becoming an MP, Munn had been a social worker and a social work manager including, in the year prior to her election to Parliament, assistant director for children's services with York City Council.

At the time the revised draft regulation was considered by the House of Commons committee, Meg Munn was chair of the Child Protection All Party Parliamentary Group. She was opposed to the proposed regulatory change. In June 2014 she is reported to have spoken against the proposals and urged the government to think again over its proposals to permit the outsourcing of children's services, and to make abuse investigations exempt from the plans ... Munn went on to warn that 'there is a big difference between providing therapeutic services to children and being responsible for the investigation of suspected child abuse'. Echoing fears voiced by academics and other senior social work professionals, she expressed concerns that outsourcing child protection work, while leaving local authorities with ultimate responsibility for its quality, would 'exacerbate risks' to young people by unnecessarily adding 'another layer of accountability, monitoring and checking'.[19]

And, as the proposals were considered in September 2014 by the House of Commons committee, Munn had an article published in *The Guardian* which said:

> Other more complex issues were not widely considered [through the government's consultation], such as independent organisations intruding into family life, and the question of data sharing between public, private and third sector organisations. The full implications of these changes to the most sensitive areas of children's services have not been explored. While many children's services are provided by charities, it would be a significant change to let them undertake child protection investigations and assessments and seek court orders to remove children from families ... An outsourced, fragmented system with long lines of accountability will put children at risk.[20]

In the House of Commons committee debate, Munn commented:

> The Minister has stated that local authorities will retain overall accountability, but once functions are delegated, how will local authorities retain sufficient expertise and experienced staff to effectively monitor the contract? Once contracted out, how will the changing pressures in children's social work be

managed? The local authority will be responsible, but will it have the mechanisms to do that? The chief social worker, Isabelle Trowler, has argued that 'For local authorities the same legal duties will apply... they will be subject to precisely the same inspection regime whether or not they choose to delegate functions. That critical thread of accountability is unaffected by anything being proposed.' Frankly, that misses the point; the local authority remains accountable but will be restricted in its ability to act. How can it show democratic accountability for processes that intrude into the lives of children and families?[21]

Another Labour MP who opposed the regulatory changes in 2014 had also been a social worker. Emma Lewell-Buck had become an MP in 2013, being elected in a by-election after David Miliband lost to his brother the Labour leadership contest to replace Gordon Brown and then resigned his seat in Parliament. Lewell-Buck had previously worked as a front-line local authority children's social worker within child protection in north east England. In October 2016 she was appointed by Jeremy Corbyn as the shadow Minister for Children and played a leading role in 2017 (as will be discussed later) in getting the Conservative government to withdraw controversial clauses in the Children and Social Work Bill.

Like Meg Munn, Emma Lewell-Buck was not appointed by Labour to the committee considering the regulatory changes in September 2014 but, like Munn, she attended the committee and spoke against the changes. In her comments she noted particular concerns about the confused accountability, and potential conflicts of interests, which could arise from local authorities contracting children's social work responsibilities to other bodies:

> Another issue that has repeatedly come up in my discussions with child protection professionals is accountability. Under the proposals, a local authority that delegates its functions remains accountable for the quality of service, even though delivery is the

contractor's responsibility. The local authority will still be required to oversee service delivery, and it will be blamed when things go wrong, but its ability to influence the quality of service will be greatly reduced.

Nor will it be clear to families who is responsible for failures. I really pity those families with a complaint or a genuine grievance who approach the delegated agency about it and are told they have to go to the local authority. Families in the child protection arena already have enough to contend with. In his letter [written to Mrs Lewell-Buck after she had raised concerns with Mr Timpson], the Minister insisted that accountability lay squarely with the local authority, but it will not appear that way to families in the system. Muddling accountability poses the danger of further damaging public confidence in child protection.

I welcome the Government's clarification that for-profit firms will not be able to take on child protection functions, but it remains the case that a for-profit company can have a non-profit arm and carry out these functions. That can create conflicts of interest—for example, if the parent company also delivers private fostering services.

I remain unconvinced that outsourcing can improve services. Serious case reviews over the decades have cited a lack of information sharing between the myriad agencies operating in the child protection arena as contributory factors in the death of children, from Maria Colwell just over 40 years ago to Daniel Pelka in 2012. Creating more agencies will not mitigate that; it will simply increase the risk of miscommunication and data loss, and provide more gaps for information to slip through, creating more opportunities for more children to suffer significant harm.[22]

Although MPs who had direct experience of being social workers and of working within child protection services spoke against the proposed regulatory change, the change went ahead and is now in place. Any organisation, including profit-making companies, so long as they have set up an (apparent) not-for-profit subsidiary, can now be contracted to take on statutory children's social work and child protection functions and responsibilities. The organisation can make its profit by requiring its subsidiary to buy from the parent company services and goods, and pay rents, at whatever price is determined by the parent company. The parent company can also set the salaries and bonuses to be paid to the senior managers of its subsidiary, and the experience of schools now within academy chains is that these rewards can be very high.[23]

The Department for Education and the private companies

At the very same time that the House of Commons committee was considering this regulatory change, the Department for Education convened a meeting attended by the big outsourcing companies to consider how to create a marketplace for statutory children's social services. The meeting was to consider how to encourage new providers to take on these services. Bearing in mind that this meeting was organised and held before the draft regulation was considered in Parliament and before it became law, it did seem to be jumping the gun and somewhat presumptive and arrogant for a government department and its civil servants to be moving ahead without, at the time, a legal mandate for what they were seeking to promote.

The meeting was chaired by Lord Warner. Lord Warner was a Labour peer[*] and former civil servant who had left the civil service to become director of social services for Kent County Council. He joined the House of Lords in 1998, and within Tony Blair's Labour government he had been a minister in the

---

[*] Lord Warner continues as a peer in 2018, but he resigned from the Labour whip in 2015 after Jeremy Corbyn was elected as Labour leader, and moved to sit in the Lords as a crossbencher.

Department of Health. It is reported that subsequently, while an active peer in the House of Lords, he was also a paid consultant and advisor to several private companies who sought access to and benefited from public service and healthcare contracts.[24]

In 2013 Warner wrote about the coalition government's proposed changes to the procurement and contracting of health services:

> The NHS faces enormous financial and clinical challenges over the next decade. The public accounts committee, under a Labour chair, has made clear that virtually every NHS trust is unsustainable in its present form. A massive programme of service reconfiguration now awaits if it is to survive the unavoidable fiscal, demographic and morbidity challenges it faces. Two acute hospital trusts have gone bust in the past few months and there are probably another 20 well on the road to the same fate. It is a fantasy to believe that we can solve the NHS's problems without the help of many new providers with fresh ideas and better management techniques. Other countries facing the same problems are doing just this. To allow new entrants from the private, voluntary and social enterprise sectors to enter the NHS market a set of fair procurement rules are required and that is what the new regulations do.[25]

In 2014 Lord Warner was appointed by Michael Gove as the commissioner for children's services provided by Birmingham City Council. This followed Ofsted reports that the services in Birmingham were 'inadequate', and a report by Sir Julian Le Grand, Alan Wood and Isabelle Trowler, whose involvement in Birmingham and elsewhere is discussed in Chapter Three.

At the time Lord Warner was seen as an advocate for creating markets for public services (although a different view of Norman Warner's positioning might be taken in 2016 when he argued against Birmingham being coerced by the government to contract out its children's services and in 2017 when he opposed the so-called 'innovation clauses' in the Children and Social

Work Bill – see Chapter Two), and this was the focus of the September 2014 DfE invitation-only seminar which he chaired. This generated an article in October 2014 in *The Guardian* by Patrick Butler. Butler wrote:

> The government's aspirations to kickstart a market in child protection services and make it easier for councils to outsource safeguarding functions continue apace. The Guardian can reveal that ministerial advisors presented detailed proposals to firms and charities last month at a private Whitehall meeting described by one attendee as a 'sales pitch'. The proposals, which would radically shake up children's social services in England, put flesh on the bone of Coalition plans floated in the summer to inject 'competition and contestability' into one of the last areas of local government not subject to market forces.[26]

Those attending the seminar included Edward Timpson, the Children's Minister, and outsourcing companies such as Virgin Care and Amey,* along with firms of management consultants. Butler provided a quote from an attendee at the seminar who described it 'as a sales pitch for privatising core children's social work activity' and also noted that 'one insider' told *The Guardian* that 'this is radically different to existing outsourcing. This is crown jewels stuff'.

In December 2014 the DfE held another meeting.[27] This time it was about creating additional capacity to improve children's social services. It was attended by, amongst others, G4S, KPMG, Mouchel and Amey. *The Guardian* article I wrote in early January 2015 following the DfE's December meeting was headed 'Plans to privatise child protection are moving at pace'.[28] It attracted considerable interest with over 14,700 'shares'.

---

* As with so many companies getting contracts for what have been the UK's public services, Amey is not UK-owned but is a subsidiary of Ferrovial, a Spanish company. The distant international ownership, and the final resort of the profits being made, is rarely advertised or publicly known.

So, in September and December 2014, while the change in statutory regulation was being introduced, the DfE was engaging in discussions with G4S, Serco, Virgin Care, Mouchel and Amey (the latter better known for building roads) as to how to generate change in children's social work services and how to create a marketplace for these services. Presumably these companies were committing money and time to engage with the DfE as they saw potential opportunities to benefit their businesses by entering and expanding into what was now being called the children's social services 'industry'.[29,30]

Alongside the autumn 2014 DfE meetings attended by the big outsourcing companies and accountancy firms, there were three other developments relevant to the privatisation journey. One was about making the children's services market more attractive for these companies. The second was to explore further how to promote this marketplace. And the third was to make progress on removing statutory children's social work and child protection outside of local authorities.

With the September change in statutory regulation already allowing other organisations to be contracted to provide these services, a further regulatory change reduced – indeed largely removed – the regulatory 'burden' from these organisations, making it more attractive and less costly for them to take on the new contracts which would now be allowed.

This was to be achieved by changes in a wide-ranging 'Deregulation Bill', of which children's social services was only a minor part. Once again, there was no formal opposition by Labour in the House of Commons to the children's social work services deregulation proposals in the coalition government's Bill. Instead it was debate in the House of Lords which highlighted the danger of deregulation. Baroness Donaghy, a Labour peer, commented:

> The Government propose that the external providers of social work services will not be inspected in their own right by Ofsted, and nor will they be registered as providers in the way that children's homes and adoption societies are. There will be no overview of their activities across local authorities where they

hold contracts and no visible assurances for the public about their financial viability, quality standards or working practices. Unison, the trade union that represents social workers, believes that the regulation and inspection of social care services are essential to safeguarding vulnerable children and their families. It also said that regulations should not be regarded as a burden in this extremely sensitive area.[31]

Baroness Donaghy continued:

Internal contract monitoring by local authorities cannot be relied on by itself to ensure that acceptable standards in the safety and quality of social work with looked-after children are upheld. By removing the separate registration of providers, the Government are relying on Ofsted to pick out issues about their fitness to operate as part of its inspections of individual local authorities. However, providers could operate across many local authority areas. Local authorities already face challenges because of funding cuts and it is likely that contracts will be held by larger private or voluntary sector contractors. Close ties with local authority teams and systems will be weakened; their interests and priorities will be different from those of the client authority. The drivers of service provision will be cost driven. Relying on local authority inspection will be inadequate and emphasises the need for a single registration point.[32]

She concluded by asking for the children's social work deregulation proposals to be withdrawn:

It also creates a lack of symmetry in the system by requiring providers of children's homes and fostering and adoption placements to be registered and inspected in their own right while providers of social work services—which are exercising major statutory functions, taking sensitive and critical decisions about placements for children—are not required to do so. How can the Government defend such inequality? Do the Government think that providing social work services is somehow less important? Are the Government confident that this act of abandonment will not lead to a lowering of standards?[33]

Despite the concerns raised in the House of Lords, the coalition government's deregulation proposals were enacted. The consequence from the two 2014 changes in statutory regulations concerning children's social work and child protection services is that any organisation can now be contracted to provide these services and they will not be required to be regulated, registered or inspected by Ofsted. Instead, it is the local authority that awards the contract that will still be held to account and be inspected and rated by Ofsted as the contract manager. The outsourced services will only be visited by Ofsted inspectors as a part of inspecting and performance grading the council and no separate report will be prepared and published by Ofsted on the organisation now providing the services.

The second development which was moved ahead in autumn 2014 was the preparation of a DfE-commissioned report on how to develop more of a market for statutory children's social work and child protection services. It followed a recommendation by Julian Le Grand, Alan Wood and Isabelle Trowler in their report on children's services in Birmingham that:

> The DfE commission a specific study on developing capacity to assist in the intervention options, involving the possible splitting of commissioning from provision, that are available to the Secretary of State in responding to a failure of a local authority to secure services which protect children and young people. The study should be presented by 30 September 2014.[34]

This recommendation appeared in a report to the Secretary of State, at that time Michael Gove, and the Minister of State for Children and Families, Edward Timpson. A DfE-commissioned study, as recommended by Le Grand, Wood and Trowler, was launched in June 2014 with the contract awarded to LaingBuisson, a market analysis company.

Le Grand, Wood and Trowler were appointed by the government as advisors to oversee the study, with it noted in the final report that 'the Advisory Panel at the Department for Education (DfE) encouraged the authors of this report to be ambitious and we have sought to be so'.[35] Indeed, as it turned out, the report was so 'ambitious' in its recommendations to create a marketplace for children's social work and child protection that it was long-delayed in its publication by the government, despite freedom of information requests about what had happened to it.[36] By the time it was published (in December 2016) there was a new Secretary of State (although Mr Timpson was still the Minister for Children), and the government distanced itself from the report and from the ambition encouraged by Le Grand, Wood and Trowler.[37] But more on this later in this chapter.

The third development in autumn 2014 was that the government motored on and increased the momentum to remove statutory children's social work services from direct delivery by local authorities.

The momentum to move services out from local authorities

In 2013 Michael Gove, as Secretary of State for Education, ordered that Doncaster Council transfer its statutory children's social services to an independent trust. This followed serious concerns about the quality of the services provided by the council as noted in Ofsted inspections and numerous case reviews. This history went back to the mid-2000s, when a combination of what seemed an idiosyncratic elected mayor and a new chief executive with no experience of public service senior management in the UK, appointed a manager with a commercial background in frozen foods as Doncaster's director of children's services. Doncaster hit the national headlines in 2009 following very serious assaults on and abuse of two boys in Edlington by two other boys.

On 1 October 2014 the Doncaster Children's Trust was launched to provide statutory children's services outside of the council. Mr Gove had decided that Doncaster Council should no longer directly provide children's social work and child protection services, following a report and recommendation from Julian Le Grand, Alan Wood and Moira Gibb.[38]

In a *Guardian* article published on the day the Doncaster Trust was launched, Patrick Butler commented that Wood saw what was to happen in Doncaster as applicable to other councils, including those councils which were currently stable:

> But although the impetus for structural reform like Doncaster's has been child protection failure, Wood is adamant that change to the commissioning and delivery of children's services is essential if performance is to be maintained in currently stable councils, not least because budgets are shrinking and demand is rising. 'There is less money; we [will not be able to] do what we do now, so can we do it differently?' ... There is enthusiasm, from Wood and the DfE, for taking Doncaster-style reform even further, using new powers of delegation to attract private and voluntary sectors, and to contract out the commissioning of children's services. Wood is impatient at what he feels is the lack of urgency with which some underperforming children's services departments have set about transforming themselves: 'We are talking about kids and families in a difficult position. You can't just dribble along.'[39]

In the *Guardian* article there was, however, a warning from Annie Hudson, who had been the director of children's services in Bristol, rated by Ofsted as 'good', and was at the time chief executive of the College of Social Workers:

> Hudson argues that it is crucial that children's services departments develop 'high-quality, innovative, responsive' children's services, but she warns against getting into 'an ideology driven, non-evidence based

debate' about how to make those improvements. There are serious issues around accountability and fragmentation that accompany the drive to outsource. Council commissioning skills are still 'embryonic', and there are questions around transparency of services, the quality of regulation and the role of profit in key decisions around children.[40]

The October 2014 transfer of Doncaster's statutory children's services outside of the council's direct delivery was not a quick fix. A year later the children's social services were inspected by Ofsted, and the council (not the trust, as the statutory responsibility was still held by the council) was rated as 'inadequate' for helping and protecting children.[41] This should not be a surprise. Much time and attention would have been given to setting up and embedding the trust arrangements, and this would have in itself created a delay in driving improvement.

A further year later Ofsted revisited the Doncaster Trust and, although this was not a full re-inspection, found 'significant progress from a low-baseline'.[42] It has been reported, however, that the council's chief executive, Jo Miller, commented:

As for children's services, Miller says she and the council did not think a trust was the right answer, but says they have worked to make sure the trust would get the best possible results – a view echoed by Ofsted in September, which praised Doncaster's 'significant progress' for children's services. But Miller thinks the improvement was in spite of the trust structure, not because of it. 'Yes, services to children have improved since the trust came along,' she says. 'But so have all the services in the council. Children's services haven't improved any quicker – and the trust costs a lot more money.'[43]

The Doncaster Trust is not the first example of a council transferring its statutory children's social work and child protection services outside of its direct control, although it is the first time (but not the last – see below) a council was forced by the government to stop direct delivery of the services.

In 2013 Kingston and Richmond Councils decided to combine their children's social services and then to set up and contract out the services to an independent community interest company which was called 'Achieving for Children', with it reported that:

> Efficiency and innovation was the initial motivation behind the recent merger of Richmond and Kingston's children's services into a single, not-for-profit body called Achieving for Children (although after the initiative had got underway, Kingston received consecutive 'inadequate' ratings from Ofsted). 'The driving force was our belief that we knew cuts in income were coming and we could do things at better value,' says AfC's chief executive, Nick Whitfield … [he argued that] AfC's operational distance from its joint local authority owners (although Whitfield remains their joint director of children's services) will enable it to 'really focus on the needs of children and families'. … Whitfield is cautious, however. He says AfC is 'not keen on privatisation' and nor will it use its autonomy to drive down the pay and conditions of new staff. 'There's no private company coming in and taking a cut,' he says, adding: 'We are not looking to do big outsourcing … We won't be contracting out major parts of our services.'[44]

It was later announced in October 2016 that Windsor and Maidenhead Council was contracting out its children's social services to Achieving for Children, with it commented that:

> Nick Whitfield, chief executive of AfC said he was 'confident' there will be mutual benefits in the long term partnership. 'We're all operating in a tough financial climate, and joining services together across Kingston and Richmond has already helped us to reduce our back office costs and improve services for

vulnerable children and young people. Any options to make further efficiencies in this area are worth looking at'.[45]

For Whitfield, it was the prospect of cuts and needing to curtail costs which was a major driver for services to be contracted by councils to Achieving for Children, and he was explicit in his concerns about privatisation. But a bridge has been crossed and a principle has been parked in that for the first time statutory children's social work and child protection responsibilities have been contracted outside the direct delivery of public services to an independent company. This may be a Trojan horse which opens the way for others to seek to provide these services outside of local government.

There are five further concerns. First, there will have been set-up costs for the new community interest company and as its only income is from the councils with which it has contracts these have to be covered by the public funds it receives. Secondly, there will be additional future cash and transactional costs, as the company will have to report back to the councils, and the councils will need to have a contract management capacity to oversee their contracts with the company. Thirdly, there is the increased complexity in accountability. The councils still hold their statutory responsibilities but no longer manage and decide on the services day to day. Fourthly, there is less transparency as an independent company is not subject to the same public reporting and freedom of information requirements as a public body such as a local authority and, if it chooses, can hide behind a cloak of commercial confidentiality. And finally, as Achieving for Children now seeks to expand to other areas of the country,[46] it distances its top management from the oversight of local services and engagement with local communities.

Many of these concerns also apply where local authorities have been forced or coerced by the government to contract out their children's services to independent trusts which have been set up specifically to take on these services.[47,48] And here there seems to be political bias and skew. As at the end of March 2017 four councils had been pushed into contracting out their children's services – Doncaster, Slough, Sandwell and Birmingham – and they are all Labour-controlled councils. No Conservative-controlled council up until 2018 had been forced or coerced by the coalition and Conservative governments to take this action, despite their Ofsted reports often showing that they were in as much, if not more, difficulty. And a further Labour council, Sunderland, where Nick Whitfield had been appointed by the government to advise on what should happen to children's services (while at the same time remaining as chief executive of Achieving for Children), was now being set off down this route:

> Nick Whitfield, commissioner for children's services in Sunderland, said: 'Sunderland is the first council to look at voluntarily transferring its services out of council control in cooperation with the Department for Education so the new company will be the first of its type in the country. The council has been very co-operative in recognising the need to do something different and that is something it deserves credit for. This is a real opportunity to deliver innovative children's services that can ensure further improvement and sustained delivery.'[49]

More recently Reading, another Labour council, has been ushered by the government in the direction of setting up a company to run its children's services, and there is now, also in 2018, for the first time, a Conservative-controlled council – Worcestershire County Council – which following government intervention is moving its children's services outside of its direct management.

How Ofsted has been used to drive the removal of children's services from local authorities

What triggers the government's sending in a 'commissioner' to advise the Secretary of State for Education and the Minister for Children on what action to take about a council's children's services is an Ofsted inspection concluding with an 'inadequate' judgement for the local authority.

I have been a part of this process, not as a government-appointed commissioner but as the independent chair of the 'children's improvement boards' which the government had required to be set up, in five local authority areas. Between 2010 and 2016 I chaired the boards, and advised on improvement, in Salford, Torbay, the Isle of Wight, Devon and Sandwell, spending two days each month, for a period of around 18 months to two years in each location.

What has concerned me about the process was the part played by Ofsted and its inspection judgements in setting in train the journey of local authorities towards having to contract out their children's services. The concern about the impact of Ofsted was shared by the Local Government Association (LGA) and the Society of Local Authority Chief Executives (SOLACE) which in 2016 stated that Ofsted had 'hindered rather than helped' children's services and that 'under the current system, councils given an "inadequate" rating for their children services are locked behind an "insurmountable barrier" to improvement'.[50]

The concerns about Ofsted were that it had been a hit-and-run inspectorate which concentrated on inspection and grading rather than service improvement and development. Ofsted's inspections had been experienced as bruising, threatening and harassing. Secondly, the consistency and reliability of its judgements had been questioned, in part because when there were terrible events concerning children, given major media coverage, Ofsted quickly moved away from the 'good' rating it had previously given to a local authority and revised and reversed its judgements (as happened with Haringey after the media's erroneous shaping of 'the Baby P story' following the death of Peter Connelly,[51] and with Rotherham after the media's exposure of child sexual exploitation[52]). Thirdly, the impact of an Ofsted inspection report, with its front-loading of what needs to improve, has generated critical press coverage even in areas which were judged to be doing well. Fourthly, Ofsted has made its standards harder and its judgements harsher (what was previously termed 'adequate' became 'requires improvement') so that more and more local authorities were rated as 'inadequate' or 'requires improvement', fewer were rated as 'good' and for a long period none were rated as 'outstanding'. The overall impression, therefore, was that local government was failing to deliver a reasonable standard of children's social services, giving ammunition to those who saw marketisation and privatisation as the way forward.

But the greatest Ofsted impact has been on local authorities and their local partner agencies when they receive an 'inadequate' rating. Confidence and morale have fallen away, triaging of incoming work has deteriorated and the service has become overwhelmed with backlogs of assessments quickly building up as other agencies have lost confidence and piled more work into children's social services partly to insure themselves against criticism. Not surprisingly, the bruised and battered children's social work workforce has imploded and disintegrated. Turnover and vacancy levels have increased, as has the dependency on transitory short-term agency social workers and managers, including senior managers. It is at this point that the government-appointed commissioner arrives to find that the situation is worse than reported by Ofsted!

In 2015 David Cameron stated that 'any children's services department rated "inadequate" by Ofsted will have a mere six months to show "significant improvement" or be taken over'.[53] My experience is that it takes 18 months to two years to rebuild and to re-stabilise after being described and denounced as 'inadequate' by Ofsted. It requires time to create a stable workforce, which inevitably will be initially skewed towards newly qualifying social workers, and to get to grips with escalating workloads and concerns about practice and performance. This all gets delayed if the government requires that time is instead spent on setting up a trust and then contracting out staff and services to the trust. This adds at least another year to the timeline!

This is a view which was shared by Roy Perry, the leader of Hampshire County Council and chair of the Local Government Association's Children and Young People Board. Perry commented that 'despite national data showing improvement in most areas of children's services since 2007, Ofsted ratings have been falling, giving more councils poor judgements which then act as barriers to improvement'.[54]

The lack of insight into Ofsted's impact was illustrated in 2013 by Sir Michael Wilshaw, who was at the time Ofsted's chief inspector.[55] He criticised the leadership of local authority children's services, and especially the high turnover of directors of children's services, but apparently with no reflection that Ofsted itself might be a major factor in driving this instability.[*]

The concerns about Ofsted's impact were longstanding, going back to at least 2009:

> Tension over the performance of the Ofsted inspectorate since the Baby Peter affair burst into the open today after an angry intervention by the child welfare expert who was sent in to Haringey at the height of the crisis. John Coughlan, who was temporarily seconded by ministers to run child protection services in the North London borough last year, accused Ofsted of 'defensiveness to the point of destruction' and openly defied its criticism of his own local authority. To loud applause and cheers from local authority chiefs, Coughlan said: 'I don't want a bonfire of the quangos, but I want the quangos to come together and lead more effectively and to stop using terms like "appalling" in public when my staff are going out to do the most difficult of jobs in the most difficult of circumstances'.[56]

Coughlan concluded:

> 'In terms of [football] terrace chants, it feels like they are telling us "you don't know what you are doing",' he said. 'Our response should be "come and have a go if you think you are hard enough".'

---

[*] In March 2018 the then new Children's Minister, Nadhim Zahawi, also commented on the leadership of children's social services, stating that 'strong leadership, rather than extra funding' (https://www.theguardian.com/social-care-network/2018/feb/28/nadhim-zahawi-leadership-key-to-turninground-failing-childrens-services) was key, this despite the Local Government Association calculating that there would be a £2 billion shortfall by 2020 in funding for local authority children's services and that the services were at 'breaking point' (https://www.local.gov.uk/about/campaigns/bright-futures/bright-futureschildrens-services/close-childrens-services-funding).

But regardless of concerns, Ofsted judgements were used by the coalition and Conservative governments as the trigger to remove children's services from the direct control of several Labour councils, whereas many Conservative councils were provided with assistance and time rather than having their children's services moved outside the local authority. And, as will be seen below, Mr Cameron as Prime Minister used the narrative of 'failing' local councils to promote his vision of a statutory children's social work and child protection marketplace.

Some councils, however, chose to voluntarily contract out all their statutory children's services. These had all been Conservative-controlled councils, including, as noted above, Kingston, Richmond, and Windsor and Maidenhead. Northamptonshire County Council also intended to move its children's services to an independent company. The motivation seems to have been an ideology in favour of the independent rather than the public sector and also an unevidenced aspiration that it would save money at a time of central government-imposed cuts:

> After five successive years of funding cuts, Northamptonshire county council believes it has seen the future of local government: it is dramatically smaller, its services are privatised, and its finances practically self-sufficient, almost entirely free of central government funding. The core services that for decades have defined what a council does, will no longer be umbilically attached to the town hall. All services, including child protection, and those for the elderly will be hived off into staff-run mutual companies, social enterprises or private firms.[57]

However, Northamptonshire County Council was soon in turmoil, with it reported by the *Daily Telegraph* that 'Northamptonshire County Council, which is controlled by the Conservative Party, has issued a section 114 notice that prohibits any new spending, apart from statutory services for safeguarding vulnerable people',[58] and with it noted in *The Guardian* that:

Northamptonshire bragged about its pioneering "easy-council" approach when it was introduced three years ago. The council outsourced every service it could, shedding all but 150 of its 4,000 staff. They were transferred to four new service providers, part-owned by the council but run like private companies, down to the payment of dividends ... It has not taken long to discover that private sector management can no more deliver adequate services on too little cash than the council can itself.[59]

In March 2018 it was announced that the council in Northamptonshire was taking back under its direct management and control all the adult social services it had previously contracted out, with the in-sourcing intended 'to save money and to simplify the delivery model'.[60] How much time, money and management attention had it cost and wasted to create this roundabout of public services being contracted out of the council and then being brought back in again? Northamptonshire's experience also belies the claim that the route to saving money is outsourcing, although this still remained the direction of travel for government policy.

The narrative makes the news

The quickening of the pace of the government's privatisation journey was not only characterised by changes in statutory regulations, statutory children's social work services being voluntarily and involuntarily moved outside of local authority direct provision, and by the big outsourcing companies being involved in discussions with the Department for Education. It was also illustrated by the narrative that had been shaped by David Cameron as Prime Minister and by Michael Gove as Secretary of State for Education.

Mr Gove has been explicitly critical of social workers and of social work education. In the midst of politically chosen policies of austerity targeting poor children, families and disabled adults, and with big cuts in public services and in the numbers and pay of public servants, he attacked social workers for being concerned about the impact of the poverty that the government, in which he was a leading minister, was creating.[61] It was reported that:

> Gove believes the [social work] profession has become too ideological – blaming social injustice rather than an individual's actions for the collapse of their lives. He will argue that the result is that 'some social workers acquiesce in or make excuses for the wrong choices' people have made in life. 'In too many cases, social work training involves idealistic students being told that the individuals with whom they will work have been disempowered by society. They will be encouraged to see these individuals as victims of social injustice whose fate is overwhelmingly decreed by the economic forces and inherent inequalities which scar our society.'[62]

Mr Gove's speech in November 2013[63] generated headlines such as 'Michael Gove [says] many social workers "not up to the job"',[64] 'Michael Gove: My life was transformed by social workers – but standards must improve',[65] and 'Gove Slams Social Work Education',[66] and provoked a negative and critical reaction from within the social work profession which highlighted that social workers were indeed aware of and concerned about the demoralising and destabilising impact of poverty on many of those with whom they had contact.[67] When in July 2014 Mr Cameron reshuffled his Cabinet and Mr Gove lost his post as Secretary of State for Education, under the headline 'Social workers will not be sorry to see Gove go' appeared the comment that:

> The Department for Education came under fire for plans that – following consultation – would open up child protection services to the marketplace, including private and profit-making companies like G4S and Serco. The controversial policies alone are enough for some to cheer his departure. Ray Jones, professor of social work at Kingston University and St George's London, has a message for Gove's

replacement, Nicky Morgan: 'I hope this will now be a time for review and reflection and that some of the potentially damaging plans Gove had will not be pursued.' These plans were 'not sensible in building strong local partnerships with local leadership to protect children', Jones says.[68]

My hope that there would be review and reflection by the government about the thrust to open up statutory children's social work and child protection was a forlorn hope, as Mr Gove's replacement, Mrs Morgan, continued – as will be seen below – and indeed intensified, the government's intention to remove children's services from local authorities, seeing the academisation of schools as the model to shape the removal of children's services outside of local councils.

Mr Gove's solution to his criticism that social workers were overly concerned about poverty and deprivation was to get Sir Martin Narey to prepare a report on social work education, which Mr Gove saw as being partly at the root of social workers' concerns, and also to launch a fast-track work-based training programme, run by an independent company, for graduates recruited from the top 'Russell group' universities who were promised quick career moves into leadership roles.

Mr Gove also, based on his personal experience of having been adopted, wanted more children to be adopted and adopted more quickly (with Edward Timpson, who continued as Minister for Children, also being a strong advocate for adoption, based on his experience of having adopted siblings and his parents fostering and adopting children[69]):

> Children are being denied loving homes because of politically correct attitudes, ridiculous bureaucracy and misguided nonsense, according to Michael Gove, the education secretary.

Gove made the claims at the launch of revised adoption guidance for local authorities.

'Thousands of children are currently in the care system waiting to be adopted,' he said. 'Every day they wait is a day they're denied the loving home all children deserve. But politically correct attitudes and ridiculous bureaucracy keep many of those children waiting far too long.'[70]

The script again is about social workers with 'politically correct attitudes', 'misguided nonsense', and 'ridiculous bureaucracy'. Hardly a ringing, or even supportive, endorsement of social work and local authority children's services.

All this was not so long after the attack on social workers led by Rebekah Brooks and *The Sun* after the death of Peter Connelly ('Baby P'). Mr Gove had at that time, in 2009, stood alongside David Cameron in targeting social workers and their managers, and like Cameron, had a social life and friendships with Rebekah Brooks and Rupert Murdoch.[71]

There was a symbiotic relationship between Mr Gove, Mr Cameron and the Murdoch-owned press – *The Sun* and *The Times*** – in their attack on social workers (and also in promoting adoption). The poor were to be blamed for their poverty, social workers were characterised as naively complicit in depicting deprivation as a major burden impinging on poor people, and the solution was, first, to get more children into adoptive homes quickly and, secondly, to recruit and train bright graduates who would see through the political correctness of the current social

---

*　The press was, however, hardly consistent in the nature and content of its attacks on social workers. All that was consistent was that the coverage was complaining and critical of social workers. At the same time in 2008/09 as *The Sun*, *The Mail* and others were lambasting social workers when a child died and social workers had not sought a court order to remove the child from their family, Camilla Cavendish in *The Times* was leading a campaign asserting that social workers were seeking to remove too many children from their families. In 2008 her campaign led her to be presented with the Paul Foot award for journalism (www.thetimes.co.uk/article/times-writer-camilla-cavendish-grabs-paul-foot-award-for-journalismwjscfzgfm38). In 2015 she was appointed by Prime Minister Cameron (with whom she had been a contemporary at Oxford University) as the head of his Policy Unit (www.theguardian.com/politics/2015/may/21/sunday-times-camilla-cavendish-head-number-10-policy-unit-david-cameron), and then in 2017 was appointed chair of Frontline, the government-favoured fast-track training programme for children's social workers.

work workforce. It was not seen as a problem that more children and families were experiencing poverty, and more severe poverty, as social security for poor families was repeatedly cut, nor that services which helped families such as 'Sure Start' children's centres were being closed down.

Mr Gove also wanted to open up statutory children's social work to the private sector:

> Michael Gove has said that more struggling children's services departments in England could be taken over by independent providers. The Education Secretary also said he was considering opening up well performing departments to private and voluntary organisations. This would be so they could innovate and improve their services, he said.[72]

This further step towards privatisation was recognised in the headline in *Children and Young People Magazine* that 'Reform proposals for social work are "privatisation through the back door"'.[73]

Mr Cameron was on the same mission as Mr Gove. A report in *The Telegraph* newspaper of a speech he gave in March 2015 is headed 'David Cameron: social workers must use "common sense" to tackle child abuse' and goes on to state that 'Child abuse is taking place on an "industrial scale" because officials are refusing to act with "common sense", David Cameron has said'.[74]

Later in December 2015 a Department for Education press release stated:

> The Prime Minister will today announce radical reforms which will mean poorly performing children's services must improve − or they will be taken over. Children's services in local authorities, which have persistently failed in the past, will be taken over immediately. Sharper triggers will be put in place so an emergency Ofsted inspection can be ordered where there are concerns about an authority's performance. This could include complaints from

whistle-blowers or evidence of poor leadership. High-performing local authorities, experts in child protection and charities will be brought in to turn children's services around – including by acting as sponsors, forming 'trusts' to take over authorities which are judged to be failing.[75]

It requires a little reading between the lines in the statement above to understand that 'experts' include private sector companies. But no reading between the lines is required in this speech from Mr Cameron in September 2015:

What energises many markets are new insurgent companies, who break monopolies and bring in new ways of doing things. We should apply this thinking to government. So many of our country's efforts to extend opportunity have been undermined by a sort of tolerance of state failure: children-in-care and prisons being two absolutely standout areas … In June, I made the case for reform of social services and child protection. We need to apply the lessons we have learned in education reform to this vital area. Just as we improved the quality of teaching by attracting brilliant new recruits, so we'll improve social work by bringing in new talent. A new programme, Frontline, has already attracted hundreds of outstanding graduates to become social workers. And just as we've replaced failing local authority schools with great new academies and outstanding free schools, so we will say to any local authority failing its children: transform the way you provide services, or those services will be taken over by non-profit trusts or other partnerships. This will be a big area of focus over the next 5 years.[76]

Then something surprising happened just after Mr Cameron made this speech. It led me to write the piece below for *The Guardian*:

And now for the strange coincidence. Two hours later [after Mr Cameron's speech], I received an email from a consultancy firm selling itself as giving 'investors a better way to access industry knowledge … helping thousands of clients get answers to their most critical questions, without leaving their desks. Rather than spending hours reading research reports, or travelling to meet people at conferences, we can connect clients directly with industry experts to hear immediate, relevant insights'. Who are these clients who want 'industry insights'? They are, according to the email I received, 'the world's finest hedge funds, asset management and private equity firms'. And what did they want from me? I was told they came across my name 'while doing some research online on social work in the UK, and wanted to see if you would be interested in a paid phone consultation with my American client'. Now, I assume hedge funds and private equity firms pay well. Just look at the multimillion pound payments received by their directors and shareholders who generate big profits from the 'industries' they cherry pick. It was a little tempting to take up their offer to be paid to advise their private investor clients. But I replied saying that I had no interest in having the conversation. Still, I suspect these companies will continue to circle child protection and children's social services and social work. And there may be others willing to advise about how and where to strike to 'energise' the market being created in children's social services.[77]

And it was these new 'market insurgent companies' which, according to Mr Cameron, would shake up children's social services, and the removal of the services from local authorities was the answer. Patrick Butler commented:

We are failing the most vulnerable children in society, the prime minister, David Cameron, admitted on Monday. He promised that this would change; he would not stand by, he promised, with the casual bluster beloved of politicians on this topic, while children are let down by 'inadequate social services'. High-performing local authorities, charities and experts will take over struggling services under government plans. It begs the question as to what exactly he has been doing for vulnerable children over the past five years. He inevitably ignored why increasing numbers of children were in such desperate circumstances that they were ending up in local authority care. His huge cuts to social security, and police and council budgets strangely didn't get a mention. Instead this was a speech for the next five years, outlining what he billed as 'one of the big landmark reforms of this parliament'. At the heart of this supposedly radical set of reforms is the belief that failing children's social services can only be rescued if they are detached from their local authority parent and their functions put out to market. So far, so Cameron. It is hard not to see this as the latest instalment of a neat cut-denigrate-privatise strategy. The cuts have been achieved. Cameron has led a barrage of criticism of social services. Yet, a full-blown market in child protection – that dream shrivelled in a blaze of public anger and expert criticism in 2014 – is on the backburner, at least for now. Cameron's model is academy schools, and the tactic will be to hustle children's services into 'academy' status. Any children's services department rated 'inadequate' by Ofsted will have a mere six months to show 'significant improvement' or be taken over. A whistleblower's complaint, or 'evidence of poor leadership' will be the trigger for an emergency Ofsted inspection. The inspectors judged 19 out of 74 children's services in England to be inadequate between February 2014 and September 2015.[78]

There were those who were in support of Mr Cameron's intentions, including Andy Elvin, the chief executive of The

Adolescent and Children's Trust (TACT).* TACT is a charity which has contracts with local authorities to provide fostering and adoption services. He wrote:

> In December 2015, David Cameron outlined plans for a more standardised system for taking over failing children's services. If a local authority shows persistent failure it will immediately be taken over by high-performing councils, charities or child protection experts, and if a service fails to show improvements in the six months following inspection, it will face a similar intervention. Children's charities must get involved in this process ... They could run these solely, go into partnership with local councils as owners of community interest companies or be the main contractor for such companies. All of these options are available under current legislation.[79]

Elvin had spoken out about against excessive profits being made by independent fostering agencies[80] and about the government's predominant interest in promoting adoption.[81, 82] But he has also been publicly supportive of the 'social work reform' measures championed by Isabelle Trowler and covered in the Children and Social Work Bill (including the government's proposals for a new social work regulator and social worker accreditation, discussed in the next chapter), writing an article which was

---

* Andy Elvin has a professional background in local authority children's social work and in the voluntary sector working with children. His professional and practice background is now something of an exception in the big national child care charities. In the 1980s I also worked in the voluntary sector as a manager for Barnardo's. At that time the big four children's social care and child protection charities in the UK – Barnardo's, Action for Children, the Children's Society and the NSPCC – were all led by top managers who had direct practice experience as social workers. None of the chief executives of the four big children's charities in 2017 had these roots or this background. Social work should have no claim to exclusivity in its commitment to care for and protect children but having a professional background and practice experience within children's social services was previously seen as particularly relevant for its top management and leadership. This is no longer so either in the voluntary sector nor, since the 2004 Children Act, within local authorities, where many directors of children's services have had backgrounds as teachers or education managers (or as management accountants).

headlined 'New reforms might be just what social workers and children want – and need'.[83]

Elvin doubts that private profit-making companies will have a route into statutory children's services:

> Are the government's much-publicised plans to introduce innovation in children's services a means of allowing private sector involvement in child protection? Some have argued so, but as the chief executive of the Adolescent and Children's Trust (TACT), the landscape looks different to me. It could be argued that the Department for Education has fudged the rules to allow private companies to sneak in under a social enterprise disguise. But I doubt any local authorities will be fooled by this over-familiar wolf in sheep's clothing. And, coming from a charity looking to work more closely with local authorities, I see a host of opportunities for innovative local authorities and entrepreneurial charities to work together to improve outcomes for our most vulnerable children.[84]

My concerns are two-fold. First, any transfer away from transparent public sector and directly locally accountable, controlled and provided statutory children's social work services adds complications and costs when what is needed in child protection investigations and decisions about the safety and care of children is clarity and clear responsibility. The fudge is that although services may now be provided by other organisations the local authority still has the statutory responsibility for the care and protection of children in its area. The very real danger here is that those providing the services are not held within the law as the body responsible and accountable for the safety and welfare of the children, and the local authorities themselves will no longer have the capacity or expertise to fulfil these functions and responsibilities.

Secondly, it is hard to see how charities will gain and sustain contracts for these services whilst maintaining professional standards, a skilled workforce and conditions of employment for social workers when private companies would be willing to constrain and cut costs whilst also generating a profit. The private companies would primarily have to do this by changing the skills mix within the workforce and reducing terms of employment. Local authorities at a time of severe reductions in funding may well look to award contracts based on costs, as much as, if not more so than, on quality. And not all local councillors and councils may see it as inappropriate or undesirable to contract out these crucial statutory responsibilities for the protection and welfare of children to private, for-profit, companies. For example, children's public health nursing services, such as health visiting and school nursing, have been transferred from the NHS to local authorities, and in some areas these are now being contracted out to private, for-profit, companies, as are child and adolescent mental health services.[85]

The government's intention that there should be new providers of statutory children's services was reinforced and made even more explicit in a government policy statement in July 2016. In the Ministerial Foreword, signed by Nicky Morgan, who had replaced Mr Gove as Secretary of State for Education, and Edward Timpson, who was still the Children's Minister, they stated that their aim was to have the services 'delivered through a more diverse range of social care organisations' and on 'governance and accountability … developing innovative new organisational models with the potential to radically improve services'.[86]

This became a focus of comment about the government's policy statement. Under a headline of 'Third of children's services to be "new models" by 2020, government hopes', Luke Stevenson in *Community Care* noted:

> More than a third of local authorities in England will be delivering – or looking to deliver – children's services through 'new models' such as not-for-profit trusts by 2020. This is the ambition set out by the government in a policy paper published this week, which claims that the current system of delivering social care services by in-house local authority teams 'is not delivering consistently excellent practice' …

The government argues new models help drive improvement by refreshing the leadership, and attract 'strong and ambitious people' to places where new ways of working are necessary. These can also provide a sharper focus on children's social care, and bring together different areas in robust structures, the paper said. However, despite a commitment to new ways of delivering services, it added that there will be 'no change' to legal arrangements which prevent local authorities delegating functions to profit-making organisations.[87]

However, as noted above, the legal arrangements did not need to be further changed to allow Mr Cameron's 'market insurgents' and the DfE's 'newcos' to be contracted to provide statutory children's social work services, as this change had already been made in 2014. It was misleading for the government to state that profit-making companies could not be contracted to provide statutory children's social work services.

In 2016 the Labour opposition in Parliament at last grasped the concerns about the route the government was taking and the journey it was on. They became more aware, alert and active when a Children and Social Work Bill was published.

Patrick Butler wrote:

Labour will call for a 'privatisation lock' to prevent a potential influx of private providers into council-run child protection services under proposed new powers to enable councils to opt-out of a raft of legal duties relating to the care of vulnerable youngsters. The move reflects concern over government proposals to allow councils to request exemption from a range of statutory obligations on the grounds that these can inhibit innovative ways of making children's services more efficient and effective. Ministers have argued that the wide-ranging measures contained in the children and social work bill will drive up standards, freeing authorities and frontline social workers to experiment with fresh ideas aimed at improving outcomes for at-risk children. A Whitehall source said: 'Too many local authorities are simply not good enough when it comes to child protection. This is about encouraging innovation. It's not about cutting red tape or cutting corners. If you need to be good, you need to innovate.' But critics argue the powers pave the way for 'academy-style' reforms of social services and threaten children's social care rights and entitlements carefully built up over recent decades, including the Children Act introduced by Margaret Thatcher's Conservative government in 1989. Sharon Hodgson, a shadow children and families minister, told the Guardian: 'We support innovation to drive improvement. Too many local authorities struggle to provide outstanding children's services. But we are not convinced that such wide-ranging powers are necessary. We are concerned that the bill could be a Trojan horse for delivering the profit motive into children's social care.' The Queen's speech promised key changes to adoption and care leaver support – but will this improve the life chances of the most vulnerable in society? A letter in the Guardian signed by 16 social care experts, including university professors and charity leaders, warns that the bill introduces a 'fast-track process for the removal of any of hundreds of local authority duties' relating to children and families.[88]

As in 2014 and the opposition to the changes in statutory regulations, it was, in part, a group letter to *The Guardian*, this time coordinated by Carolyne Willow[89] of children's rights group Article 39, which triggered the news coverage, and this time the Labour opposition were also engaged in raising concerns about what the government was proposing. This is the subject of the next chapter.

TWO

Creeping political control: the Children and Social Work Bill and anti-professionalism

In May 2016 as a part of its intention to reframe and reposition social work, especially in the context of children's social services, the government introduced its Children and Social Work Bill. It was described in the professional press as 'promising an overhaul of social work' in England.[1] The overriding concern was that the Bill was a badly drafted mishmash of widely varying topics. Its route to becoming law took a series of zig-zags before going down a number of cul-de-sacs leading to quite dramatic U-turns. This route was caused by the government accelerating and gaining speed without seeing the chicanes of opposition ahead. The parliamentary debates on the Bill were described as a 'magical mystery tour'[2] as the government time and time again altered and added new clauses to the Bill.

This was not unusual for the government at the time, with U-turns becoming a quite common political manoeuvre when David Cameron was Prime Minister of the Conservative government in 2016,[3] and continuing in 2017 with Theresa May as Prime Minister.[4] The U-turns ranged from quick volte-faces on tax measures just announced in the 2017 Spring Budget to the even more shocking change to stop lone child refugees entering the UK.[5] U-turns are a sensible manoeuvre when you are going in the wrong direction but even better not to set off on the wrong course in the first place so that others have to get you to change route and correct the plan. Yet this is what came to characterise the passage of the Children and Social Work

Bill. The genesis of the Bill, and the lack of consultation which preceded it, was commented upon in Parliament, first by Lord Watson in the House of Lords, and then by Emma Lewell-Buck in the House of Commons:

> ... the Government continue to rush out Bills that lack proper thought or preparation. That is evidenced in this case by the fact that the noble Lord, Lord Nash, has himself introduced more than 150 amendments, several of them containing new clauses. The Government could have avoided much of the pain that they have suffered had they undertaken meaningful consultation with the relevant, very interested sectors which have contributed behind the scenes to the Bill's progress.[6]

> I [Emma Lewell-Buck] would like briefly to echo some comments made in the other place [the House of Lords] about the rushed pace and hurried nature of the Bill. Noble Lords expressed concern that the Bill had not been carefully thought out; they were right, of course, because thanks to their diligent work the Bill before us is markedly different from the one that was introduced. The legislation appears not to have been made in response to any particular burning issues or needs—nor, despite its being a Bill about children and social workers, does it appear to be built on extensive consultation with children or social workers ... Since Second Reading last week, I have been inundated with expressions of concern that the Bill has progressed so rapidly to Committee without any sittings to take evidence from the sector or agencies that work closely with vulnerable children. Neither the Opposition nor the sector and the agencies working in the field feel particularly comfortable about the Bill's passage through Parliament.[7]

Part 1, Chapter 1 of the Bill was about children, and especially children looked after by local authorities and children and young people leaving care. Much of what was proposed was welcomed and viewed as largely uncontentious with its focus on corporate parenting,* 'a local offer for care leavers', and the education of looked after children (including extending responsibilities to academy schools). There was some comment about the additional attention being paid in the Bill to promoting and supporting adoption whilst there was nothing in the Bill about helping families and parents to care for their children.[8] There was also a more general concern about what would happen when the good intentions in this part of the Bill hit the reality of local authority funding cuts,[9] but overall there was agreement and support for much of what was proposed for children in care.

The 'exemption clauses'

But tension and trouble arose when Part 1, Chapter 2 of the Bill was considered. There was a considerable consistency in this section of the Bill and what followed. The intention was to give wide executive powers to the Secretary of State for Education over children's legislation and children's services.

In Part 2 of the Bill, which is discussed below, this intention that political control should be held by the Secretary of State for Education was also prominent and paramount. Part 2 of the Bill was about social work and social workers. It was not primarily or exclusively about children and children's services, which are within the remit of the Secretary of State for Education and the Department for Education. It might have been expected, therefore, that the more general social work proposals would have been included within a separate social work Bill to be presented jointly by the relevant social care minister in the Department for Health as well as the Department for Education. However, as with so much of the recent government drive towards

---

* Although, as more and more of the foster care and residential care of children is contracted outside of local authorities – and with the 2014 regulatory changes allowing that even social workers for children may no longer be within and employed by the council – how councils as 'corporate parents' were to stay in touch and engaged with children in their care is becoming more difficult and problematic.

privatisation and the marketisation of social work, it had been led and energised within the Department for Education rather than in the Department for Health.

The most publicly contentious intention within the Bill was to give whoever was the Secretary of State for Education at the time the power to take executive decisions, without parliamentary debate and changes in statute, to set aside legislation giving rights to children and responsibilities to services. This would be a fundamental constitutional change, a 'subversion of Parliament's constitutional position',[10] allowing one minister to override and overrule primary and secondary legislation.

The 'exemption clauses' would, on an application from a local authority, have allowed the Secretary of State to exempt local authorities from statutory requirements and responsibilities for up to six years. It was stated that this would encourage and enable local authorities to innovate, and the clauses in the Bill were then described as the 'innovation clauses'.

There was widespread concern that these powers in the hands of the minister would lead to an 'increasingly threadbare patchwork quilt'[11] of rights for children and responsibilities for services which would vary between local authority areas. Not only would there be a 'postcode lottery' of what legislation was in place depending on where a child lived, but carefully crafted legislation such as the 1989 Children Act might over time be unwound step by step without parliamentary scrutiny and without any tracking and painting of the new legislative canvas which would emerge.

Over 50 organisations formed a Children's Coalition to oppose the 'exemption clauses in the Bill, with Article 39 and its director, Carolyne Willow, taking a lead coordinating and campaigning role, as did Children England (led by its chief executive, Kathy Evans), an umbrella organisation for smaller voluntary organisations and community groups concerned for children. The British Association of Social Workers was active with its membership in contacting MPs to oppose the government's proposals. Many of the voices heard in opposition to what the government intended came together in a coalition 'Together for Children'[12] and they ranged from the Association of Lawyers for Children, the Care Leavers' Association, Children's Rights

Alliance for England, National Association for People Abused in Childhood, and Women's Aid. Other organisations which expressed concerns about and opposed the proposed 'exemption powers' included Action for Children and the NSPCC,[13, 14] the Royal College of Paediatrics and Child Health[15] and the National Children's Bureau.[16]

Over many months there were letters in *The Guardian*[17, 18, 19, 20, 21] and *The Times*,[22] and over 100,000 people signed a petition[23] against the proposals in the Bill. The overwhelming view was that the government's proposals were misconceived. The energy and effectiveness of the campaigning in opposition to the 'exemption clauses' was impressive.

Not all, however, were opposed to the 'exemption' powers being given to the Secretary of State. Isabelle Trowler, the Chief Social Worker for Children, was in favour.[24] Local authorities through the Local Government Association (LGA)[25] and individually, as with Leeds City Council[26] and Hampshire County Council[27] (both councils rated as 'outstanding' and 'good' by Ofsted, and with much respected children's services senior managers), along with the president of the Association of the Directors of Children's Services,[28] saw benefits in being able to set aside children's legislation so that they could be more innovative. There were also profit-making companies (such as Foster Care Associates[29]) and not-for-profit charities and companies (such as Barnardo's and The Adolescent and Children's Trust [TACT]) which supported the government's proposals.

Andy Elvin, the chief executive of TACT, specifically addressed the concern that the 'exemption clauses' might be attractive in setting aside legislation which might deter private companies to pitch for statutory children's social services contracts:

> Timpson assures us that: 'There is absolutely no intention of allowing the delegation of child protection functions to profit-making organisations'. I believe this is not only true but that G4S et al would not want to run child protection even if they were allowed. The experience of Circle Holdings in its disastrous running of Hinchingbrook hospital

[see Chapter Eight] shows that the private for-profit sector falters where unlimited demand is at play. Circle was sunk by the continual demands placed on A&E, it couldn't get the financial model to work for it as it was overwhelmed by demand and so was facing significant losses. Similarly, any given local authority cannot control the numbers of children in its area requiring statutory intervention; demand is not controllable as it is if you are running a children's home or a prison with a fixed capacity. So fears that clause 15 is a gateway to privatisation are misplaced … Social work as a profession is all too often seen as suspicious of, and hostile to, innovation and change. Many local authorities have shown this need not be the case over the past few years through the delivery of excellent new ways of working, some funded by the DfE innovation fund. Alongside this, Frontline (of which I am a board member) and Step-Up have brought new, and successful, innovations to social work recruitment.[30]

Although (after the government amended the 'exemption clauses' to enhance the consultation to be undertaken before legislation could be set aside, and after the government excluded some statutory duties from the scope of the 'exclusion clauses') the LGA did not oppose the clauses, there had been concern expressed by Richard Watts, the LGA's co-chair of the Children's Services Improvement Board, who 'strongly opposed' another of the Bill's clauses 'that gives the Education Secretary very wide-ranging powers to force individual councils in intervention to take some flexibilities'. Watts continued: 'We do worry what that is a back door to. A lot of councils see that as potentially a backdoor to mass privatisation of children's services.'[31]

Even if it was the explicit intention of ministers to introduce the 'exemption clauses' to introduce and allow authorities in turn to set aside statutory duties and this was seen as a positive by some local authorities and other providers of children's services, there was the very real danger, as with the removal of statutory children's social work services to independent trusts and community interest companies, that this could be the thin end of a wedge. It could be a Trojan horse which could later be expanded and exploited by any future government and Secretary of State to cut back on children's rights and service responsibilities either to save money or to make a commercial marketplace less onerous and more attractive to 'market insurgents' and 'newcos'.

There was also a very real danger that there could be a considerable cumulative impact from separately taken but then aggregated decisions by the Secretary of State to set aside statutory duties. This was a scenario I submitted in January 2017 to the House of Commons Children and Social Work Public Bill Committee based on what were being suggested and canvassed as duties from which local authorities might get exemptions and which could leave children in care without the current legislative protections.[32]

The 'exemption clauses' were debated and then voted down in the House of Lords in autumn 2016 but then the government re-entered the clauses in January 2017[33] when the Bill was considered in committee in the House of Commons. En route the government introduced changes about how and with whom the Secretary of State would have to consult before setting aside legislative duties to protect and assist children, but the fundamental constitutional concerns of principle, and practical concerns of what it could mean for the safety and welfare of children, remained unchanged, with Lord Watson, the Labour lead on the Bill in the House of Lords, commenting:

> What matters is that the children's services are delivered comprehensively, effectively and safely, and that these services are available across the country. The standard may vary, though that can and must be addressed when it arises. The nature of the services provided should be, as near as possible, uniform across the country. This is about defending children's social care rights. The alternative is a postcode lottery ... the Chief Social Worker for Children and Families asserts: 'We must be enabled to use our professional judgment in flexible and creative ways, rather than having to follow a procedural path or series of legal

rules'. For the chief social worker to seek to avoid having to follow 'legal rules' is worrying at the very least and invites the question as to whose side she is on; some have recently questioned whether the answer is vulnerable children. If local authorities are unable to provide a full and effective service in social care, then the main reason is usually a lack of resources, especially in terms of staffing. I think it is pertinent to ask: why is the chief social worker not using her position of influence to campaign for more resources to enable her fellow social workers to do their job to the best of their ability, rather than undermining and demoralising the profession as many social workers feel that she is doing?[34]

In the Commons committee Emma Lewell-Buck, the shadow Children's Minister, linked the proposed 'exemption clauses' with fears that it would 'pave the way for the privatisation of child protection services', stating that 'companies such as G4S, Serco and Virgin Care have all attended meetings with the Department to consider how they can play a role in delivering and shaping statutory children's social care services. It is little wonder that very few trusted the motivation behind the original clauses or that fears persist that behind this power is an insatiable appetite for breaking up children's social care'.[35]

She then issued a challenge that 'if the Minister really means what he says about profit and child protection, he should be seeking to prohibit subsidiaries of profit-making companies from delivering social care functions'. The minister, however, did not take this opportunity to rescind the 2014 changes in statutory regulations which allowed profit-making companies to enter the market being created in children's social work and child protection services.

But in March 2017 the relatively new Secretary of State for Education, Justine Greening, did decide to withdraw the 'exemption clauses' from the Bill, with this being described by the BBC as the 'Ministers' U-turn over "bonfire of children's rights"'.[36] What was it that led to this turning point? The Labour shadow Children's Minister asked in Parliament: 'Can the Secretary of State explain her U-turn in signing Labour's amendments to scrap her own innovation clauses in the Children and Social Work Bill? Since her Minister and Chief Social Worker were the key protagonists of those strongly opposed and dangerous clauses, will she explain how she can possibly remain confident in their ability to protect our most vulnerable children?' It was the Children's Minister, Edward Timpson, who replied, saying 'It is very simple: we were unable to build the consensus required to take forward the power to innovate'.[37]

There can be little doubt that the campaigning over the previous eight months, and the strength and quality of opposition in Parliament, will have had an impact. And in February 2017 there was the impact of two leaders in social work, Professor Eileen Munro and Lord Laming, making known their opposition to the 'exemption clauses'. Herbert Laming, who had led the 2002 inquiry following the death of Victoria Climbié,[38] made his concerns known in a meeting with the Secretary of State. Eileen Munro, who had undertaken the coalition government-commissioned 2011 review of child protection in England,[39] made her concerns publicly known through a letter to MPs.[40] It was especially powerful as previously she had been quoted as being in favour of the 'exemption clauses',[41] and Edward Timpson, the Children's Minister, had claimed in Parliament that Munro supported the government's proposals.[42] Both Lord Laming and Eileen Munro had been contacted by those concerned about the 'exemption clauses', and what may have been of some impact in changing Eileen Munro's position was a briefing she received on the extent to which the 'exemption clauses' would give powers to the Secretary of State for Education to pause and put aside key legislation protecting the rights of children.

It was also of significance that Tim Loughton, the Conservative Children's Minister who had been removed from his post by Mr Gove and replaced by Mr Timpson, was instrumental and central to getting the government and the new Secretary of State for Education to back off from pushing forward on the 'exemption clauses'. Loughton had been much respected across children's organisations and by social workers, both as a long-standing shadow minister and then as Children's Minister, spending time with social workers and ensuring he was well briefed and informed about social work with children and families.* His opposition to the 'exemption clauses' was crucial and he arranged a meeting with Justine Greening as the new Education Secretary which preceded her abandoning the 'exemption clauses' in the Bill.[43, 44]

Local Safeguarding Children Boards

But it was not only the 'exemption clauses' which would give the Secretary of State greater direct control of social work and children's social services. This also was to be enabled through the proposals in the Bill on serious case reviews (SCRs) and changing the requirement that every local authority area be covered by a local safeguarding children board (LSCB).

These proposals in the Bill followed a review undertaken by Alan Wood of existing guidance and requirements on multi-agency working in child protection. Alan Wood had frequently been commissioned by the Department for Education to undertake reviews. He was also, for example, commissioned to undertake a review of youth custody for the Department of Justice when Mr Gove was its Secretary of State. The findings of this review commented on the role of the private sector in providing secure training centres for young people:

> The introduction of for-profit providers in the running of STCs has not been without controversy. The appalling situation at Medway and the decision of G4S to sell its remaining STC contract indicate that these arrangements have not played out as intended. It raises questions as to the capacity to manage contracts and suggests the contracting arrangements are insufficiently flexible to deal with

---

* In 2016 Tim Loughton became one of the three patrons of the Social Worker of the Year Awards; the others – both former social workers – were Emma Lewell-Buck, the shadow Children's Minister, and Baroness Howarth, a cross-bench peer and a former director of social services and chief executive of Child Line. Each was active in the debates on the Children and Social Work Bill.

underperformance, ensure high quality provision and effective recruitment and retention of skilled staff.[45]

The Wood proposals were that new arrangements should be piloted for the management of the two new, government-proposed secure schools and that 'this would require a very clearly different approach to the current YOIs, and not be run according to Prison Service rules or instructions. It would not restrict the option of inviting other providers (including from the commercial sector) to run secure schools once the pilot had been assessed'.[46]

So there was a recognition here of major failings by the private sector in providing custody for young people, significant limitations in the management of the contracts awarded to the private companies, a recommendation that there be a pilot of new provision and that the pilot should exclude the private commercial sector, but that, post-pilot, the commercial sector might be contracted again to run the services.

A teacher by professional background, as director of children's services for Hackney Alan Wood had been the senior manager of Isabelle Trowler and Steve Goodman before Trowler and Goodman left Hackney to set up their private company Morning Lane Associates. The next chapter reflects on the networks of a small number of key players who have been frequently associated and active within the government's agendas for social work and child protection.

In his review of LSCBs, Wood argues that LSCBs are largely ineffective yet costly, although Ofsted's analysis of its inspections of LSCBs and of councils found that LSCBs performed slightly better overall than local authorities.[47] Wood recommended instead that there should be locally determined multi-agency arrangements determined by 'health, the police and local government' and that 'they should draw up a plan that describes how their services, in partnership with other agencies, will deliver the new statutory framework' albeit in the context of a new statutory framework.[48] This is a radical proposal when set in its historical context. David Jones, a social worker, previously a NSPCC manager and general secretary of the British Association of Social Workers (BASW), and a former DfE civil servant who led on child protection, who was in 2016 chair of the Association of Independent LSCB Chairs (AILC), said that 'the review represents the most fundamental change to children's services since 1970'.[49]

LSCBs were established after the Victoria Climbié inquiry, which reported in 2003.[50] LSCBs were a requirement set for every local authority with statutory children's social services responsibilities by section 14 of the 2004 Children Act, which followed the Climbié inquiry, and by the Local Safeguarding Children Boards Regulations published in 2006. When the statutory guidance on protecting children was revised in 2015 it was reaffirmed that LSCBs were to 'coordinate what is done by each person or body represented on the Board for the purposes of safeguarding and promoting the welfare of children in the area; and to ensure the effectiveness of what is done by each such person or body for those purposes'.[51]

Since the mid-1970s, and following the inquiry into the death of Maria Colwell,[52] there have been government-specified requirements to structure multi-agency working to protect children. First there were area review committees (ARCs), then area child protection committees (ACPCs), and since 2004 LSCBs. Each iteration has sought to strengthen multi-agency and multi-professional partnership working to protect children, and the scope has been much wider than the three statutory partners specified by Wood. It included, for example, schools, the variants which now exist of what was the Probation Service, and voluntary and community organisations. It is also difficult to see which one organisation and which health service chief officer would now be able to span commissioning, community and mental health services, and hospitals.

The proposal to abolish the requirement for LSCBs in each local authority area was attacked by a solicitor who had represented girls and young women who had been sexually abused in Rotherham. He wrote:

> Let's recall what LSCBs are for: to coordinate local attempts to safeguard and promote the welfare of children, and to monitor and ensure the effectiveness of what its member organisations do, both individually

and collectively. They scrutinise local organisations to ensure they are fulfilling their statutory obligations and, where mistakes are made, that lessons are learned. Importantly, LSCBs are independent of the agencies they coordinate. Even more importantly, LSCBs have drawn in partner organisations not previously involved in local safeguarding arrangements: sexual health services, youth offending teams, probation services, the voluntary sector and schools. This has been crucial; it is only recently, for example, that schools have started to become fully involved in tackling child sexual exploitation. Under the regime proposed in the new bill, I fear there may be no involvement of schools outside the local authority orbit – such as academies and free schools – and no effective monitoring of their safeguarding work where they do participate ... Looking at Wood's report, which among other things highlighted the cost of LSCBs, it is difficult to escape the conclusion that their abolition is austerity driven.[53]

Wood's proposal fits within an intention to declutter and reduce child protection prescription and procedures which have built up incrementally over the past 50 years. The government has sought to do the same with the statutory 'Working Together' guidance. Less bureaucracy and less proceduralisation, as argued by Munro, should be welcomed. But amid the increasing complexities of fragmented services, many of which – for example within the health services, probation and schools – are now owned and managed by organisations with no local roots and with distant senior managers, it might be argued that there need to be stronger rather than looser requirements in terms of multi-agency working.[54]

Serious case reviews

The Wood review also focused on SCRs, which had to be undertaken after a child died or was seriously harmed as a consequence of abuse or neglect. The review recommended that

SCRs should be discontinued. This should be welcomed. Since 2011 SCRs – with few exceptions – have had to be published in full, exposing children and adults within families to media-promoted local voyeuristic and vigilante interest. This led to an initial drop in the number of SCRs being authorised by the independent chairs of LSCBs.

SCRs had also become a mechanism for allocating 'accountability' to workers and agencies when a child died or was seriously injured, with reviews being rejected by the minister if they did not apportion accountability, as happened when Edward Timpson rejected the first SCR following the death of Hamza Khan in Bradford and then required that another review be undertaken.[55]

SCRs prepared after something terrible has happened to a child, along with Ofsted's more demanding inspections, with more demeaning judgement labels ('adequate' becoming 'requires improvement'), have provided the government with the ammunition to claim that councils are not competent to directly provide children's social services.

In 2014 the coalition government set up a so-called 'national panel of independent experts' (although those who formed the board – a journalist, a barrister, a former head of the Big Lottery who became the chief executive of the NSPCC, and an air accident investigator – had no direct experience of front-line child protection work) to push for more SCRs to be done and published in full, and to report on whether those which were undertaken were adequate and whether they took the assumption that workers and agencies had failed.[56]

The panel was successful in delivering what the government wanted. It put pressure on LSCBs and their independent chairs to undertake, and to publish in full, more SCRs, with the panel's first annual report showing that it made the prior assumption that there must have been agency and worker 'failure' and 'mistakes' if a child or young person had been significantly harmed or had died as a consequence of abuse or neglect.[57, 58]

SCRs have been skewed by their focus on one case, and often one incident, with all the benefit of hindsight of now knowing that something terrible has happened but with little or no account taken of the context of other work and working conditions in which the workers at the time were immersed. SCRs have become feared, as well as costly and distracting, with the completion of the SCR becoming the goal in its own right before moving on to another SCR sometime in the future.[59]

What Wood proposed would give the Secretary of State for Education the responsibility to set up an independent national body, reporting to the Secretary of State. Here lies the primary concern. When Wood's proposals were integrated into the Children and Social Work Bill with the intention that a 'Child Safeguarding Practice Review Panel' be established by the Secretary of State for Education, it was stated that the panel would 'identify serious child safeguarding cases in England which raise issues that are complex or of national importance, and where they consider it appropriate to arrange for those cases to be reviewed under their supervision'.[60] The chair of the panel and its members would be appointed by the Secretary of State. The response of the AILC was that:

> This is of great concern to AILC. It is critical for the authority and credibility of this Panel that it is demonstrably independent from ministerial control, and can pose the difficult questions about policy which may emerge from national reviews that are complex and important.[61]

This is not an unreasonable concern expressed by the LSCB independent chairs. As noted above, when the government set up a 'national panel of independent experts', none had experience in front-line child protection or its direct management. A similar scenario arose when the Secretary of State in 2016 appointed Amanda Spielman as the new Ofsted chief inspector for Education, Children's Services and Skills. She had no teaching or children's social care experience. Instead her background was as a merchant banker and chair of the Office of Qualifications and Examinations Regulation (OFQUAL). She had also worked as Director of Research and Policy at ARK schools, a multi-academy trust, with the government's flagship education policy being that all schools should become academies outside the control of local authorities (a policy which was enhanced further by Theresa May who, when she became Prime Minister, wanted to establish academy grammar schools).

Amanda Spielman's lack of experience in any of the professions, or of the direct management of the services that Ofsted inspects caused consternation to the Education Select Committee and its Conservative chair who advised against the appointment.[62] The government still went ahead. This was shortly followed by the resignation of the government's recently appointed chair of Ofsted, also a former city banker, after he spoke about schools on the Isle of Wight and called the island a 'ghetto' characterised by 'in-breeding'.[63]

A lesson which might be drawn from these 2016 Ofsted experiences is that having been a city or merchant banker had, according to the government, greater credibility for inspecting schools and children's social services than having been a teacher, head teacher, social worker or children's services director. It is not surprising, therefore, that the AILC should comment:

> We are disappointed that the [Children and Social Work] Bill fails to take account of the necessity to specify that this new [Child Safeguarding Practice Review] Panel must include members with frontline safeguarding experience.[64]

When the membership of the national Child Safeguarding Practice Review Panel was announced in June 2018[65] there was some relief that its membership did include those with a wide-ranging and embedded experience of child protection across social services, health, schools and the courts. However, the panel is to be chaired by Edward Timpson, the former Minister for Children who lost his parliamentary seat at the 2018 general election and who had led for the government on the Children and Social Work Bill with its proposals to undermine the rights of children and increase the political control of social workers.

A consistent theme

From all of the above a theme can be seen to have emerged of increasing central government's intended political control of children's social services. This is of a different nature from Parliament debating and setting legislation which gives duties and powers to local authorities and others to assist, and when necessary protect, children and which gives rights to children. What was proposed and intended by the government through the 'exemption clauses' was that an individual politician should have the power to set aside legislation and to determine who he or she wants to have control over serious case reviews. This is a combination of the centralisation of power and the creeping politicisation of children's services.

Social worker regulation, education and accreditation

These themes were repeated and reinforced in the clauses in the Bill which referred to the registration of social workers, how they should be educated, and how they were to be accredited (which would determine whether or not they would be able to be employed in specific roles).

Here is the justification given by Lord Nash,* the Schools Minister who led for the government on the Bill in the House of Lords:

> Almost one in four councils inspected under Ofsted's current inspection framework has a judgment which indicates that its practice is inadequate. In the light of that startling statistic, it is critical that the Secretary of State is able to bring forward improvement activity that she believes will help raise the standard of social work practice by making clear what standards are expected of children and family social workers and assessing social workers against those improvement standards.[66]

---

* There is another continuing theme evident here of bankers, venture capitalists and management accountants dominating and determining the future of social work. Baron Nash had a background as a venture capitalist setting up private equity companies and was a major donor to the Conservative party and sponsor of academy schools. Justine Greening, the Secretary of State for Education, had previously been an accountant for, among others, PricewaterhouseCoopers.

As Andy McNicoll commented in *Community Care*, 'In other professions, we might expect a professional body to undertake that work but, for now at least, there is no such body for social workers.'[67] Why is there no such body for social workers? In 2012, with the support of the coalition government and with Tim Loughton, as Children's Minister, a champion for its development, a College of Social Work was founded, following the recommendations of the Social Work Task Force.[68] Despite warnings to the contrary, its founding embryonic board whose composition had been determined with considerable influence from ministers and civil servants, decided right from the beginning on a costly infrastructure for the College based on assumptions about a rapidly growing paying membership. The consequence of this was that it was dependent on government funding and this dependence ran well beyond its initial set-up period. This challenged any view about the independence of the College,[69] and was reinforced when those initially appointed to key roles within the College decided that there would be a pause for several years before the membership would be able to elect the College chair.

The College then hit the financial buffers when the Department for Education decided to award a £2 million contract to KPMG, the international company of management accountants, to develop a national accreditation process for children's social workers. This role should have been central to the remit of the College, and the failure to get this contract, set alongside the high operating costs of the College, led to the College being financially unsustainable, and within a few months in 2015 it closed.[70]

It may, rightly, be noted that the government and civil servants, in influencing how the College was initially structured and then later through the routing of money to a commercial management accountancy company rather than to the College, were complicit – and indeed central – to the College's quick demise. It may seem somewhat disingenuous, therefore, when the minister in the Lords argues that the government should determine and control the assessment of social workers (in England) because there is no social work body to fulfil this task, especially when it is reported that 'the government [had] concluded in 2015 that the College was an organisation "that was no longer wanted or needed"'.[71] It is also of note how Ofsted and its ratings of local authorities was used as a vehicle and justification for the government to take control of the social work profession and social workers.

Social work regulation

So what was proposed by the government in the Children and Social Work Bill? First, on social worker regulation in June 2016, the Department for Education and the Department for Health jointly published a policy statement in which it was stated that:

> The current regulator, the Health and Care Professions Council (HCPC), has an approach designed to maintain minimum standards of public safety and initial education across a range of professions, rather than drive up standards in any one profession. The need to drive up standards in social work is, though, vital for a profession where the safety of our most vulnerable people is inextricably linked with the highest standards of practice. In addition, it has not been possible in social work to create a sustainable professional body which could play a decisive role in raising standards. A distinct social work specific regulator will have the expertise and standards oriented approach essential to this drive for improvement. Given the need for reform, the desire to effect change quickly and the links to its wider reform programme, Government believes that the most appropriate course of action at this time is for regulation to move closer to Government.[72]

So it was clear that the new regulator (Social Work England) was to be 'closer to government', with the implication of greater political oversight, interference and influence.

Unlike the other UK administrations, which have maintained a consistency in the arrangements for regulating social workers, there had been rapid churn and change in England. In 1998 the then Labour government published a White Paper on 'Modernising Social Services', which included the proposal to establish a General Social Care Council (GSCC) to register (and when necessary to deregister) those working in social care, including in particular social workers, and to oversee their education and training. 'Social worker' would for the first time become a protected title to be used only by those who were appropriately qualified and registered, and social work was to be a graduate profession.[73]

The GSCC was established in 2001. In 2012 it was closed by the Conservative and Liberal Democrat coalition government as a part of its austerity drive by reducing the number and costs of quasi-autonomous non-governmental organisations (QUANGOs). The GSCC functions were integrated into the Health Professions Council, which was renamed the Health and Care Professions Council (HCPC). The cost of the GSCC closure and the transfer of social work regulation to the HCPC was stated to be £17.9 million, with it estimated that the transfer would save each year £13.5 million.[74] It was a surprise, therefore, that only four years later the government had a change of mind and wanted to establish in England a regulator for social work only, albeit one which was much closer to, and in the control of, the Secretary of State for Education. This new regulator would determine who could and could not be a social worker and how they were to be educated and trained, by whom, and what was to be the content of their education.

The move to a separate stand-alone specialist regulator for social workers might be seen as positive by the social work profession but there were concerns about the costs of the new regulator and how these might lead to higher registration fees for social workers. Primarily, however, the concern was about the proposed government control of the social work profession.

The proposal for greater government control of social work and social workers was supported by the two Chief Social Workers, who wrote:

> The policy statement confirms that government will initially establish the new regulator as an executive agency. It will be jointly supported by

both the Department of Health and Department for Education. We know that this closer relationship with government will cause some concern but believe that this is the right model to deliver the changes that we all want to see as quickly and efficiently as possible.[71]

Isabelle Trowler, the Chief Social Worker for Children, in an interview in July 2016 reinforced her support for government-controlled regulation of social work and social workers:

Trowler acknowledged the plan was contentious but said giving social work 'a closer relationship' with government was necessary and offered an opportunity to get ministers to understand, invest in and promote the profession. She said: 'When push comes to shove it is the best chance all round to get us to a position of rebuilding public confidence in the social work profession. No matter how unfair you think it might be that this is the public narrative – that we need to get better – we are stuck with it until we do something about it.'[76]

This comment from the Chief Social Worker for Children in 2016 echoes her comments in 2014 that:

As a profession we have long argued to be allowed professional autonomy, for society to trust our judgment and let us get on with the job. For this to happen, and with such a chequered recent history, we have to earn that public trust before we can expect to be given the professional freedoms we crave.[77]

The intention to have a government-controlled regulator of social work and social workers, however, was widely rejected by social workers,[78, 79, 80] and by directors of children's services and the Local Government Association:

The Local Government Association said the new regulator 'must have guaranteed independence' and lent its support to an amendment to the bill that would require this. Dave Hill, ADCS president, told *Community Care*: 'We think it ought to have independence. When you imagine an executive agency of government making judgments about individual social workers' permission to practice, it seems to us a very odd position to find ourselves in. This may not happen in practice, but in theory it means [children's minister] Edward Timpson, or [education secretary] Nicky Morgan or whoever is in the government at the time, could directly have a role to play in decisions about an individual social worker. Say there is a serious case review and someone was being critical of the social worker in that scenario. We just think it cries out for that to be arm's length from the government.'[81]

In the face of concerted and widespread opposition to the intention that the social work profession and social workers in England should be within the control of the Secretary of State for Education, and despite this being championed by the Chief Social Workers, the government dropped this proposal. Instead, there was an acceptance by ministers in October 2016 that the new social work regulator should not be located within, or within the direct control of, government after 'fierce criticism from several sector bodies has prompted a rethink, with the British Association of Social Workers (BASW), the Association of Directors of Children's Services and the Local Government Association among those who insisted that any new regulator must have independence from government'. The Secretary of State for Education would, however, determine who was to be the chair and chief executive of the new social work regulator.[*, 82, 83]

---

* There was relief and reassurance when it was announced that former social workers had been appointed as the chair (Lord Patel) and the chief executive (Colum Conway) of Social Work England (https://www.basw.co.uk/media/news/2018/jun/new-chief-executive-social-work-england-urged-work-basw-england-promote).

Social work education

At the last moment in February 2017 as the Children and Social Work Bill was concluding its progress through Parliament, and therefore avoiding much further comment and debate, the government introduced new clauses which would still give the Secretary of State for Education control over the education and the accreditation of social workers. The government may have moved back from its initial intention for there to be direct political control of the social work regulator but its last-minute manoeuvre still means it has found a new route to exert political control of social work and social workers, as noted by Thoburn, Featherstone and Morris:

> The last minute introduction of new clauses on, and the wording of, ministerial powers and duties relevant to social work education (replacing section 67 in the 2000 Act) also raise concerns. This could open the door to the minister holding untrammelled powers over qualifying education. Finally, [a new clause inserted into the Bill] empowers the minister to take full responsibility for the assessment and accreditation of qualified social workers working in statutory child and family social work. This offers an unprecedented level of control to a government minister over a key aspect of post-qualifying development and opens the door very explicitly to political control. It is important that an area such as social work education is not subject to the whims of any government whatever its political hue.[84]

The government's proposals, shaped and led by the Chief Social Worker for Children, for the accreditation of children and families social workers and managers (working in statutory services) had caused concern because, as noted by the Association of Directors of Children's Services, they posed 'a serious risk ... to unintentionally, destabilise and demoralise the workforce'.[85] There had also been concern that the government was requiring and supporting too-early specialisation by social workers, rather than a generic initial education and training, followed by post-qualification more specialised education and training.

The government's preference for fast-track social work education and training programmes, and especially the training provided by the Frontline company for student children's social workers and social work managers, which in 2017 announced that it would now deliver its education programmes on its own and not through universities, also generated concern that it was taking social work education away from being embedded in universities and from its links with research and knowledge generation.[86]

Frontline is a controversial vehicle for the education and training of social workers. It was set up by Josh Macalister, a teacher educated through the fast-track Teach First programme who left his short career in teaching to set up the Frontline company to parallel Teach First in social work. It is based on the premise that new entrants to social work should be recruited from graduates from top-ranking 'Russell Group' universities in the United Kingdom, and should undertake a foreshortened social work education which focuses on children's social work and especially child protection. Frontline students receive a salary, unlike most social work students who instead have to pay fees for their social work education. Frontline students spend most of their time working in local authority children's services with short periods of education outside of their service agency. They are promised fast promotions into leadership roles in social work (or within, for example, the civil service). Both Conservatives and Labour political groups have given support to, and favoured, Frontline over other routes for the education and training of social workers.*

The concerns about Frontline and how it is developing have been expressed by the House of Commons Education Select Committee[87] and by Professor Donald Forrester, the first academic director of Frontline.[88] There was concern that

---

* The Department of Health has spawned a similar programme to Frontline, called Think Ahead, for mental health social workers. Neither of its co-chief executives are social workers. Both have backgrounds as civil servants, including leading on the government's policy agenda for the academisation of schools, taking them outside of local authorities.

too early specialisation failed to recognise the core professional competencies required of all social workers and that unhitching social work education from universities with their knowledge generation as well as knowledge transmission functions would undermine social work research. There was also concern that the generous government resourcing of Frontline and its students, at the same time as university social work education and social work students were seeing funding and bursaries cut, discriminated against (what was still) the majority of social work students.[89]

The financial support of Frontline by hedge funds also caused concern, with it noted that:

> Frontline's founding partners include international children's charity Ark, which was set up by a group of hedge-fund financiers and runs 34 academy schools, the Boston Consulting Group and the Credit Suisse financial services group. In addition to £3.7m of government funding (£6m if student bursaries are included), [Frontline] says it has received £1.2m in 'support from elsewhere'. Sam Baron, chair of the Joint University Council's Social Work Education Committee, says: 'One of our chief concerns is that social work education must remain in the public sector where there is accountability and transparency. Frontline is premised on the idea of private funding and that leads to a disparity of resources between the different [training] routes.'[90]

There was concern about how Frontline might easily slot within a future of privatised children's social work services, with Frontline-trained social workers and managers as the new cadre within privatised services[91] overseeing a practice workforce increasingly made up of those who were not professionally qualified social workers (a pattern which would replicate what has already happened in what was the Probation Service). This concern was reinforced by Deloitte's, the international management accountancy firm, providing training on leadership within the Frontline programme,[92] and the constitution of the Frontline board replete with bankers and those with their professional backgrounds in international finance and consultancy.[93]

There is also concern that the government's funding and marketing preference for Frontline and other fast-track social work training programmes will undermine the two- and three-year degree programmes provided by universities. It was only in 2002 that social work in the United Kingdom became a graduate profession. Since that time several universities – including the Russell Group universities favoured by the government – have closed their social work degrees. These include Oxford, Exeter, Reading and Southampton Universities and the London School of Economics and Political Science. There is a danger that without a coherent national plan for social work education some regions and areas could find themselves without a regional or local university where students with local ties and links might undertake their social work education.

One of the major means of building a stable social work workforce is to support local people to become social workers. They are more likely to stay in the area, as this is where they have their roots, identity and family commitments. This will be undermined if there is no geographically accessible university. Unless there is coherence in the strategic planning of social work education decisions will be taken institution by institution, as is now happening. For example, Durham University in 2017 looked to close its social work degrees stating that it was informed in part by 'the launching of new fast-track schemes' in north east England,[94] although following campaigning, social work education at Durham University is set to continue.

The commitment of universities to providing social work degrees is not helped by three factors. First, it is getting more and more difficult in some areas to arrange placements within local authorities as they have already committed themselves to provide student placements through Frontline and these students are given priority. Secondly, the government in 2016 caused great concern, and showed great disrespect to social work students and educators, by leaving it until the beginning of August to give information about student bursaries for students due to start their degree programmes in September.[95] Thirdly, whilst giving a commitment to the (increased) future funding of fast-track programmes largely provided outside of universities, the government has left uncertain and vulnerable the future funding of students undertaking, and universities providing, two- and three-year social work degrees.[96] Funding has already been reduced and courses have been closing, with the number of social work courses falling by 7% in 2014/15 alone.[97]

In the 2017 general election political manifestos, both the Conservative party and the Liberal Democrat party gave an explicit commitment to support Frontline and Think Ahead fast-track training programmes with no mention of the other routes to social work qualification. The Labour manifesto, in contrast, stated:

> We will continue to support all training routes for social workers, including initial social work training provided within or accredited by a higher education institution. We will also prevent the private sector and subsidiaries of private companies from running child protection services. We will deliver earlier protection to victims of abuse by strengthening mandatory reporting, and guaranteeing allegations will be reported and action taken to make children safe.[98]

The first two Labour manifesto commitments might be supported by many social workers. The third commitment to 'strengthen mandatory reporting' of child abuse would lead to an overwhelming flood of new referrals to children's social services from other professionals in, for example, schools and the health services who might take what would be a sensible personal strategy of reporting every instance of a bruise or any other concern to social services whether or not the concern had any foundation. Families would be drawn into a rapidly widening net of investigations and intrusion, and children who needed protection would be lost from sight. To quote Eileen Munro, who undertook the government-commissioned review of social work and child protection in 2011,[99] widening the net ends up looking for a needle in a haystack with the haystack getting bigger and bigger.[100] Mandatory reporting, along with introducing an imprisonable criminal offence of wilful neglect for social workers and others, were proposals from Mr Cameron's Conservative government which were abandoned in 2018.

The roots of the political support for Frontline go back in part to the review of social work education commissioned by Michael Gove when he was Secretary of State for Education and where Mr Gove again drew on Sir Martin Narey, who had previously been active for Mr Gove and the DfE in championing adoption (and when Mr Gove moved to become Secretary of State for Justice, Narey also moved to become one of the advisors to Mr Gove's new ministry). Martin Narey recommended that 'universities should be encouraged to develop degrees for those intending to work in children's social work'.[101]

Narey's call that there should be separate and specialised initial education for social workers who might want to work in (statutory) children's services (albeit with implications for later restrictions on cross-national and career movement for social workers into and out of children's services) ran counter to the argument of David Croisdale-Appleby's more extensive and evidenced review commissioned by the Department of Health that initial social work education and qualification should be generic, and followed by post-qualifying specialist education and continuing professional development.[102] It was the Croisdale-Appleby review, and how it was undertaken and informed, which was applauded within the social work community.[103]

Sir Martin Narey also called 'for the current requirement that all registered social workers must have a degree in social work to be scrapped. Child protection should become a two-tier profession made up of graduates and a new cadre of "social work assistants".'[104] The dangers of down-skilling the overall social work force – as has happened for probation officers in what had been the Probation Service since it was largely opened up to the commercial marketplace (see Chapter Nine) – were now on the table.

In 2017 it was reported that the social work regulators in Scotland and Northern Ireland would place restrictions on social workers in England qualifying through Frontline:

> Social workers trained by the Frontline fast-track programme will face restrictions on practising outside

of England. The social work regulators in Scotland and Northern Ireland have concluded Frontline's course is not generic enough to arm social workers with the skills to work with all age groups. As a default, the regulators will only register Frontline graduates on the condition they work in children's services or take on extra training. The move is unprecedented and means changes are likely to be made to a longstanding agreement designed to help social workers move between UK countries.[105]

In 2015 Sir Martin Narey was still canvassing support for his report and his proposals, and noting that 'his call for the shift in social work training came from meeting graduates from the Step Up to Social Work and Frontline training programmes'.[106] The way these programmes receive preferential treatment by government in 2017 indicate that Narey's proposals have largely been accepted by the government. The government funding differential between different social work education routes is startling:

> The unit costs to government are significantly lower for the traditional routes. The cost is lowest for the undergraduate route (£14,675) with the postgraduate (MA/MSc) route 58% higher at £23,225. The lowest accelerated unit cost route is Step Up, which at £40,413, is 12% lower than Frontline (£45,323). The most expensive accelerated route unit cost is approximately three times higher than the lowest cost traditional route.[107]

Isabelle Trowler, the Chief Social Worker for Children, has consistently been a strong advocate for Frontline despite the concerns about its impact on the coherence of the social work profession, not to mention its high costs at a time when social work services are experiencing financial cuts generated by government.

Knowledge and Skills Statement

It was the Chief Social Worker for Children who also took the lead in creating and promoting the Knowledge and Skills Statement (KSS)[108] for statutory children's services social workers, a task which Sir Martin Narey in his report on social work education had argued should be allocated to her. As with so many government-generated changes for social work in England in the 2010s, the drive has been initiated within the Department for Education, with the Department of Health having to respond to ensure that social workers working with adults are not left outside of the government's script. It was not until October 2014 that a consultation on a KSS for adult social workers was launched,[109] several months after the publication of the draft KSS for children and families social workers.

The KSS are intended to define the knowledge and core skills to be required by social workers working in statutory children's, and separately adults', social services, with social workers to be tested against the standards set by the government. This will then govern who will be allowed to hold social work posts within local authority (and outsourced) statutory services.

There are many concerns about the development and advent of the KSS for children's and adults social workers. First, the KSS are divisive, separating social workers into children's or adults' social workers from the earliest stage of their social work career rather than providing a competency statement which would apply to all social workers. Secondly, they undermine the Professional Capabilities Framework (PCF) developed through the Social Work Task Force by those within the social work profession, which provides a career-long progression framework applicable to all social workers. Thirdly, the KSS have been generated with little engagement with social workers or the social work profession, and their genesis, development and ownership is within the government. Fourthly, the initial consultation process on the KSS for children was launched on 28 July 2014 and closed on 1 September 2014. It is hard to think of anything less credible and more disrespectful than giving only the holiday month of August as the timeframe for a national consultation.

But possibly most surprisingly, the initial draft KSS statement prepared and published by the Chief Social Worker for Children included the statement that social workers should 'demonstrate positive relationships and attitudes towards politicians'.[110] The original draft KSS consultation document containing this statement that social workers should have a positive attitude to politicians was no longer traceable on the government's websites in 2017. It is shocking, however, to think that it was ever proposed that social workers should be required to hold and to demonstrate a positive relationship and attitude to politicians regardless of the policies, actions and impact of the politicians.

Social worker accreditation

The KSS is of particular significance as it will shape the future education curriculum for children's social workers (which, as a consequence of section 43(2)(b) of the 2017 Children and Social Work Act, can be determined by the Secretary of State for Education) and it provides the foundation for the government-owned and -controlled accreditation process being introduced for children's social workers working within statutory children's services.

In January 2016[111] the then Secretary of State for Children, Nicky Morgan, also noted that the KSS would be used as the foundation for the government's compulsory scheme to accredit children and families social workers and their managers, and through the scheme to decide who would be able to be employed in statutory children's social work services.

The contract to develop the accreditation process for children's social workers was awarded by the government in March 2015 to a consortium led by KPMG in partnership with Morning Lane Associates, the University of Leeds and LEO (a digital learning company),[112] with it being noted that:

> KPMG, one of the four largest professional services companies in the world, is expected to share the contract with Morning Lane Associates – the consultancy jointly set up by Isabelle Trowler along with former Hackney assistant director Steve

Goodman after they developed the Reclaiming Social Work model. Trowler resigned from the company when she became children's chief social worker in September 2013. The company's public accounts show she handed over her shares in the August before she took up her post.[113]

It was the letting of this contract to KPMG rather than the College of Social Workers which brought the College to an end. The PCF had been within the remit of the College and it was transferred to the British Association of Social Workers when the College closed. In 2017 it was being reviewed and revitalised by BASW,[114] albeit with the government still ploughing ahead with its separate Knowledge and Skills Statements for different employment groups of social workers.

KPMG's leading role in developing a government-controlled accreditation scheme for children's social workers and their managers working in statutory services was illustrated in April 2017 when at a conference organised by a company named 'Policy Communications' it was a director and a manager from KPMG who were billed as speaking on the 'national accreditation system for child and family social workers'.[115]

The government's plans to introduce a government-controlled national scheme of accreditation for children and families social workers[116] caused considerable concern. The British Association of Social Workers surveyed its members, and it was subsequently reported that:

> BASW, which represents more than 22,000 social workers, said the accreditation system planned by the Department for Education was 'unjustifiably' costly and poorly designed, risked worsening the profession's recruitment and retention problems, and marked a further step towards breaking the link between adults and children's social work. The association urged the DfE to rethink the 'flawed and unpopular' plans and work with the profession to develop an ongoing CPD framework for all social workers. The DfE's lack of sector involvement in the

development of accreditation was a 'significant failure' ....The association said the plans also added to wider fears over the way the knowledge base for social workers in England is being developed, with concerns the DfE is favouring profit-making firms over sector bodies and universities for projects that are key to shaping social work. The department awarded a £2m contract to develop accreditation to a consortium led by management consultancy giant KPMG and social work firm Morning Lane Associates. Global consultancy firms Mott MacDonald and Deloitte have also won DfE contracts to oversee other key planks of social care reform.[117]

The public sector trade union Unison also surveyed its social work members and 'almost all (99%) said the system would place more pressure on individual social workers, yet a similar proportion (94%) felt the assessments would not assess practice standards fairly or accurately ... Asked what the government's priorities for social work should be, most respondents (58%) said more funding for social services, followed by action to help limit caseloads (30%). The introduction of accreditation was cited by 2%.'[118] Unison called for the government's accreditation proposals to be withdrawn.

But it was not only social workers through their professional association and trade union who opposed the government's accreditation scheme. It was also of concern to directors of children's services, the top managers of local authority statutory children's services. Through their Association in May 2016 they issued a 'position statement' on the then still embryonic government proposals, commenting that there was:

a serious risk that this reform agenda will, unintentionally, destabilise and demoralise the workforce ... ADCS acknowledges that in implementing these two statuses, we are as a sector forcing specialisation in statutory child and family social work from an early postqualifying stage in a social worker's career. We consider that there may be

unintended negative consequences as a result, which
we should be alert to and prepared to address. There
is also a risk that the implementation of these two
statuses may hamper the continuous professional
development and potentially therefore the retention
of social workers who wish to gain a breadth of
experience and knowledge across several domains
of social care practice ... There is a further danger of
creating a second class social work profession – those
that fail to become accredited in statutory child and
family social work remain registered and move into
non-statutory child and family social work (e.g.
early help) or worse, that adult social work comes
to be perceived as the Cinderella service for those
who fail to become accredited. This is not only a
concern about how the social work profession as a
whole is perceived, but it is a concern that the link
between adult and children's social work is broken.
ADCS firmly believes that in order to address the
needs of vulnerable children and young people in an
holistic and sustainable way, that a systemic approach
is required which includes breaking the cycle of adult
disadvantage, much of which is driven by the impacts
of alcohol or drug dependency or poor mental health
on adults' ability to parent their children.[119]

Almost a year after expressing their concerns in this position
statement, in March 2017 the ADCS issued further warnings:

Government plans for children's social workers to
take accreditation tests offer poor value for money at
a time frontline teams are under 'considerable strain',
directors have warned. The £23m cost of setting up a
national assessment and accreditation system (NAAS)
would be better spent on frontline social work and
early help services, the Association of Directors of
Children's Services said.[120]

These concerns were repeated and reinforced by Alison Michalska, the new incoming president of ADCS in May 2017.[121] The concerns of children's services directors about fragmenting the social work profession from the very early stage of a social worker's career, and about adult social work becoming 'a Cinderella service' when it was the behaviour of adults which had a major impact on the development and safety of children, were echoed by the president of the Association of Directors of Adult Social Services.[122]

But what of those who had been involved in the KPMG pilots of the accreditation process, and what was found through the pilots? Here is the conclusion of a social worker who volunteered to take part in the testing of the KPMG-generated accreditation tests:

> So, what was my feeling about the whole experience after helping shape the future testing of social workers? Somewhat disheartened. And most certainly disengaged. I am not closed off to the suggestion of a rigorous, national standard for child and family social workers. Indeed, I am all in favour of social workers getting used to being observed more as qualified practitioners, and to receiving greater feedback on their practice than they might currently do. However, my reasoning for doing so is constructive, not destructive. It is to build up social work skills and to develop the 'confidence in practice' from the public that the DfE has so euphemistically named this whole charade. The great irony here is, I don't believe it will win the confidence of the profession … The sad result is that this process, with its potential for promoting higher standards, feels imposed on the profession and linked to a continuing governmental rhetoric of social work failure with a desperate need for change.[123]

In addition to the concerns noted above from a participant in the accreditation pilot testing, the pilot found that older and black and ethnically minority social workers scored less well in the accreditation testing and the difference was statistically highly significant,[124] suggesting a bias in the testing process which disadvantaged those who might have more, and more relevant, professional and personal experience.

There was a particular issue that it was the role play assessment, or what was called the 'simulated practice observation', which led to a fifth of all the social workers in the accreditation pilot failing the assessment.[125] This could be a considerable deterrence for those who might have considered seeking to become children's services social workers. At the 2016 Association of Directors of Children's Services annual spring conference it was reported that:

> The failure rate triggered some concern among children's services directors at the conference. One asked if directors should prepare for employment tribunals if the pilot results meant that 20% of their workforces could fail the assessment. Speaking on a panel at the ADCS conference, Isabelle Trowler, the chief social worker for children, said she was 'not surprised' by the failure rate. She said: 'I think is it is going to give us a push to make sure the social workers that we are employing, and continue to employ, are doing a really good job'.[126]

However, if one in five children's social workers should fail to be accredited and then not be allowed to work in statutory children's social work services this would have a dramatic and immediate effect on the viability and capacity of children's social services and on the future recruitment and retention of children's social workers.

The House of Commons Education Select Committee was also concerned about the uncertainties and dangers being generated by the government-led accreditation process for social workers working in statutory children's social services, stating that 'there are still too many unanswered key policy questions for a programme which has the potential to destabilise an already fragile workforce. Subjecting social workers to rapid reform and possible upheaval may have severe consequences.'[127]

The concerns of the MPs' Select Committee in 2016 were shared by Emma Lewell-Buck in 2017 in the House of Commons debate on the clause injected very late (so it received little scrutiny) into the Children and Social Work Bill which would give the Secretary of State for Education the power to set the accreditation standards and processes for social workers:

> The new clause attempts to reassert the role of the Secretary of State in setting standards and developing assessment benchmarks post-qualification.... I cannot help thinking that there is an attempt to do something else with the new clause, especially as it has been introduced once again without any consultation or discussion with the social work sector.[128]

So, there are significant fears from social workers, directors of children's services and of adult's services, and Members of Parliament, that the intention to introduce the KPMG-developed and government-controlled accreditation process with its significant cash cost at a time of service cuts will cause confusion and potentially destabilise the statutory children's social work workforce. It is a workforce which is already experiencing high turnover, instability and a skew towards workers with little experience. The accreditation process for children's social workers also has the danger of undermining social workers working with adults who may come to be seen as having a lower status.

Despite these risks, the government committed itself to testing over 30,000 children's social workers by 2020, since revised down to 1,200[129] and then with further revision limited to social workers in only five pilot local authorities.[130]

The continuing abject failure in 2017 to engage with and listen to the social work profession, and the directors of children's and adults' social services, belied the message of Justine Greening, who in 2016 had replaced Nicky Morgan as Secretary of State for Education, about 'wanting to work with the social care sector in delivering reforms'.*

So in 2017 the government had taken upon itself the power to set professional and improvement standards for social workers and to assess and accredit social workers against these standards.

There may be another dimension of the political control of social work which is relevant to this book. If and as social work, including social work in statutory children's services and child protection, is opened up to a commercial marketplace how are standards to be set and enforced? One way is for the government to have control over the assessment and accreditation of the social work workforce, regardless of whether they are employed as public servants by a local authority or as employees of subsidiaries of G4S, Serco, Virgin Care or any other private sector contractor.

The government-controlled national accreditation of social workers reduces local authorities' capacity to decide who they can employ, or continue to employ, as social workers. It means, for example, that someone who is viewed as an experienced, competent and much respected social work practitioner or manager by the local authority and its local partners may fail the national accreditation assessment and no longer be allowed to continue in their role and employment. It is a high-risk strategy for the stability and future capacity of the social work workforce in children's and adults' services.

The journey towards privatisation which had now reached the point at which statutory children's social work and child protection services were starting to be moved outside of local authorities, with increasing explicit political control not only of the tasks performed by social workers but also of the social

---

* I am writing the first draft of this section on 8 June 2017, the day of a general election with the Conservatives, led by Theresa May, promising continued austerity, the selling off of publicly owned assets, and more cuts in funding for schools, the NHS, local authorities, welfare benefits, and public servants' pay, and Labour, led by Jeremy Corbyn, with a platform of investment in public services and holding back on and reversing some privatisations of public services. The stark contrasts between the main political parties highlight the dangers and difficulties of social work, social work education and social work standards being politically determined and controlled by whoever forms the government of the day … and now it's a day later, 9 June, and Edward Timpson, the Children's Minister, and David Mowatt, the Social Care Minister, have both failed to be re-elected, showing the volatility of politics and politicians to which the profession of social work is now being exposed.

work profession, has had a long trajectory, and this trajectory is tracked in Part Two.

The next chapter highlights one characteristic of the recent journey – the interrelationships and networking of quite a small number of key people who have been central to the agendas which have been described and recounted in the first two chapters.

THREE

The key players and their networks

As the controversy about the Children and Social Work Bill reached a crux and crescendo,[1] with the government apparently doing a U-turn[2] to water down some (but not all) of its intentions to politically control the profession of social work, and with the House of Lords voting against the (subsequently abandoned) plans that the Secretary of State for Education should be able to decide to set aside key parts of children's legislation, it is timely to reflect on who has been advising ministers and advocating for government policy. So here is a Who's Who of many of the key players. What is notable is how few there are, how widely they network with each other, and overall how little experience they have in social work practice or its direct management.

The Chief Social Worker

Isabelle Trowler is the Chief Social Worker for Children and Families and the primary professional senior civil service advisor to the government on social work with children. She was appointed in 2013 after the preferred candidate, following a full extensive and elongated civil service recruitment process, was not accepted by ministers. Michael Gove was Secretary of State for Education at the time. The recommendation of the government-commissioned and social work-led Social Work Task Force, and of the Munro review of child protection, was that there should be one chief social worker for England to advise government about social work and to be a social work champion. Ministers decided in 2013, however, to split the chief social

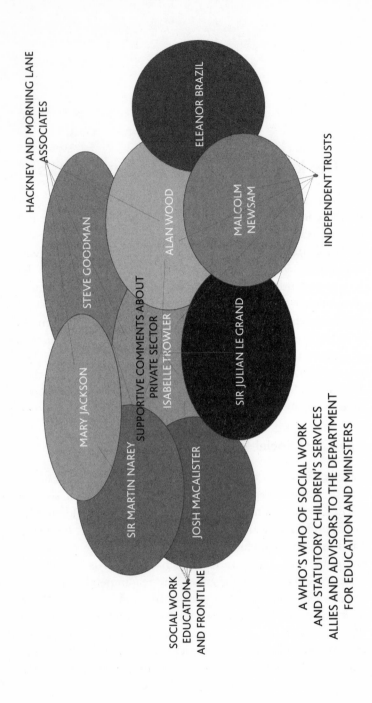

HACKNEY AND MORNING LANE ASSOCIATES

ELEANOR BRAZIL

STEVE GOODMAN

ALAN WOOD

MALCOLM NEWSAM

INDEPENDENT TRUSTS

MARY JACKSON

SUPPORTIVE COMMENTS ABOUT PRIVATE SECTOR

ISABELLE TROWLER

SIR JULIAN LE GRAND

SIR MARTIN NAREY

JOSH MACALISTER

SOCIAL WORK EDUCATION AND FRONTLINE

A WHO'S WHO OF SOCIAL WORK AND STATUTORY CHILDREN'S SERVICES ALLIES AND ADVISORS TO THE DEPARTMENT FOR EDUCATION AND MINISTERS worker role, and that there should be two separate chief social workers, one in the Department for Education (DfE) and one in the Department of Health. This caused subsequent concern to the House of Commons Education Select Committee:

> Despite the confidence of the Minister and the Chief Social Worker for Children and Families, we are concerned that the DfE and DH agendas are not coordinated, and the profession is being pulled in two different directions. There is a pressing need for greater coordination within Government on the future of social work in England. The splitting of the profession into two separate strands has been unhelpfully divisive. The appointment of two Chief Social Workers, apparently against the wishes of the profession, has exacerbated the problem ... We recommend that there be one Chief Social Worker sitting outside departmental structures, as proposed by the Munro Review. One Chief Social Worker would unify the profession at a national level and encourage joined-up thinking within Government.[3]

Isabelle Trowler was formerly assistant director for children's services in Hackney. Her actions as Chief Social Worker have not been without controversy. As noted in the previous chapter, she has introduced a competency and accreditation framework, based on the Knowledge and Skills Statement (KSS) for Child and Family Social Work,[4] which was separate from the career-spanning and profession-wide Professional Capabilities Framework[5] that had been carefully constructed by the Social Work Reform Board, with considerable contribution from across the social work community, and promoted by the College of Social Work (TCSW). Isabelle Trowler was based within the Department for Education, which in 2015 awarded a £2 million contract[6] to develop a national accreditation process based on the KSS for (statutory) children's social workers to KPMG, an international financial accountancy and auditing commercial company, and to Morning Lane Associates (MLA), at the time a small company which Isabelle Trowler had founded with a former colleague from Hackney, Steve Goodman, before she became Chief Social Worker. TCSW's failure to gain this contract led in part to its quick demise although the business plan drawn up by the College's board and management led to significant and unsustainable financial deficits.[7, 8]

Although a civil servant, Isabelle Trowler has frequently been the public spokesperson promoting government policies for social work rather than ministers. She has supported increasing private sector, for-profit participation in the provision of statutory children's social work services, tweeting that those who opposed this commercial marketisation are like the animals in *Animal Farm* who saw 'four legs good [the public service sector], two legs bad [the private, profit-focused, sector]'.[9] She was right. Those opposing private, for-profit, companies delivering statutory social work and child protection services did see a clear difference of principle, as well as motivation, between crucial decisions about the welfare and safety of children being taken on behalf of the state by non-profit, publicly accountable, public service organisations, and commercial companies whose primary and foremost concern is making money having a part in this process.

Isabelle Trowler has also said that social workers have yet to earn public trust if they are to have professional freedoms.[10] She has argued that it is 'essential' that social work regulation at this time is controlled by the government,[11] rather than social work being regulated as an independent profession. And she has also been a champion for Frontline, a fast-track education programme discussed in the previous chapter, which is very well financed by the DfE for a small minority of social work students and is now to be provided outside of universities.

Frontline and Josh Macalister

Frontline is led by Josh Macalister, briefly a teacher, after being trained through the Teach First programme.[12] He has also had a wider presence commenting in support of government policies. The Chief Social Worker for Children, who is prolific on Twitter (@isabelle trowler), publicly tweeted on 3 March 2017 to Frontline's chief executive on his birthday 'Josh Macalister may the sun always shine on you',[13] which might be seen as a little unusual as a public message from a senior civil servant to the chief executive of a company with which her department had significant contracts and which was receiving large government payments.

Frontline has considerable potential to undermine university social work courses and a unified and integrated social work profession. It has expanded into Firstline, a social work management development programme, with MLA as a major DfE-funded partner, and with Mary Jackson as Firstline's leadership development director. Jackson, who is not a social worker but has worked in change management, recruitment and communications, was previously working in Hackney and then became a shareholding director of MLA (alongside Steve Goodman and Isabelle Trowler who, as well as being the founding directors and shareholders of MLA, had been colleagues together in Hackney).[14, 15]

Morning Lane Associates and Steve Goodman

Morning Lane Associates was formed as a private company in 2010 by Goodman, Trowler and Jackson. Isabelle Trowler resigned her shareholding and directorship on 31 August 2013 when she became the DfE's chief social worker. Mary Jackson also resigned on 31 August 2013 from her MLA directorship when she was appointed as a director of Frontline prior to becoming a director of Firstline.

The concerns about the potential conflicts of interest for Isabelle Trowler and MLA, and the allocation of DfE funding to MLA, were reported on in 2015[16] and were rather exceptionally the subject of a specific investigation and report in October 2016 by the National Audit Office (NAO).[17] The NAO report states that when Isabelle Trowler was appointed as Chief Social Worker to the board of the DfE's Innovation Fund, she disclosed that she had a 'close and personal relationship' with the remaining founding MLA director, Steve Goodman. Before she became Chief Social Worker, the NAO reports that no DfE or government contracts had gone to MLA. From the DfE's

Innovation Fund alone, since September 2013, MLA with its partners have now received over £4.4 million.

The money going to MLA from the DfE's Innovation Fund, which was the focus of the NAO inquiry, is, however, only one source of government money which has been received by MLA over the past three years and which it continues to receive. It has also had, among other public funding sources, government funding as a DfE improvement and intervention advisor,[18] for 'Children's Social Care Services Advice, Support and Challenge'[19] and for the social work education and accreditation[20] developments that Isabelle Trowler has been championing. Steve Goodman, MLA's director, is also Frontline's professional advisor.[21] It may be that MLA, as a small private consultancy which previously had no government contracts, has received nearly, and maybe more than, £10 million of DfE and other public funding through a range of routes since September 2013.

The MLA company accounts filed for the year ending 30 September 2016 (as of March 2018, the most recent accounts filed with and published by Companies House) showed 'shareholders funds' of £1.97 million.[22] The company has one shareholder – its director, Stephen Goodman.[23] There was consternation in October 2017 when Steve Goodman tweeted: 'The only people responsible for increased children in care are the ADCS – don't blame austerity – adopt the Reclaim Social Work model!'[24] This denial of the impact and significance of the government's politically chosen policies of austerity targeting the poor and public services caused Twitter exchanges expressing shock that the director of MLA shifted the blame to directors of children's services for increasing numbers of children in care and sought, at the same time, to promote his own company's product – the 'Reclaiming Social Work' organisational model (see Chapter Six).

Steve Goodman was awarded an OBE in 2014, with the citation noting he was Director of Morning Lane Associates and that the OBE had been awarded for services to child protection.[25]

Sir Alan Wood

Alan Wood was Director of Children's Services (DCS) at Hackney Council, and in 2011 he was awarded a CBE for services to education and local government, in part as recognition for his success in improving schools in the borough.[26] In 2017 he was made a knight.[27]

While Sir Alan was Hackney's DCS, Steve Goodman and Isabelle Trowler were, respectively, deputy director and assistant director of Hackney Council's children's services where they created and introduced their 'Reclaiming Social Work' model.[28] Goodman and Trowler left Hackney Council to set up Morning Lane Associates (Morning Lane was the address of the children's services office in Hackney) to promote the model more widely, a process which was now supported by the DfE's Innovation Fund, with £4 million allocated to MLA and five local authorities in 2014,[29] although the way in which the model was being implemented in at least two councils led to 'inadequate' judgements by Ofsted.[30]

Isabelle Trowler and Alan Wood were original members of the five-person 'Innovation Fund's programme investment board', which had the brief to 'provide rigorous advice to the Minister on what projects the Department should invest in'. The three other board members were from the financial sector, investing in and managing hedge and investment funds.[31] The Innovation Fund itself was managed by the Spring Consortium, which was led by the international management accountancy firm Deloitte.[32]

Alan Wood's professional background was as a history teacher who became Hackney's director of education and then DCS.[33] In 2013–2014 he was president of the Association of Directors of Children's Services (ADCS). There was outrage when, in an interview as the incoming ADCS president, he called newly qualifying social workers 'crap' and was also reported as being 'unperturbed by government proposals that child protection providers might be charitable arms of for-profit providers'. Wood was described in the report of the interview by *The Guardian* as the government's 'go-to fixer for child protection'.[34]

Wood has also, in combinations alongside Isabelle Trowler and Julian Le Grand, been deployed by the government to review local authorities where Ofsted has judged them to be 'inadequate', with Doncaster[35] and Birmingham[36] having now been forced and coerced by the government to transfer their statutory children's social services outside of the public sector to independent trusts, in what has been seen as a potential Trojan horse manoeuvre taking the services outside of the public sector en route to privatisation.[37]

Since having retired as Hackney's Director of Children's Services, Wood has been commissioned to undertake a number of government reviews, including a review of the national policy of local safeguarding children's boards and serious case reviews, and of secure training centres for young people (see Chapter Two). In June 2016 he was asked by the Secretary of State to lead an Education Advisory Board for the Department for Education on the review of the role of local authorities in relation to education and children.[38] In 2017 he continued as the government's go-to person when he was appointed to the Youth Justice Board[39] and also as the chair of the Children's Residential Care Leadership Board,[40] a board which was formed to deliver the recommendations in a review undertaken in 2016 by Sir Martin Narey.[41] In 2018 Sir Alan was appointed by the government to chair the What Works Centre for children's social services, which has been awarded £20 million of government funds.[42]

Sir Julian Le Grand

Alongside Alan Wood and Isabelle Trowler in reviewing local authority children's services judged as 'inadequate' by Osfted has been Sir Julian Le Grand. He was made a Knight Bachelor in the 2015 New Year's Honours List 'for services to social science and public service'.[43]

Le Grand is the Richard Titmuss Professor of Social Policy at the London School of Economics and Political Science (LSE). The LSE closed its social work education courses many years ago. Le Grand is not a social worker and has no experience as a social work practitioner or manager of practising social workers.

Le Grand had been an advisor to Blair's New Labour governments, and had a key role in the shaping of policies introducing academy schools, foundation hospitals, and social work practices (to be discussed in the next chapter). The latter were set up to be independent companies, owned by social workers or others (including within the private, profit-making, sector), to deliver contracts from local authorities for parts of statutory social work provision, such as services for care leavers. They have not been a success, as they were separate and stranded from other council services, such as legal, human resources and finance services, on which they still needed to draw,[44] and five of the six pilots in children's services were discontinued.

Le Grand is also a board member of Think Ahead,[45] the government-created and -sponsored adult mental health social work education programme which in many ways parallels Frontline, which he also helped to shape.

A report of a recent interview with Le Grand stated:

> Julian maintains there is a 'genuine commitment" to improve services within government. He describes the current reforms as a 'flailing around to find the best way to do it'. 'It is creative turmoil. And the thing about turmoil is it is very difficult to predict what the outcome will be. I know what I would like. Whatever the outcome is I am certain it will be better.'[46]

It probably does feel like 'turmoil' to the social work workforce although they may not be so confident that the outcome of the 'flailing around' will certainly be better for children and families or for social workers.

Le Grand, Trowler and Wood were appointed by the DfE to form the 'Advisory Panel' in 2014 which was tasked 'to provide insight, guidance, and advice around the findings and options for consideration' to the LaingBuisson review and report[47] on how to 'develop the capacity and diversity of provision of children's social services in England' (see Chapter Two). This is essentially a report on how to further promote the marketisation, commercialisation and privatisation of children's social (work) services. The publication of the report was delayed by the government for over two years, maybe because the recommendations of the report, overseen by the DfE's appointed advisory panel, were too politically hot to handle. On the same day that the government published the report, when Justine Greening was the relatively new Secretary of State for Education, it also published its response,[48] distancing itself from major recommendations in the report. Media headlines following the publication of the report included that it 'revealed private sector appetite to run "full range" of children's services'[49] and the report described as proposing the '"forced privatisation" of child protection services'.[50]

Sir Martin Narey

Sir Martin Narey is another key government advisor who is not a social worker and does not have practice or management experience within the statutory children's social services he has been appointed to advise on. Sir Martin had a career in prisons management, became head of the prison service, and was an advocate for market testing of all prison provision in the UK and for greater provision by the private sector.[51] In 2015 there was a concern when he supported G4S in challenging Ofsted inspection findings about a young people's secure training centre which was run by G4S. There was some consternation when it was subsequently reported in *The Guardian* that Sir Martin had previously been paid as a consultant by G4S.[52]

When he retired from the prison service Sir Martin became the chief executive of Barnardo's, one of the four largest children's social care charities in England.* Sir Martin has been an advocate for the private sector to be involved in providing statutory child protection services.[53] He has also been the government's 'adoption czar'[54] at the time when Mr Gove, who had been adopted,[55] and Mr Timpson, whose parents had adopted and fostered children,[56] were ministers wanting more children to be adopted and to be adopted more quickly.

---

* As noted earlier, previously each of these leading children's charities was led by a social worker or by someone with their primary career experience in children's social services. None are now led by social workers or those with children's social care as their primary previous experience.

Sir Martin was commissioned by Mr Gove in 2014 to provide a report on the education of social workers, which was discussed in Chapter Two.[57] Separately, surprisingly, and wastefully, another central government department, the Department of Health, also commissioned a report on social work education.[58] This might be seen to have pre-empted a conclusion, which was drawn by Sir Martin for the DfE but not by Professor David Croisdale-Appleby who authored the DH report, that social work education should be separate for those who would work with children and those who would work with adults (somewhat ignoring the reality that children and adults live together[59]).

Sir Martin shared Mr Gove's views[60] that social workers and social work education gave too much weight to the impact of poverty and deprivation, a view which is challenged by the recently confirmed evidence that poverty and child protection concerns are linked and that it is more difficult to parent well when very poor.[61, 62, 63] The conclusions in Sir Martin's report, which has been criticised for its dependency in part on unattributed anecdote and on 'observations' not 'evidence',[64] would have given encouragement to the increasing DfE funding of Frontline, which introduced separation and a specialisation for children's social work within social workers' initial qualifying course, which had been one of Sir Martin's recommendations.[65]

More recently Sir Martin was commissioned by the government to provide a report on children's residential care. In his review he recommended that the DfE 'consider how they might encourage alternative providers from the voluntary and private sector to enter the secure care market'.[66]

Sir Martin, however, was more wary and concerned about the growth and impact of private, for-profit, foster care agencies. In the report he was commissioned to write on foster care it was noted that local authorities had been weak in their commissioning from private foster care companies and that independent foster care agencies can meet needs which local authorities cannot meet.[67] In the report by Narey and Owers, there was concern, however, about the financing of private foster care agencies:

Historically, as IFAs [independent foster care agencies] have been bought – and sometimes after a relatively short period – sold again, investor returns realised upon the sale of the business have been very high and, in our sample, ranged between 23 and 38%. This is significantly ahead of returns from both mainstream stock markets and private equity fund returns during the same period. In short, although day-to-day operating profits, which currently average around 10% may not be excessive, previous investors have obtained very high returns from selling IFAs and the debt burden of those IFAs is now, consequently, high. Servicing that debt must, we assume, contribute to the prices charged by the operating businesses. To put it another way, prices in some of these larger providers appear to be inflated by the burden of very large profits taken by investors when businesses have been bought and sold.[68]

Taking statutory children's social work and child protection outside of local authorities

Two former social workers who have been directors of children's services, Malcolm Newsam and Eleanor Brazil, have been centrally involved in reviewing and making recommendations to ministers about local councils. They have also had key roles where it has been decided that the council should transfer its statutory children's services to independent trusts, including in making recommendations to ministers and in setting up the trust arrangements. They were both involved in Doncaster, where the council was required by the government to set up an independent trust to provide its statutory children's services,[69, 70] and other recent roles include as government-appointed commissioners in Slough[71] and Sandwell,[72] with both councils required to set up independent trusts to run statutory children's social services. Brazil was awarded an OBE in 2017 and Newsam a CBE.[73]

Nick Whitfield has also been central to statutory children's social services being moved outside of local authorities. A former teacher and then schools inspector in Richmond in 2008, he became director of education and children's services for the London Borough. In 2012 he led the transfer of children's services from Richmond and Kingston upon Thames councils into the newly created community interest company 'Achieving for Children'. He subsequently was appointed by the Secretary of State for Education to advise on the future of children's social services in other councils which had been rated as 'inadequate' by Ofsted. Within his role as chief executive, Whitfield had a specific remit to expand and grow the organisation he was leading. He negotiated for children's social services in Windsor and Maidenhead also to be transferred to Achieving for Children. Whitfield was also appointed by the government as 'children's commissioner' in Sunderland,[74] and in Reading[75] he has had a leading role in advising the Secretary of State. Both councils are now transferring their children's services to newly formed companies. He was subsequently appointed to oversee the transfers. Nick Whitfield was awarded a CBE in 2017.[76]

Whitfield, Brazil and Newsam have not been advocates for the privatisation of children's social work services (indeed the reverse). And each has been much respected within their previous roles as senior managers and leaders within children's services. However unintentionally, their recent roles present the danger that having crossed the rubicon of moving children's social services outside of local authorities it has created the Trojan horse which others might use to achieve their ambitions and intentions to create a commercial marketplace for the services.

What conclusions?

What conclusions can be drawn from the Who's Who above? First, there has been a relatively small number of people who are especially engaged in advising ministers and civil servants (who rarely themselves have any practice or management experience in children's social services) about shaping and changing children's social services and their move outside of local authorities.

Secondly, many of these advisors have no professional experience in social work practice. Their motivation to improve and enhance children's social services and social work is not in question, but the initiatives and changes they have spawned are contributing to the concerns about the direction in which these services and social work are being taken.

Thirdly, the advisors appear time and time again across councils or linked through networks. For example, in January 2018 Josh Macalister, along with Edward Timpson, the former Children's Minister, was appointed to the five-person advisory board to the Children's Commissioner for England, of which Sir Martin Narey was also a member.[77] This frequent networking has been particularly noticeable in relation to those who worked in Hackney and have been associated with Morning Lane Associates (see the Who's Who chart).

Fourthly, there has been the notable absence and marginalisation of organisations such as the British Association of Social Workers (BASW), ADCS, the Local Government Association (LGA), APSW (the Association of Professors of Social Work) and JUCSWEC (the Joint Universities Council for Social Work Education), who have often been outside the ring of DfE advisors despite the responsibilities, experience and expertise held within these organisations about social work, its education and practice, and the management and delivery of statutory children's social services.

Fifthly, this may all go some way to explain the disconnect which occurred between the government and the DfE and those providing children's social services, and the discontent felt about being disengaged from central government and detached from the shaping of policies and priorities. The Education Select Committee, for example, urged that there should be more engagement by the government with those delivering children's social services.[78]

Only a few years ago the Social Work Task Force[79] and the Social Work Reform Board[80] – which the government notes it disbanded[81] when the Chief Social Workers were appointed in September 2013 – had extensive engagement from across the social work community. Both were ably chaired by Dame Moira Gibb, who ticked all the experience and expertise boxes – she was a social worker who had chaired BASW's Children and Families Committee, was a former director of social services and president of the Association of Directors of Social Services, and was, at the time she chaired the Task Force and Reform Board, a local authority chief executive. The powerful initiatives they promoted – the Professional Capabilities Framework, the College of Social Work, improvements in social work education and the selection of student social workers – have been marginalised or consigned to history by the DfE. But what has been happening over recent years has had a long history, and this is recounted in the next part of the book.

Part 2
The long haul

FOUR

The formation of the welfare state and its 1980s rejection by Thatcher

The 2014 Children and Social Work Bill and the thrust towards opening up statutory children's social work and child protection to the private sector have not emerged in isolation or in a vacuum. They are creatures of their time, and indeed, when compared to the developments and changes elsewhere, might be seen as behind the times.

What is being jettisoned?

The transfer of what were publicly owned assets and public services to a privatised commercial marketplace has been a fundamental change of principle and process. It is now the interests of the owners and shareholders, rather than the interests of the community and of service users, which are legally the first priority for those running privatised public services, including children's social services, which are now described as an 'industry'. Wealth trumps well-being and welfare as the legally required first concern of the companies now interested in the marketplace for these services which the government has wanted to create. What a change from the history embedded in much of the past 50 years.

1945–48 and through to the mid-1970s: the welfare state consensus

William Beveridge in his 1942 report[1] provided the argument and the framework for the soon-to-come welfare state with its plans for a comprehensive system of social security and the intention to tackle the 'five giants' of want, disease, ignorance, squalor and idleness.[2] As Hennessy noted:

> The essence of the Beveridge Report was the abolition of poverty by attacking its multiplicity of causes – illness, unemployment, old age – from a variety of angles with a comprehensive array of instruments. To change metaphors, it turned a patchwork of provision into a quilt.[3]

It was the 1948 National Assistance Act which first and formally noted the demise of the Poor Law. The first sentence of the 1948 Act states that it is 'an Act to terminate the existing poor law', a law which Beresford noted was built on principles of discrimination and deterrence.[4] First established in the Elizabethan era in 1601, with subsequent amendments, it had a lifespan of over 350 years before it was substantially replaced by a new moral and policy framework and a new nationwide legislative and service infrastructure.

Once established by Attlee's post-war Labour government, the commitment to a welfare state had cross-political-party backing running through the 1950s and 1960s and into the 1970s.[5] The Conservative manifesto, for example, for the 1951 general election,[6] where the Conservatives gained a majority and Churchill was returned as Prime Minister, gave an explicit statement of support for the newly created welfare state.* There was, however, a harbinger of what was to come 30 years later:

> Margaret Roberts (the future Margaret Thatcher) insisted, in more or less blatant disregard of her party's accommodation [in 1951] with the post-

---

*   What may be of some surprise in the 2010s is that the welfare state in the United Kingdom was established at a time of austerity following the economic costs of the 1939–45 Second World War. In 2010 the Conservative and Liberal Democrat coalition government used the banker-induced and -created financial crisis of 2008 to introduce a politically chosen campaign of austerity aimed at cutting back and cutting out the welfare state, targeting the poor for greater poverty, and seeking to take public expenditure back to the proportionate levels of the mid-1930s.

war settlement, that Labour's policies of universal welfare were 'pernicious and nibble into our national character far further than one would be aware at first glance'.[7]

The cross-party commitment to the welfare state even had its own phrase – Butskillism, a combination of the names of Butler and Gaitskill, leading Conservative and Labour politicians in the 1950s and early 1960s.[8] Electricity, gas and water supplies were supplied through nationalised companies. Schools, health and policing were all maintained and developed as universal public services available to and for the benefit of everyone. Council housing, social security and care for older people and for children were public services to be accessed and provided selectively when they were needed. All were within an ideology and framework of public good as a state responsibility to plan, fund and deliver.

For social work and the personal social services, the late 1960s and early 1970s were probably the pinnacle. A combination of the 1969 Children and Young Persons Act, the 1970 Chronically Sick and Disabled Persons Act, and probably most significant of all, the 1970 Local Authority Social Services Act, together gave greater legislative recognition and responsibilities to social workers.

It was the Local Authority Social Services Act, based on the 1967 Seebohm Report,[9] which led to an integrated and generic profession of social work with one professional qualification (the Certificate of Qualification in Social Work), which was introduced in 1972 by the new Central Council for the Education and Training of Social Workers (CCETSW). This was matched by the development of an integrated professional association for social workers across the United Kingdom, the British Association of Social Workers (BASW), with social work to be embedded as the lead profession in Social Services Departments (Social Work Departments in Scotland) located within local authorities.

1974–79: The wearing away of the welfare state consensus

In 1970 Harold Wilson's Labour government was replaced by a Conservative government led by Ted Heath, and Alan Clark, who became a Conservative MP in 1974 and a minister in the 1980s, noted:

> [Heath's government] failed to overturn the orthodoxy of the previous six years of Labour rule. But it went further, building upon what Wilson had put in place. There was a very small amount of privatisation, the travel agents, Thomas Cook, and some pubs in Carlisle. But other industries were nationalised, like Upper-Clyde Shipbuilders and Rolls Royce. On balance, the Heath government nationalised a larger share of economic activity than had its Labour predecessor. While the Tories had criticised the growth of public expenditure during the Wilson years, over the winter of 1972–3, public spending was accelerated.[10]

But the shared ideology and commitment to public services and the welfare state started to noticeably break down in the mid-1970s at a time when the national economy started to struggle. International financial forces hit the UK hard, and industrial and employment relationships had become strained and contentious. In the midst of industrial unrest and frequent strikes, Ted Heath, the Conservative Prime Minister, called a general election in 1974 with 'an appeal summed up in a simple three-word phrase – a phrase that became a symbol of the decade. "Who governs Britain?" But the answer was not what Heath was expecting.'[11] The replacement of the Conservative government with Labour-led governments in 1974 and in 1976 did not resolve the industrial and economic crisis – indeed, the economic crisis was about to get much worse, with significant implications for the cross-party consensus in support of the welfare state and public services, as noted by Nicholas Timmins:

Very slowly, but very surely, one of the key conditions of an affordable and effective welfare state – full employment – was being eroded. It was soon to receive a much more dire blow. In October 1973 the Yom Kippur War between Israel and the Arabs broke out. On 8 October, Sheikh Yamani, the Saudi Arabian oil minister who would soon be dubbed 'Yamani-or-your-life', met his counterparts in OPEC, the Organisation of Petroleum Exporting Countries, in Vienna. The outcome was a four-fold rise in the price of oil, the most dramatic and economically damaging global price rise in history. In Britain it produced the three-day [working] week and the rash of industrial actions which included the power workers, the railwaymen and the second miners' strike which finally brought [prime minister] Heath down ... If there was one turning point for the welfare state after 1945, this must be it. It took time and Labour's attempts to spend its way out of the trouble for the full effects to be rammed home in 1976 with the visit of the IMF [International Monetary Fund]. In future there would be plenty of expansion, not just contraction, in the field of Beveridge's five giants, and it would be far from all doom and gloom. But it would never again be quite such a glad, confident morning for the welfare state.[12]

With inflation and unemployment both high, the incoming Labour government in 1974 borrowed £5 billion from the IMF to try to ride out the oil price shock and continued to invest in public services. It had only a small parliamentary majority and was always vulnerable. In 1976 the Chancellor of the Exchequer, Denis Healey, applied to the IMF for a further loan of £2.3 billion to prop up the value of sterling. The IMF terms were that there would be more cuts of £1 billion in 1977/78 and £1.5 billion in 1978/79, beyond the £2 billion cuts in public expenditure which were already being applied.[13]

But, as noted by Dominic Sandbrook, the story was not quite as it was told at the time:

The biggest irony of the IMF crisis, though, was that it was based on dodgy figures. In an almost unbelievable twist, it transpired that the Treasury had been far too pessimistic about Britain's position. Instead of borrowing almost £11 billion a year, Britain was borrowing only £8.5 billion, which meant that Healey only needed half of the IMF money and was able to repay it more quickly than anybody had expected. Some observers have even concluded that the whole crisis was a nefarious plot by 'right-wing' Treasury officials and grasping American bankers to drag Britain away from socialism. But this is nonsense. There was no Treasury plot, not least because Healey's senior officials were so divided about the right course. The exaggerated borrowing figures were the result of a cock-up, not conspiracy.[14]

While all this was unfolding, the Parliamentary Conservative opposition were sitting waiting in the wings, with Margaret Thatcher having replaced Ted Heath as party leader in 1974.[15] In 1979, following a 'winter of discontent' characterised by strikes and other industrial action, especially across public services and by public sector workers who were experiencing the brunt of the public expenditure cuts, the Conservatives won the general election. This was the start of 17 consecutive years of Conservative governments, with major ramifications for public services.

The 1980s: Thatcherism and the push to privatise and minimise

On 4 May 1979, Mrs Thatcher became the United Kingdom's new Prime Minister. In her speech to the media outside 10 Downing Street she used a quote attributed to St Francis of Assisi:

Where there is discord, may we bring harmony.
Where there is error, may we bring truth.
Where there is doubt, may we bring faith.
And where there is despair, may we bring hope.[16]

Never can a stated aspiration have been so failed in its follow-through. Thirty-four years later when Mrs Thatcher died there were celebrations in some areas, especially the mining communities decimated in the mid-1980s, and the Wizard of Oz song 'Ding Dong! The Witch is Dead' reached number two in the music charts.[17] Despite Mrs Thatcher's inaugural Downing Street address it has been stated that 'without doubt, the great imperative was the political will to curtail public expenditure, and to wean the British people away from what the Government saw as the "dependency culture" created by an over-lavish welfare system'.[18]

The undermining of and retrenchment from the welfare state in the late 1970s was undertaken with a zeal and energy by Conservative Thatcher-led governments throughout the 1980s. It was also a time of deregulation, increasing inequality, and indeed of greed from those who already were affluent, including the bankers whose selfishness and recklessness were to undermine the national and international economies 30 years later based, in part, on the platform they created in the 1980s:

> The City became a draw for American investment banks that were going through a stage of aggressive expansion, backed by a [Reagan] US administration as keen on deregulation as Mrs Thatcher ... It is often suggested that the 1980s, or at least their second half, were years of rampant greed, let off the leash by a government that encouraged people to grab what they could and enjoy it. Mrs Thatcher had staked out her position when she was first elected leader of the Conservative Party. She declared that 'the pursuit of equality is itself a mirage ... opportunity means nothing unless it includes the right to be unequal and the freedom to be different'.[19]

It takes some imagination to see being poor, destitute and homeless as a right.

Within four years of being elected as Prime Minister in 1979, Mrs Thatcher had cut redistributive direct taxes, and especially higher rates of tax for those with the biggest incomes, but had increased VAT, which impinges disproportionately on those with the lowest incomes. Her mission to cut public expenditure, however, was in difficulty as the previous Labour government had already made significant cuts and the policies of the Conservative government were increasing the numbers of people unemployed and, despite reductions in benefits rates, this was creating an increase in expenditure on social security.

As Sir Ian Gilmour, one of the increasingly disenchanted one-nation Tory ministers, noted in 1998, 'Mrs Thatcher was irritated by the welfare state, telling one of her ministers that she thought Britain would have to return to soup kitchens',[20] and in 1992 that 'public provision was frowned upon; individualism was all ... so far from market forces proving benign in social matters, citizenship was devalued and society damaged'.[21] Mrs Thatcher, who died in 2013, did live long enough to see the introduction and expansion of food banks (and of charitable baby clothes banks), alongside soup kitchens and school breakfast clubs, as the contemporary response to increasing poverty and hunger for children and adults.

This terrible indictment of the Conservative governments of the 1980s, written as the decade ended, is all the more trenchant for being authored by a Conservative senior minister who was an insider in the early days of these governments.[*] It flags up not only the move to abandon the welfare state, public services and collective well-being, but to replace them by giving primacy and priority to largely unrestrained competitive commercial markets.

---

[*] Another account from a critical insider is to be found in Alan Clark's (1998) *The Tories: Conservatives and the Nation State 1922-1997* (London, Weidenfeld and Nicolson), pp 338-389.

FIVE

Thatcher's levers and mechanisms to promote marketisation and privatisation

A number of levers were pulled by the Thatcher government to generate the changes needed to open up public services to a competitive commercial marketplace, and these will be examined in turn in this chapter. First, there was the creation of a purchaser–provider separation within services as an initial step on the way to the fragmentation and carving up of services.

The purchaser–provider separation

The person who pulled this lever within the National Health Service and within adult social care was Sir Roy Griffiths. It might not be a surprise that his recommendations for the NHS and for social care within two government-commissioned reports were to create internal markets en route to the opening up of external markets for these services. Why no surprise? Well, Griffiths had been the managing director of Sainsbury's supermarkets with a background in retail and supply chains for groceries.

Along with the creation of a market culture, primacy was to be given to managers, who would be the new breed to drive the market processes – in effect, the next iteration moving on from the Poor Law administrators of the pre-1940s and the welfare state professionals post-1940s. This became called 'managerialism' within public services (overtaken in the 2000s by rise of the accountants who came to dominate within the increasingly privatised former public services).

For the NHS:

> The outcome was a reorganisation that separated the 'purchaser' from the 'provider' within the NHS's new 'internal market'. The main 'purchasers' were the GP practices, which were allocated budgets that they used to 'buy' hospital care. The hospitals became self-governing trusts, selling their services to GP practices and other primary care organisations. There was a veritable explosion in the number and the pay of NHS managers, as every trust needed its separate accounts department, personnel department, and so on. In five years, from 1985-1990, the cost of administering the NHS rose, after inflation had been taken into account, by 23 per cent.[1]

Even GPs as 'purchasers' of health care were to be in competition with each other:

> The aim was plainly to stimulate competition for patients amongst GPs, getting them to enter something more like a market in which patients have more choice and GPs would have to be more responsive.[2]

Griffiths was also let loose on adult social care. His 1988 report, *Community Care: An Agenda for Action*,[3] argued that local authorities, through the social workers they employed, should be 'the stimulators, facilitators, enablers and monitors – but that they did not necessarily need to provide services themselves. They could buy in much of what was needed from the private and voluntary sector[s], gaining the benefits of competition and flexibility'.[4] He especially recommended that local authorities should expand the involvement of the private sector and that 'The onus in all cases should be on the social services authorities to show that the private sector is being fully stimulated and encouraged and that competitive tenders or other means of testing the market, are being taken'.[5]

He was also critical of the track record of local authorities and argued that:

> Nothing could be more radical in the public sector than to spell out responsibilities, insist on performance and accountability, and to evidence that action is being taken; and even more radical to match policy with appropriate resources and agreed timescales.[6]

Griffiths' proposals were to be achieved by social workers and others becoming 'care managers', who would undertake assessments of individual needs, and discuss with people using social care services how within the available funding they wanted their needs to be met and who they wanted to provide them with the assistance they required. The local authority should devolve its care budget and decision-making to front-line workers and teams close to service users, set and publish eligibility requirements for services, and have a strategic role in analysing local needs and stimulating local care services through establishing a Community Care Plan and contracting for services with voluntary and private care providers.

Case management, which was to become known as care management, as a concept and process had been piloted and evaluated in Kent[7] and Gateshead[8] in the late 1970s and 1980s, and in Darlington[9] in the early 1990s, with older people. It was reported that it was cost effective in reducing admissions to residential care and hospital admissions, better matched levels of need and resources, and stimulated and harnessed a wider range of assistance. Social workers became care coordinators, supporting and advising others who were providing help to the elderly person as well as themselves assessing and counselling the older people. In essence, case management was seen to move away from the process of slotting older people into a limited and pre-ordained range of services, such as home care, day care and residential care, towards creating and drawing on wider family, neighbour and community resources.

One stumbling block for the Griffiths Report was that it recommended that local authorities should remain as the main agency delivering social care responsibilities, and indeed with the transfer of social security funds to local authorities this would mean an expanded responsibility. This did not meet with the approval of Mrs Thatcher, who was suspicious of and antagonistic towards local government in general and Labour-controlled councils in particular, which led to a delay in accepting and then (partially) implementing the Griffiths proposals.[10]

The Griffiths Report and the subsequent 1990 NHS and Community Care Act led to many local authorities introducing a 'purchaser–provider' separation within their adult social services. At the time I was deputy director of social services, and director of operations, within Berkshire County Council. In 1991 there was a reorganisation and I became 'senior assistant director (purchasing)' with a responsibility for all the social work teams, alongside a senior assistant director (service provisions) with all the foster care, home care, day and residential services within her remit, and a senior assistant director (strategy) who had responsibility for planning and also an arms-length management responsibility for the chief inspector and service inspection unit which at that time was within the council. A colleague in another local authority (Ted Unsworth in Cambridgeshire) with the same new job title as mine was often heard to comment that he was now in charge of 'shopping'!

It is hard to see how introducing the additional transactional costs of contract management and contracting out to companies who would take a (10–15%) slice of what they were paid as profits was going to generate savings and efficiencies, but this was the argument that was made then (and now). In addition to the profit-take for the owners of these companies, their chairs, boards, chief executives and senior managers were paid more than the local authority councillors and managers, who they were not replacing but duplicating, as the councillors and managers were still required to be in place to let and supervise the contracts.

The intention was to challenge and change the dominance within public services of what were seen as national and local public sector monopolies, professional protectionism, and an assumed lack of concern for costs, but the remedy to address these stated concerns – the contract culture and privatisation – was itself costly in terms of cash and of increasing complexity, as will be noted below in this chapter and also in Chapter Nine.

The 1990 NHS and Community Care Act with its focus on a purchaser–provider split within adult social services led to the separation within social services departments of adult services from children's services (where the 1989 Children Act had not driven such a split). This separation was later to be taken further through the 2004 Children Act, with children's social services being placed with local authority education services within a department of children's services, and adult services becoming lodged in a separate adult social services department.

Rigging the market

This 'mixed economy' of care in adults' social services which already existed prior to the 1980s was now to be expanded. It was, though, to be promoted in a rigged market. Following the 1990 NHS and Community Care Act, in 1992 local authorities were allocated by central government a cash-capped and reducing 'special transition grant' (STG) as they took on the responsibility for funding adult social care services, which included the money formerly available from the national social security budget for paying for residential care and nursing home care.

At this time local authorities were themselves major direct providers of these residential care services although the private sector had been growing quickly during the mid-1970s and through the 1980s following a decision that those entering care could receive their care costs through social security payments but only if they were in a non-local authority care home.

Post-1992 it remained financially preferential for local authorities to place younger and older disabled people in independent, mainly private sector, homes as there was still a social security subsidy, albeit reduced, per person towards the cost of their weekly care home fees for those living in a non-local authority care home.

The market was also rigged through a second manoeuvre. The newly set national standards concerning space and facilities requirements for care homes meant that many needed to be upgraded but the government imposed stringent restrictions on local authority capital borrowing and expenditure which made it very unlikely that local authority care homes could be upgraded while provided and managed by local councils.

Across the country many local authorities in the mid- and late 1990s and beyond either closed their care homes or transferred the homes to independent trusts or to private and voluntary care providers. Few new local authority care homes were built and the expansion in the care home market continued to be largely, indeed for older people almost exclusively, in the private and not the voluntary sector.

As the director of social services in Wiltshire in the late 1990s I led on the transfer outside of the council of 19 care homes for older people – although in the context of what was a hung council with no overall political majority the transfer was to a not-for-profit independent care trust rather than to the private sector care home companies, as the Conservative administration needed the support of the Liberal Democrat and Labour councillors who were unwilling to see the privatisation of the homes. Private companies were also seeking to get the contracts for outsourced home care services as they expanded quickly by taking on the ownership and control of local authority care homes.*

Another change introduced by the Thatcher governments of the 1980s was also to have a long-lasting impact on the care home market and on local authorities' influence over the market and market prices (as well as a significant lasting legacy in hampering councils from tackling homelessness). The right-to-buy policy which allowed, indeed encouraged, council house tenants to

---

* One of the unintended – or at least never publicly acknowledged – consequences of the purchaser–provider separation and the outsourcing of care services, is that, as a director of social services, my opportunity and ability to see and find out for myself what was happening within these services by calling in when passing and speaking with residents, relatives and staff and managers, became less possible as I no longer had a management responsibility or right of access to the services. And when, a little later, service inspection and registration units were transferred outside of local authorities to national inspectorates I lost access to the immediate information and intelligence about the independent sector services which had been available from the local authority chief inspector and inspectors who were within my management remit. I was now less informed and aware of what was happening within the care services within my area and for which I still felt an overall responsibility.

buy their council properties at preferential rates meant that many more people became home owners. Thirty or so years later when they might need residential care, the value of their property was taken into account when assessing whether they should pay for the care themselves. This, along with the occupational pensions from the pension reforms of the 1960s and 1970s, meant that many older people had more financial assets and led to more being self-funders when they needed residential (and home) care. This too has stimulated a greater private sector share of the care market, where local authorities themselves are now almost absent in some areas as either providers or purchasers of residential care.

But it was not only public sector health, care and housing services which were moved into an increasingly commercialised and competitive marketplace during the 1980s and into the 1990s. The push to privatise publicly owned services was seen as 'the jewel in the crown' of Thatcher's domestic policies.[11] Privatisation was also the fate of what had been nationalised public utilities such as the railways, telecommunications and essential supplies such as water.[12]

Nicholas Ridley was one the architects of Thatcher's push to privatisation.* He was an Old Etonian and the brother of an earl. In 1988 he published a pamphlet with the title 'The Local Right':

> Its argument was that local authorities should be stimulators, facilitators, enablers and monitors – but that they did not necessarily need to provide services themselves. They could buy in as much of what was

---

* Someone else who was also active in the privatisation push in the mid-1980s, and who was to be at the centre of the continuation of this push in the 2010s, was Oliver Letwin. He was the 'minister for policy' in the 2010 Coalition and the 2015 Cameron governments (https://www.theguardian.com/politics/2015/may/11/davidcamerons-new-cabinet-full-lineup). In the mid-1980s he was co-author of a pamphlet with John Redwood arguing for greater private sector involvement with the NHS (https://www.cps.org.uk/files/reports/original/111027171245-BritainsBiggestEnterprise1988.pdf) and the author of a book titled *Privatising the World*. Another former Etonian, when he became a government minister in 2010 he had to resign from his non-executive directorship of the merchant bank NM Rothschild Corporate Finance Ltd, where he had worked in the mid-1980s in its international privatisation unit (https://www.theguardian.com/politics/2003/oct/07/interviews.conservatives2003).

needed from the private and voluntary sector, gaining benefits of competition and flexibility.[13]

The personal social services were not be left out of this prescription for public services. Norman Fowler was the Secretary of State for Health and Social Security. Speaking in Buxton in 1984 at the annual national social services conference he set out a vision for the personal social services as enabling and not providing services and promised a Green Paper, which was never produced, on how this vision was to be taken forward.[14]

While Thatcherism was still steaming ahead in 1989, Mike McCarthy, who had been head of research for a trade union, then an assistant general secretary of the British Association of Social Workers, and is now a regional director of Retirement Securities Limited (a company providing sheltered private housing for older people), wrote:

> The government clearly saw a number of advantages in dismantling and narrowing existing [personal social services] arrangements. A wider conception of social services offered the opportunity to reduce expenditure and shed responsibilities; it would shape and control expectations; it would provoke new ideas and new initiatives; it would offer an opportunity to compare practice and policy between sectors; and it would strike a curiously popular chord, finely tuned to the Thatcherite emphasis on freedom, self-help and responsibility, which would enable tens of thousands to 'give something back to their own community by participating in social support'. Ultimately, society would come to recognise the family as the frontline of care, that the closest circle of support should be friends and neighbours and that voluntary organisations and charities should step in thereafter. The social services department would be firmly recast in the mould of 'enabler' rather than direct provider, facilitating and perhaps co-ordinating the efforts of these other sources of support.[15]

This does not seem unlike Mr Cameron's 2010 vision of a 'Big Society' of voluntary and community action replacing the role of the state in funding and delivering services,[16, 17] but in the 1980s it would have been difficult to give it this label when Mrs Thatcher had stated 'there is no such thing as society, only individuals and families'.[18]

For Fowler in the mid-1980s the focus was on promoting more of a marketplace of mixed providers for the personal social services but based on voluntary and charitable organisations rather than private companies taking on social services' responsibilities, and especially services for children. To give it impetus several central government specific grants were made available, but only charities and not local authorities were allowed to bid for these grants.

There was the 'Under Fives Initiative' funding, which the big children's charities used to develop family centres at the time the charities were moving out of providing children's homes and special boarding schools for disabled children. There were the 'Opportunities for Volunteering' grants, which funded volunteer programmes run by charities to provide help to families and disabled and older people. And there was the 'National Intermediate Treatment Fund', which again could only be drawn on by voluntary organisations and charities and which was used to develop 'IT centres' in the community for adolescents who had offended. And in Wales there was funding for the 'All Wales Strategy on Mental Handicap', which supported the development of community resources such as special fostering and respite care services as a part of the process of closing what were then the long-stay mental handicap hospitals.

At this time I was a divisional manager in South West England and Wales for Dr Barnardo's (previously Dr Barnardo's Homes and now Barnardo's). Barnardo's, as with the National Children's Homes (what had previously been the Methodist Homes for Children and is now Action for Children) and the Church of England Children's Society (previously the 'Waifs and Strays Society', now The Children's Society), was capital rich as these big national children's charities in the 1980s had sold off the sites of their children's homes and special boarding schools for children with special needs, because specialist fostering and inclusion within mainstream schools reduced the demand for residential care and segregated education. Looking to reposition their resources and reputations, they sought to expand into family and community services, drawing on the government's specific grants and in a context where growth within local authority services was drying up as government funding to councils slowed down.

There was an explicit negotiating position I was expected to take from within Barnardo's with local authorities. First, Barnardo's had uncommitted capital funding which it was willing to bring to the negotiating table to adapt or build new family and IT centres, with the ownership of the sites as an investment for Barnardo's (which could be reclaimed in the future by the charity if the contract with the council ended or the service closed). Secondly, I could negotiate that Barnardo's would contribute up to (but preferably less than) 40% of the revenue cost of the new service, which would be in the control of and managed by Barnardo's and provided through a contract to the council. But, thirdly, as a matter of principle, the new services were to enhance and enrich, but not take over or replace, the statutory responsibilities and services of the local authority.[*] So, for example, Barnardo's centres were developed to provide assistance to families within large isolated post-war council housing estates on the outskirts of Bristol, but would not replace the social work teams within the social services department. This is a different approach and principle to what is now the position, with the statutory responsibilities of councils allowed, and already in places required by the government, to be contracted outside of the local authority.

But this encouragement of a (non-statutory services) marketplace through the government making specific funding available only to voluntary organisations and charities was not the most powerful of the levers that the government created in pursuit of its polices of privatising public utilities and services. And here it was Nicholas Ridley, as Secretary of State at the Department for the Environment (which included responsibility

---

[*] It was also at this time that the NSPCC stopped using its powers to have 'inspectors' directly investigating allegations of child abuse and initiating care proceedings to seek the removal of children from families, with these actions recognised as being essentially a statutory responsibility of local authorities and not a role for a charity.

for central government local authority funding), who came to the fore again.

Compulsory competitive tendering

Ridley's particular contribution to the changing role for local government was as the author and advocate of the process of compulsory competitive tendering (CCT) for public services, one of the key processes to remove these services from collective public ownership and provision.[19]

Along with CCT as the process to drive much of the privatisation agenda, the narrative attacking public services included the mantra of VFM (Value for Money), and the 'three Es' of economy, efficiency and effectiveness, all of which, it was argued, would be enhanced by moving services into a commercial competitive marketplace. What was missing from the three Es were the Es of equity and equality, as evidenced by the second target (alongside public services) of Thatcherism – the poor. The poor were also in the firing line from reduction in access to and the amount of social security benefits. For example:

> Grants to the very poor for one-off necessities they couldn't afford were replaced by a Social Fund oriented towards loans rather than grants. At the furthest perimeters of society, the squeeze was now discernibly applied against a disease long identified in Thatcher rhetoric as the 'dependency culture', but hitherto thought too dangerous to try and cure by deprivation.[20]

Hugo Young in his overall conclusions to his 1989 biography of Margaret Thatcher noted that:

> One of the prime objectives of the Thatcher Government, repeated from a thousand platforms and rehearsed in scores of policy documents, was to reduce the role of government itself in the life of the nation. This was seen as a matter of economic efficiency: believers in market liberalism held as an

axiomatic principle that state intervention in what markets did to the economy should be held to a minimum.[21]

However, although the Conservatives won a majority in three general elections with Mrs Thatcher as their leader and then as Prime Minister, this was with a minority (about 40%) of the votes cast in the elections. As Ivor Crewe, a political scientist and analyst, noted in 1988:

> Mrs Thatcher believes in holding down government spending in order to facilitate tax cuts. But the electorate disagree: they want an expansion of public expenditure. The Gallup poll has asked at regular intervals whether, if forced to choose, they would prefer tax cuts – even at the expense of some reduction in government services such as health, education and welfare – or for these services to be extended even if this means some tax increases. In May 1979, when Mrs Thatcher entered Number Ten, there were equal numbers of tax-cutters and service-extenders. By 1983 there were twice as many service-extenders as tax-cutters; by 1987 six times as many.[22]

How to solve the enigma, then, that, although out of step with the views of most of the electorate, Thatcher was re-elected as Prime Minister throughout the 1980s? Here's Crewe again:

> So Conservative success remains a puzzle. Voters oppose the Government on a vast array of specific policy initiatives. They say they prefer Labour on the issues that matter. Their economic values are solidly social democratic, their moral values only half Thatcherite, and on both fronts they have edged to the left since 1979 ... [and Mrs Thatcher] is both intensely admired and deeply loathed ... not much liked as a human being, she is grudgingly respected as a leader ... Therein lies her electoral appeal, and it offers a clue to solving the electoral puzzle ... For

policy-based party preferences to be translated into votes, a prior condition is probably crucial: the party in question must be regarded as 'fit to govern'. In [the general elections of] 1983 and 1987 both Labour and the [Liberal and Social Democrat] alliance fell at this first hurdle, allowing the Conservatives to win because the voters judged that indeed There Was No Alternative [what at the time was known as TINA].[23]

There was a recognition in the early years of the Thatcher governments that the selling off of public assets and utilities and the privatisation of public services was not necessarily popular with the electorate. Writing in 1984 about what might now be called media and political spin, Michael Cockerell, Peter Hennessy and David Walker, three leading television and newsprint journalists, noted that in 1982 at a meeting of a government cross-departmental committee chaired by Mrs Thatcher:

The Minister of State at the Treasury, Mr John Wakeham, raised the question of how best to sell the government's privatisation policies to the electorate. He feared that the public totally misunderstood the government's motives and believed that it was selling off national assets in order to balance the books. His colleagues argued that although their 'policy concept was clear and convincing, the language lacked appeal; privatisation was an ugly word'. It was decided that the Conservatives' newly appointed marketing director, who had spent a lifetime promoting pre-packaged food and soap powder for the company that produces Mars Bars, 'should advise on a more appealing presentational approach of the government's privatisation policies'.[24]

It was not only of note, however, that Mrs Thatcher's political philosophy and privatisation programmes were not shared by all. The intention that privatisation of what were seen as public sector monopolies would drive efficiency through competition was also often not delivered, as noted by Jonathan Aitken, who was a Conservative MP in the 1980s and a minister in John Major's government in the early 1990s:

> Margaret Thatcher's personality played its part in both the strengths and weaknesses of privatisation. Strength came from her instinctive understanding that the programme was not just a series of commercial transactions; it was an important plank of her personal philosophy that the frontiers of state socialism should be rolled back. 'Privatisation is at the centre of any programme of reclaiming territory for freedom', she asserted. By 1989 she was able to claim, 'Privatisation: five industries that together were losing over £2 million in a week in the public sector, now making profits of over £100 million a week in the private sector'. Yet she did not do as much as she might have done to promote freedom of competition within the architecture of privatisation. The Electricity industry [for example] simply became a series of regional monopolies, with their ownership ending up in the hands of foreigners [a fate which also befell water and rail amongst others].[25]

Margaret Thatcher ceased to be Prime Minister in 1990, her term of office ending when the Conservative MPs turned against her, fearful of the next election and of public dissent against the poll tax (the regressive council tax which Thatcher had introduced and imposed). John Major became Prime Minister and went on to win the 1992 election. He continued the privatisation journey which Thatcher had launched, privatising British Rail, electricity generation and supply, and concluding the privatisation of the coal mines (although the intention to privatise the Royal Mail and Post Office was seen as a step too far at the time following public opposition – it was achieved by the Coalition government in 2013). Major also continued the undermining of local government, with central government imposing more controls and restrictions.[26]

In 1993, at the time Major was Prime Minister, Bob Holman, a community worker and social worker who had previously been a professor of social administration, wrote about the impact of the continuation of Thatcherism:

> Legislation to impose internal and external markets, the sharp restriction on statutory spending, the doctrine of management supremacy plus, [and] it must be added the underclass dogma which condemns many of the users of the services, have combined to mould the environment, values and practices of social welfare. In my judgment, the outcomes are – or are likely to be – serious, adverse and regrettable.[27]

Holman also noted how what was happening elsewhere to public services was now starting to be applied to children's social services:

> So far, the Government has not legislated that SSDs [social services departments] must contract out its work with families and children, although some have begun to do so in regard to adoption and fostering placements, day nurseries, the running of centres for alleged child abusers, the overseeing of child protection cases and the supervising of after-care of children who are the responsibility of local authorities. Moreover, at a 1993 conference entitled 'Child Care and the Contract Culture', the Government minister, Tim Yeo stated: 'Local authorities and the independent providers have much to gain from a whole-hearted embrace of the contract culture.' The Government then established a Support Force for residential child care with a particular brief, to make use of the private sector. Clearly, the Government is giving the green light for the welfare of children to be put out to tender.[28]

Holman was prescient in 1993 in flagging up an alert about how the welfare of children would be caught and captured in the contract culture privatisation net 20 years later. It is why we should be concerned now about the building blocks that have been put in place, and which are discussed in Chapter Two, such as the 2014 changes in statutory regulations allowing statutory children's social work and child protection responsibilities and services to be contracted outside of local authorities. Once the bricks for the foundations are in place, at any time in the future the building can be brought to completion. For children's services the foundations of privatisation are now in place and the transfer of responsibilities outside of local authorities has begun through community interest companies and the government-required independent trusts.

'Choice' as an argument for creating markets

Along with the Conservatives' focus on controls, competition and contracting there was a fourth 'c' which characterised the pressure applied to public services. Choice was also a part of the mantra which was used to drive the move of public services out of public ownership. Those who used public services were recast as consumers no different from shoppers in a retail marketplace and it was argued that if they had greater choice of services and providers this would generate a more responsive market which would drive improved quality and lower costs. But, as noted by Knapp in 1989, it was not quite so simple and straightforward:

> A common and potentially strong argument for contracting-out is that it increases the available choice to consumers [assuming, of course, that the move is not from a public to a private sector monopoly or dominant player in the market] ... But what happens when governments contract out to promote choice? We must remember that governments often take responsibility in the first place because they are not happy to leave the service to market forces. In social policy contexts, the government takes responsibility partly because the users of services – school pupils,

hospital patients, old people's home residents – might not be able to act with sufficient competence or power as consumers. They often cannot make their own views known and cannot easily move to another supplier. So on the one hand, the government wants to promote choice, but on the other hand it must recognise that the consumer may find it difficult to exercise choice. It must regulate the quality of service.[29]

These concerns would be of particular relevance to the 'consumers' of personal social services, who may be needing and seeking assistance and services at a time of personal crisis when their lives are disrupted, and/or who may have limited capacity, and/or who – as with some of those in contact with children's or mental health services – may not be choosing to have contact with the services but the contact is a consequence of concerns about their behaviour and its impact on themselves or on others.

The regulation of the quality of services was also noted by Knapp to have an impact on the diversity of services and on choice:

The problem is that [in 1989] there is now enough evidence to suggest that government regulation of private and voluntary producers of services can greatly interfere with their patterns of working. In particular, the government will require that they meet certain standards. In the extreme this makes the non-public producers more and more alike, and more similar to the government's chosen style, quality and orientation of service.[30]

The result is more standardisation rather than variety and diversity of services between which to make a choice. In essence, the packaging may look different, but the product is very similar. But there was a further concern:

[Government regulation to set and enforce standards] is also likely to encourage faithful adherence to those

> practices which are readily subjected to monitoring
> to the neglect of other objectives or activities. In
> other words, government regulation of quality can
> *reduce* choice and variety.[31] (emphasis in the original)

Regulation and its enforcement having the unintended consequence of distorting, distracting and damaging services has been forcefully felt within, in particular, children's social services in the 2010s. Being on the knife edge, waiting for an inspection, created a state of 'frozen watchfulness' within some services, and showing that rules and procedures had been followed became the primary focus and task.

Direct (cash) payments

The concept of choice was promoted especially in adult social services, first, through the 1987 Griffiths Report and the 1990 NHS and Community Care Act (discussed above) and, secondly, through the 1996 Community Care (Direct Payments) Act.

Griffiths held back from proposing that local authority care funding should be allocated as cash to disabled people so that they could decide on and purchase their own care. This was seen in the late 1980s as a step too far in enabling choice and control for disabled people. He had, however, given this some consideration and noted that:

> There is no reason why, on a controlled basis, social
> services authorities should not experiment with
> vouchers or credits for particular levels of community
> care, allowing individuals to spend them on particular
> forms of domiciliary care and to choose between
> particular suppliers as they wish.[32]

The 1990 NHS and Community Care Act which legislated many of Griffiths' recommendations did not give the power to local authorities to conduct such experiments or to transfer resources, or decisions about how they should be used and deployed, direct to service users (or, as they were called by Sir Roy Griffiths, 'consumers of community care').

Disabled people themselves, however, campaigned for such a power and process, with Jane Campbell and Michael Oliver noting in 1996:

> There is a final area where the [disabled people's] movement has succeeded in producing new legislation, and that is in the promotion of independent living by making it legal to pay disabled people cash to purchase their own personal assistance services ... Direct payments to disabled people, which have been illegal since the National Assistance Act of 1948, will be legalised in 1996, and that is solely attributable to the disability movement.[33]

Several local authorities – Hampshire, Kingston upon Thames and Wiltshire (where I was the social services director) – acted ahead of any intention by the government to allow direct payments of cash to disabled people by circumventing the existing legislation. These local authorities transferred through grants a proportion of their community care budget to a third party voluntary organisation which was then able to make cash payments to disabled people so that they could decide on and arrange the assistance they needed and wanted. These 'indirect payment' schemes were the herald and forerunner of the direct payment schemes which were allowed by the 1996 Community Care (Direct Payments) Act and which went on to become mandatory and expanded as a part of 'personal budgets'.

The intention to enable more choice and control by disabled people has been increasingly compromised, however, by the over-proceduralisation and bureaucratisation of the processes of assessing individual need within increasingly stringent rationing criteria.[34]

In effect, 'personal budgets' and 'direct payments' have been promoted and colonised by the government and compromised by bureaucracy. They allow cuts in funding and assistance to be made on an individual-by-individual basis and unseen by the wider public (unlike, for example, the closure of a care home),[35] with disabled people left with the role of rationer of the help they need and want.

But as the long run of Conservative governments in the 1980s and 1990s was brought to an end in 1997, would this also be the conclusion and end of the thrust towards marketisation and the privatisation of public services, including personal social services for children and for adults? Well, not quite, as will be recounted in the next chapter.

SIX

Blair and New Labour's continuation of the journey towards privatisation

The 1997 general election ended 17 years of Conservative governments and heralded 13 years of Labour in power. Tony Blair became Prime Minister, with Gordon Brown as the Chancellor of the Exchequer. But there was continuity as well as change from the Conservative to New Labour years, with Simon Jenkins titling his 2007 book on the transition and New Labour 'Thatcher and Sons', and writing:

> Tony Blair had [already] changed the British Labour party beyond recognition. On 2 May 1997, he set out to 'change Britain'. His objective was not achieve any great policy upheaval. He had shown no interest in reversing the Thatcher revolution and in power respected it. Just as the post-war 'welfare settlement' had held sway through the governments of both parties for thirty years, so now the Thatcherite settlement assumed an equal bipartisanship. Debate was how to make it work.[1]

Part of making it work was the focus on the modernisation rather than the abolition of public services. Thatcher had seen public services as wasteful. Creating competition was promoted as the means to drive value for money. The consequence was that more services were delivered through a commercial marketplace by private companies, public servants became the makers of contracts, and managers, rather than professionals, became more powerful and controlling.[2] The contract culture and managerialism had come to dominate the public service agendas. These were all trends which were continued by the New Labour governments from 1997 onwards.

The journey continued, but some of the jargon and processes were reset. Value for money and the focus on the three Es was rebadged as seeking and demanding 'Best Value' from public services. There was to be a move away from the Conservative government's enforced compulsory competitive tendering of public, and especially local authority, services. Instead there was to be a national requirement that *all* local authority services (there were to be no exceptions so all social services and social work services were captured within this process) were to be opened up to a 'Best Value' analysis and appraisal which was to be based on the 'four Cs' of compare, challenge, consult and compete.[*,3]

The context for the 'Best Value' requirements introduced in 1999 by New Labour was described by Tony Blair:

> I was learning how complex the institutions of public service were, how multiple their pressures, how vast their demands, and how great the expectations were of what could be done and in what period of time. The millennium may have been an exceptional moment in the calendar, but the 1999/2000 NHS 'winter crisis' came with the monotonous predictability of death and taxes. And two and a half years in [to the New labour government], people expected better ... I had an increasing worry on health and education, which was that while the Tory reforms may have been badly implemented and badly explained, their essential direction was one that was in fact nothing to do with being 'Tory', but to do with the modern world. These reforms were all about trying to introduce systems

[*] In Wiltshire, where I was the social services director, we added three further Cs to our Best Value social services reviews – community, cooperation and collaboration – with community involvement and community engagement of services provided in collaboration with each other seen as having value in driving local commitment and contribution, and in promoting coherence across and between services. This variation and enhancement of the required 'Best Value' review process was not challenged by the District Auditor who, at the time, oversaw for the government locally undertaken Best Value reviews.

where the money was linked to performance and where the service user was in the driving seat ... I could see a trend that was about breaking down centralised and monolithic structures, about focusing on developing tastes of consumers, about ending old demarcations in professions; and this trend seemed to me to be related to how people behaved, not how government behaved. The precise shift in the way the private sector was organised and managed seemed, and not unnaturally, to have its echo in the challenges facing the public sector.[4]

In addition to the 'Best Value' requirements, with their focus on competition and potential outsourcing, Blair also initiated a unit[5] to drive improvements within public services:

We established a [public sector change] Delivery Unit ... It was an innovation that was much resisted, but utterly invaluable, and proved its worth time and time again. It was a relatively small organisation, staffed by civil servants but also outsiders from McKinsey, Bain and other private sector companies, whose job was to track the delivery of key government priorities. It would focus like a laser on an issue, draw up a plan to resolve it working with the department concerned, and then performance-manage it to solution.[6]

But, as explicitly noted by Blair, the changes being introduced and enforced for public services were also about opening up the services to the private sector:

I have described a journey. At first we govern with a clear radical instinct but without the knowledge and experience of where that instinct should take us in specific policy terms. In particular, we think it plausible to separate structures from standards, i.e. we believe that you can keep the given parameters of the existing public service system but still make fundamental change to the outcomes the system produces. In time, we realise this is wrong; unless you change structures, you can't raise standards more than incrementally. By the beginning of the second term [of the New Labour government from 2001], we have fashioned a template of the reform: changing the monolithic nature of the service; introducing competition; blurring distinctions between public and private sector; taking on traditional professional and union demarcations of work and vested interests; and in general trying to free the system up, letting it innovate, differentiate, breathe and stretch it limbs.[7]

The third way

So this was to be what was called 'the third way': a blurring of the differences and boundaries between public and private sectors. The direction of travel, however, was always away from direct public service provision towards private sector growth, facilitated by, for example, the public–private finance initiative (PFI) where private sector capital investment (with big returns over 25 to 30 years to the investors) was being used to fund the building of new hospitals and schools.

The financial costs of PFI to the public and to public services were highlighted by the National Audit Office (NAO) in 2018. The NAO reported that 'overall cash spending on PFI projects is higher than publicly financed alternatives'. It found that 'data for one group of schools shows that PFI costs are around forty per cent higher than the costs of a project financed by government borrowing ... a similar analysis in 2011 ... estimated the cost of a privately financed hospital to be 70% higher than the public sector comparator'.[8] The consequence has been hospitals and other public services becoming increasingly financially unviable within the funding they have been allocated because of the debt repayment burden they now hold, and this is used to characterise the services as being high cost. The private sector gets a significant financial return on its investment plus a reputational return as the public sector is seen as expensive and inefficient.

PFI had been introduced by John Major's Conservative government, with Anthony Sampson commenting:

To attract private capital and professional management [into what had been public sector services], the Treasury had introduced in 1992 the system known as PFI, which subcontracted public services to private companies under Treasury controls. Sir Steve Robson, the Treasury knight who insisted there was no such thing as a public service ethos, explained that Whitehall could not itself cope with these major industries. 'The public sector is averse to improvement. Improvement requires necessary change. Change necessarily involves risk. The public sector is risk averse'. After Gordon Brown took over the Treasury in 1997 he committed himself to extending both PFI and PPP (public–private partnerships) into more areas.[9]

But, as Sampson noted when reflecting on accountability:

> The responsibility becomes more confused as civil servants delegate still more activities to private companies and subcontractors. Those who complain about shortcomings in hospitals or schools find themselves confronting subcontractors for maintenance, cleaning and other services who are remote from government control.[10]

It was not only accountability, however, which was made more confused and complicated by PFI. It also added to costs in the longer term, costs which over 20 years later are still having to be met by, for example, hospitals and schools, with profits being taken from the public purse, and this at a time when the reductions in public services funding have cut deep. *The Guardian*, for example, gave a summary of a report published in August 2017 about the continuing costs of PFI to NHS hospitals:

> Companies that have built NHS hospitals under the private finance initiative have made pre-tax profits of £831m over the past six years and are poised to make almost £1bn more over the next five years.

Large sums that could have been used for patient care have instead gone into the pockets of a handful of PFI companies at a time when the health service is starved of funding, according to the Centre for Health and the Public Interest.[11] Its analysis, published on Wednesday, found that if the NHS had not been paying pre-tax profits on PFI schemes between 2010 and 2015 inclusive, the deficits in its hospitals would have been reduced by a quarter.[12]

But profits for the private sector are not only made by the PFI charges levied on public sector services. They are also made by making big cuts in the costs of the facilities management and maintenance contracts, such as for cleaning, which the private sector companies are awarded as a part of the PFI deals. These profit-generating cuts then impinge heavily on the low-paid privatised workforce the companies employ, as Polly Toynbee noted in 2003 in a book she called 'Hard Work'. It might also have been called 'Tough Luck' as that must be how it seems for many of those employed in private outsourcing companies making big profits. Toynbee wrote:

> The words are 'outsourcing', 'subcontracting', 'market testing', 'best value', 'externalisation – for people working on the bottom rungs of the public sector, all these words have meant just one thing: lower pay, worse conditions, less security. It has reduced the idea of public service to a cheap and expendable commodity. The public ethos of these private companies is negligible: profit and avoiding litigation is everything. There is no loyalty to the staff they hire, nor any expected from them. The surprise is that the staff give so much anyway.[13]

Making profits out of paying low wages and cutting back the workforce was also noted by Sampson in 2006, who again commented on how the investment banks (the same banks which within a year were to be exposed for their high risk-taking incompetence in the drive for more profit and riches) were the real winners from privatisation:

> The most obvious beneficiaries of privatisation were the investment banks, led by Rothschilds which had close links with the Tory government and found itself collecting unprecedented fees [for advising on the privatisation of public utilities and services]. And the real controllers of the new corporations were the small groups of chairmen, chief executives and directors favoured by Thatcher, who had prepared [the public utilities and services] to be profitable in the market-place and organised their transformation. These people were awarded with sudden opportunities for enrichment that would soon help to change the British social landscape and power-structure. Many of them were more autocratic than their nationalised predecessors: they were freed from the controls of the Treasury, and they were able to face down the much weakened trade unions [weakened by legislation introduced in the 1980s] and cut back their workforces. They were experienced in finance, with close connections to the City, advised by finance directors who were becoming much more important. They were rewarded handsomely, as entrepreneurs who had transformed their companies – though they were not genuine entrepreneurs who had risked their own money to build innovative new industries. They became more detached from the management of the utilities as they grew more internationalised. Many private companies became closely linked with foreign groups, if they were not owned by them, while many chief executives would come from outside Britain.[14]

As Mark Drakeford, a professor at Cardiff University of applied social studies – a discipline he then deployed as Minister of Health in the Welsh Assembly, commented:

The Thatcherite preference for privatisation, in the narrow sense of services privately funded, purchased and provided, was halted during the Blair years. Yet 'modernisation', in the broader sense, entailed the onward march of marketisation and privatisation across the whole welfare frontier. It amounted to a sustained, interconnected and comprehensive paradigm shift away from public services and responsibilities and in favour of private welfare.[15]

Rightly, and not surprisingly as a minister in the devolved Welsh government, Drakeford notes that this is a comment on what has been pursued primarily in England and has not been replicated in the three other UK administrations.

This 'third way' as an ideology and political strategy was developed and deployed by Clinton's Democrats in the USA and Blair's New Labour in the UK as an alternative and antidote to the right-wing governments of Reagan and Thatcher. One of its primary academic advocates was Anthony Giddens, who was director of the London School of Economics and an advisor to New Labour. During New Labour's first year in government in 1988 he wrote one of the seminal books on the 'third way'.[16] Then in 2007 reflecting back on 10 years of New Labour government, Giddens wrote:

> The 'first way' was traditional social democracy – in the context of this country [the UK], Old Labour – based on an unswerving faith in the state, Keynesian demand management and reliance upon the working class as the main basis of voter support … It was a defining political standpoint for other parties too, because it set the terms of political debate. The 'one-nation Tories' accepted the importance of the welfare state and much about the mixed economy … The 'second way' was Thatcherism, or free market fundamentalism. Thatcherism was founded upon a belief in the primacy of markets, the need to reduce the scope of the state and minimise taxes, and upon a relative indifference towards social justice.[17]

But what of the 'third way'? Giddens noted it required that:

> The customary suspicion of markets must be dropped, since a healthy economy is the basis of effective social policy. The state and government will have important roles to play, but they themselves must be reformed to make them more efficient and responsive to the needs of citizens (p 17) ... People should be free to live their lives as they choose, but freedom carries personal and social responsibilities (p 21) ... Invest in public services, above all health and education, but only on condition that they are reformed quite radically (p 22) ... [and] efficiency, but also choice and voice, are of crucial importance in public services. Centralised delivery by the state is by no means always the best way of delivering these objectives. Third sector groups or commercial organisations, if properly regulated, can sometimes be more effective than direct control by the state. We have to decide in all instances which combination most effectively creates public goods. It is gratuitous and wrong to counter-pose, as many critics do, 'public' (state-based) services and 'private' (not-for-profit or commercial) ones. The real test is which serves the public interest best in any specific context (p 22).[18]

The consequence of embracing markets as the means of delivering state responsibilities which had previously been delivered through public services was that the public sector shrank and became minimised and marginalised. And to encourage and promote the market, regulation was reduced, with the prime example being in the banking sectors (of which more below).

The 'third way' might have been called the 'half-way', somewhere between the 'first' and 'second ways' ('a middle ground between old Labour on the left and the Thatcherites on the right'[19]). One difficulty was that it followed the years of Reaganomics and Thatcherism. It inherited the platform which had been left as an inheritance and legacy and, as such, was prone to continue the trajectories Reagan's and Thatcher's governments had set, fuelled and powered up. There was investment in public services by New Labour, but the direction of travel continued to be the fragmentation and outsourcing of these services.

In addition to Giddens, another LSE academic, Professor Julian Le Grand (see Chapter Three), generated for New Labour specific proposals about how to introduce more competition, a purchaser–provider separation, and marketplace dynamics within public services and, in particular, how services might be taken outside of direct delivery by local authorities. Le Grand's 2006 proposals for independent social work practices outside of local councils was commented upon in Chapter One. He also shaped the move to foundation hospitals and academy schools, both introduced by New Labour and energetically and eagerly promoted and pursued by the post-2010 Conservative-led governments.

Writing in 2003, Le Grand commented:

> In most countries, the state has historically played a major role in both the finance and the delivery of social services such as education, health care, housing, and social care. Often this role has taken the form of some kind of state bureaucracy actually providing the service ... During the 1980s and the early 1990s, there was something of a revolution in this kind of social policy. In several countries where a combination of state provision and state finance had been the norm, the state, while retaining control of finance, began to pull back from provision. Instead of providing the service through monolithic state bureaucracies, provision became competitive with independent providers competing for custom in market or 'quasi-market' settings ... The growth of these quasi-markets had a number of causes. A major factor was the fiscal pressure leading governments to search for new ways of using increasingly scarce resources efficiently. However, underlying the whole movement was a fundamental shift in policy-makers' perceptions concerning motivation and agency.[20]

What was this fundamental shift? Le Grand wrote about 'knights and knaves, and pawns and queens'. Public servants had, he argued, been accepted as 'knights' serving the public but had, post-1979, been seen as self-serving and self-protecting 'knaves':

> The assumption that knightly behaviour characterised those who worked within the institutions of the welfare state proved vulnerable. Fuelled in part by people's experience of both dealing with and working within the welfare bureaucracies, many politicians and policy analysts grew increasingly sceptical of the view that bureaucrats and civil servants necessarily operated in the public interest, and that professionals were only concerned with the welfare of their clients. Instead there was an increasing acceptance of the argument of the public choice school of economists and political scientists that the behaviour of public officials and professionals could be better understood if they were assumed to be largely self-interested.[21]

What was the implication of this changed perception of the knights now being seen as knaves? It was to make the 'pawns' whom they had badly served into 'queens', who would be empowered by being given choice between services in a marketplace. Advised by Giddens and Le Grand, this was to be integral to New Labour's 'third way' policies.

Bill and Charlie Jordan, writing in the early days of 2000 about social work and the 'third way', commented:

> Like the public sector generally, this profession [social work] and these [social services] agencies are tainted, in New Labour's eyes, by the involvement in the policies, practices and political cultures of the period 1948–79, when the public sector was the dominant one in policy and politics, when its expansionism threatened the market and civil society, and when the Thatcher reaction against all this began. Furthermore, they are tainted by association with the resistance of local authorities

and the public sector generally during the Thatcher-Major period – with a culture of rule-bending and 'banditry' in favour of very disadvantaged service user groups, such as the poor, ethnic minorities, asylum seekers and homeless people. They are paying a high price for their ambiguous and ambivalent activities under Conservative governments. This is because New Labour takes forward many of the themes of Thatcherism-Majorism, but under the banner of moral revival and social inclusion. The instruments of Thatcherism – a strong central state, regulating the professions, trade unions and public sector interests for the sake of taxpayers and 'customers', favouring commercial and voluntary providers or public-private partnerships over local or central government agencies, and using new initiatives (zones, projects and new agencies and services) to subvert the established power of the large public sector organisations, through the creation of new sets of actors and professionals who owe no allegiance to those interest – are brought to bear on the new issues given priority within the Third Way.[22]

Ten years later, two years after the beginning of the banking crash which started to get attention in 2007–08, and when Blair and Brown's New Labour governments were replaced in 2010 by a Conservative–Liberal Democrat coalition government led by David Cameron, Bill Jordan pronounced the 'third way' a failure:

The ultimate failure of the Third Way has been a moral one, and this has stemmed from an inadequate and incoherent analysis of how ethical principles can be applied to the workings of a market economy exposed to global forces ... In retrospect, it was always unlikely that a regime that cherished conspicuous affluence, cut-throat trading, media celebrity and instant gratification would also foster distributive equity, social well-being and sustainable lifestyles.[23]

And in the same year, 2010, in a book on 'the rise and fall of New Labour', Andrew Rawnsley looked back on the 'third way':

> The 'Third Way' was debated at earnest summits abroad and giggled to death at home. Blair often seemed more about style than content ... New Labour was a hybrid of both right-wing and left-wing. It accepted the Thatcher economic settlement. Markets were unrestrained, the money-changers lightly regulated, and the rich indulged. The animal spirits of the City were allowed to rip. New Labour believed this was necessary to sustain the consumer boom that kept voters content and produced the tax revenues for investment in public services and quiet redistribution of resources to the poor.[24]

Toynbee and Walker gave a similar summary of New Labour's 13 years in government, arguing that 'Labour's leaders had convinced themselves that the electorate was essentially conservative-minded ... Labour convinced themselves that progressive policies could only be pursued by stealth and must be offset by populist Tory gestures on choice and "reform".'[25]

On public services, Toynbee and Walker commented:

> Margaret Thatcher campaigned against the state, pretending to be an outsider cutting government down to size, calling its employees parasites. But she had an ideological commitment to shrinking it. Surely Labour would champion the value and virtue of government? Instead, led by Blair, they copied the Tories: he made a remarkable speech about 'the scars of my back' from his dealings with public servants.*

---

* It is noteworthy that Blair's comments on the public sector and public servants that he had scars on his back after two years of seeking to reform public services were made in a speech in 1999 which he gave to the British Venture Capitalists Association, by whom they were probably well received. He said: 'People in the public sector are more rooted in the concept that "if it's always done this way, it must always be done this way" than any group of people I've come across' (http://news.bbc.co.uk/1/hi/uk_politics/388528.stm).

Toynbee and Walker noted that:

> Tax and regulation were 'burdens'; nobody did it
> better than businesses; firms, social enterprises they
> said, anything but bureaucracy ... [Blair and Brown's
> programme of public sector reform] was a mixed
> bag: contracting out, American theories of 'the new
> public management', more choice among services.
> The state was a shop and the citizen was a consumer,
> not a participant in a collective endeavour.[26]

The 2007–08 banking crash

What dramatically and specifically undermined New Labour with
its 'third way' commitment was the national and international
banking crisis which emerged in 2007 and 2008. Its roots were
within the policies of reducing regulation as a part of limiting
state involvement and interference with the market, and, in
particular, deregulation of the financial markets and of banking.

Deregulation had a history throughout Thatcherism and New
Labour. It was intended to reduce or remove the burden and costs
of regulation – presented as 'red tape' – which, it was argued,
hindered the workings and efficiency of the marketplace.*
However, it contributed to (and largely caused) the international
banking collapse in the late 2000s amidst the unrestrained bonus
culture and reckless greed of bankers who invented investment
vehicles which were high risk but so complex that the risk was
hidden and not recognised.[27, 28]

Gillian Tett, with a PhD in anthropology and who became a
journalist with the *Financial Times*, used her academic research
training to interview the bankers who had been involved in
generating the financial crisis. The title of the book she then

---

* Gordon Brown applied the general commitment to reduce the costs of regulation
specifically to social work and social care in 2006 when, within a lengthy report
following his budget speech, he announced that the Commission for Social Care
Inspection, which regulated children's and adults' social services, was to be abolished
as a financial saving and that its responsibilities would be split and integrated into
what were two existing inspectorates: the health service inspectorate (the Healthcare
Commission) and the schools inspectorate (Ofsted).

wrote in 2009 sums up what had happened. The book was titled 'Fool's Gold: How unrestrained greed corrupted a dream, shattered global markets and unleashed a catastrophe',[29] and she noted how by the late 1990s:

> Free-market ideology was winning minds over more and more of the globe. Innovation, competition, efficiency and deregulation were the rage, not just in finance but in other spheres too. Pundits, politicians and bureaucrats alike argued that globalisation was inevitable and to be embraced: the product of the increasingly unfettered forces of a new and improved capitalism.[30]

Tett wrote about the 'greed' of bankers. Joris Luyendijk, another financial journalist who interviewed bankers after the crash, titled his book 'Swimming with Sharks: My journey into the world of the bankers'.[31] Luyendijk's book was published in 2015, which suggests that not a lot had changed in the attitude and behaviour of bankers since Tett's book appeared in 2009. And it was not only financial journalists who saw the national and international economic crisis as the consequence of the behaviour of the bankers. Vince Cable, the Liberal Democrat's chief economic spokesperson, writing in 2009 commented that it was the 'individual and collective stupidity, greed and complacency' of bankers and within the banking system that had created the crisis and then the crash.[32]

It is hard not to conclude that it was the bankers, with their high salaries and bonuses (which continued even after the crash) and their reckless behaviour, who were the self-interested knaves, to use Le Grand's terminology, rather than the public servants who were soon to suffer the politically chosen consequences of the banker-created economic crisis.

Here is a prescient prediction, written in 2007 by Robert Peston, then the BBC's business editor, at the time of the early exposure of the banking crisis, and which, 10 years later as this book is being written, seems to have remarkable traction:

Here is a possible United Kingdom in ten years, on current trends. Public services would be creaking for lack of investment, as the burden of tax fell on a dwindling number of private sector employees [including those who had been out-sourced from the public sector] whose skills weren't quite rare enough or valuable enough to take them to the top league of globally mobile earners. And year after year, the real disposable income of the majority would be squeezed ever so slightly, because that would be the only way they could keep their jobs in the climate of intense international competition endured by their respective employers. Meanwhile, the plutocrats who own these businesses would shuttle from London to Monaco to Moscow and Mumbai to Shanghai and Rio and back again, refusing to pay the subscription price to belong in any meaningful sense to any nation or community, except the global community of the super-wealthy. In that world, elected politicians would seem less and less relevant to the daily lives of the majority. The potentates would be the stateless plutocrats.[33]

What had, in part, driven this rise in riches for those already rich was the unrestrained and largely unregulated reshaping of businesses and the growth of ownership through private equity, with Toynbee and Walker writing in 2008 that:

Flooded with capital [and, it might be said, cheap borrowing and rampant tax avoidance], equity funds stalked plc [public limited company] boardrooms during the go-go years of the economic cycle that started shuddering in 2007. But the takeover boom inflated rather than punctured the growth of top earnings. Private equity turned out to be a sleight of hand … most of the capital needed to buy the companies was borrowed on the security of the victim's assets, requiring it to generate income to service the debt for years to come. Private equity deals mostly sell off a company's assets for the sake of a quick win.[34]

As will be shown in Chapter Ten, this is exactly what has happened to care homes for older people, bought on borrowed money by private investors who asset-stripped the homes to make a quick profit.

SEVEN

Cameron, the coalition and the Conservatives: 'Cambornism' and enhanced Thatcherism

One consequence of the banker-created economic crisis, which was presented by the Conservatives in the 2010 general election as an exemplar of New Labour's financial mismanagement of the economy, was that a new government was elected. The Cameron-led Conservatives failed to get a parliamentary majority but, rather surprisingly to those who had voted tactically for the Liberal Democrats to stop Conservative MPs being elected, they were able to persuade the Liberal Democrats, led by Nick Clegg, to form a coalition government.

Alistair Darling, who had been New Labour's Chancellor of the Exchequer from 2007 to 2010 (after Tony Blair had been replaced by Gordon Brown as Prime Minister), throughout the emergence and management of the banking collapse, wrote:

> A new government can blame the outgoing government for whatever crisis or misdemeanours it chooses ... The Conservatives' main priority was to cut public spending; they wanted rapid and deep cuts to eliminate the structural [economic] deficit during the course of a parliament. From the Tory viewpoint, they were landed with an unexpected political windfall, brought about by going into coalition with the Liberal Democrats. They could cut faster and harder than they would ever had they secured a majority on their own. And if growth is a

lot lower for longer, that will mean even deeper cuts. Faced with criticism from within, David Cameron can blame the Liberals for stopping him from serving up the red meat his party's right wing demands ... Reducing the deficit was a convenient excuse that provided the Conservatives with cover to make the kind of deep public spending cuts many of them were wanting for ideological reasons. Their message was simple: things were worse than they thought; if we didn't cut now, we'd end up like Greece; Labour was entirely to blame. They were wrong on all three counts.[1]

Darling wrote as a self-identified 'centre ground' politician. Here is a statement which may be somewhat stronger, written as it is by Owen Jones, a newspaper columnist and author, about the banking crisis and how it was used as the rationale by the post-2010 Conservative-led governments to justify politically chosen austerity:

In the City, Britain's financial sector, you can find the mentalities of the Establishment expressed in its purest form. The sector is permeated on the one hand by a passionate resistance to the state, characterised by a reluctance to pay taxes and an acute hostility to any form of government regulation ... The City abounds with rampant dog-eat-dog individualism; an intimate familiarity with political power; and an all-to-common indifference to the lives of those who lose out from the status quo. And – perhaps most strikingly – a sense that there is one code for those at the top, and another rule for everybody else. The state bail out of the banks following the 2008 financial collapse came with few government-imposed conditions, and with little calling to account. But in the austerity programme which followed, by contrast, state support for those at the bottom of society has been increasingly stripped away.[2]

There are three key issues about the credibility of the austerity programme politically chosen by the post-2010 Conservative-led governments. First, it did not achieve its stated aim. George Osborne, the Chancellor of the Exchequer, set a target of removing, through the austerity policies, the national financial deficit by the end of the coalition government. He failed. Secondly, there was a more successful alternative, in part followed by President Obama in the US, to stimulate the economy to promote growth. This was Keynesian economics, in contrast to the post-1979 monetarism. Thirdly, the argument that there was no choice but to introduce austerity in the UK is also not true, as noted by Alistair Darling:

> The [coalition government's] claim that they had no choice but to make deep and rapid cuts, stands even less scrutiny. A growing number of commentators have become more sceptical about whether the new government can deliver on austerity plans and, equally important, express concern that the cuts to public spending will prevent economic growth.[3]

It was in his first budget of autumn 2010 that Osborne mapped out the austerity route of severe and prolonged welfare and public spending cuts which, in 2018 with Theresa May as Prime Minister and Philip Hammond as Chancellor, were still being enacted and enlarged. In a 2012 *Guardian* newspaper piece captioned 'The Bullingdon boys want to finish what Thatcher began', Seamus Milne (who in 2016 became the director of communications for the Corbyn-led Labour opposition) wrote:

> The savagery unveiled today by George Osborne doesn't only amount to the deepest programme of public-spending cuts since the 1920s. As the chancellor's fog of spin started to clear, the scale of the political ambition behind them also became apparent. The Tory-led coalition is using the economic crisis not only to rein in the state, but to reorder society. This is to be Britain's shock therapy. It is the culmination of the Conservative project to dismantle

the heart of the welfare state – or, as Osborne put it today, to 'reshape' public services – that began more than thirty years ago … Coalition leaders have used the absurd claim that the country is on the brink of bankruptcy to force through an array of sweeping changes, any one of which would normally be the focus of a prolonged political debate … Now the brutal reality has been spelled out. Government departments will in fact take an average hit of 19% over the next four years. The heaviest cut, however – of at least £18 billion – is to welfare, targeted on the poorest of the country … It is women, families and the sick who, it turns out, will be picking up the bill for the bank-triggered meltdown, along with low-income teenagers and public sector workers in their millions – while Cameron and Osborne are hoping local authorities will take the blame for their 30 per cent cut [a cut which was soon to become 40%].[4]

In essence, the financial crisis created by the bankers was used as the 'shock' to allow unpalatable and largely unopposed policies to be promoted and enacted, and to further the push to privatisation and corporate profits.

Naomi Klein, writing in 2007, noted how in the US (and replicated in the UK) privatisation moved to encompass what had been core state responsibilities:

By the time the Bush team took office [2001], the privatisation mania of the eighties and nineties (fully embraced by the Clinton [and Blair] administrations as well as state and local governments) had successfully sold off or out-sourced the large, publicly-owned companies in several sectors, from water and electricity to highway management and garbage collection. After these limbs of the state had been lopped off, what was left was the 'core' – those functions so intrinsic to the concept of governing that the idea of handing them back to private corporations challenged what it meant to be a nation-state: the military, police, fire departments, prisons, border control, covert intelligence, disease control, the public school system and the administering of government bureaucracies. The earlier stages of the privatisation wave had been so profitable, however, that many of the companies that had devoured the appendages of the state were greedily eyeing these essential functions as the next source of instant riches.[5]

Naomi Klein eloquently but horrifically described in 2017 how major crises and disasters – both natural, such as the impact of global warming and Hurricane Katrina, and manufactured, such as the war in Iraq and other recent wars – have been used to push and promote radical neoliberal policies, but added that:

> The most frequent midwife [delivering the shock] by far has been large-scale economic crisis, which time and again has been harnessed to demand radical campaigns of privatisation, deregulation, and cuts to safety nets. But in truth, any shock can do the trick – including natural disasters that require large-scale reconstruction and therefore provide an opening to transfer land and resources from the vulnerable to the powerful.[6]

Klein was prompted to quickly write her 2017 book by the election of Donald Trump in the US, and she also refers to the referendum in the UK, which had triggered the process of withdrawal from the European Union. In an account of what led to Brexit, Tim Shipman wrote that 'in the hands [of the right-wing Europe sceptics in Britain and elsewhere] the tone of politics could change', and he quotes the leading funder of the Brexit campaign, Arron Banks, as saying 'we use a bit of sense of humour, we use a bit of shock and awe. We changed the rules a bit'.[7]

It was just this type of use of shock and awe to which Klein and Banks refer that was taken advantage of by the post-2010 Conservative governments to take Thatcherism to a further extreme, winding back public spending to the pre-Second-

World-War levels of the 1930s, and seeking to wipe out much of the post-war welfare state.

The Cameron-led coalition government's intention to push ahead on the privatisation and marketisation of public services was made explicit in a 2011 White Paper, with Toynbee and Walker writing:

> If you wanted a three-word badge for Cameron's first half [of the coalition government's term of office] it would be Any Qualified Provider. The Open Public Services white paper published in July 2011 expresses their radicalism. It was to have been published in February that year but a scandal at Winterbourne View, a long-term private residential hospital [for people with learning disabilities], provoked alarm at private profiteering. Undeterred, Letwin and Maude, Gauleiters for the policy, went ahead and published the master plan a few months later. The default position for all public services is private provision, and not even the military or policing is to be exempt. Most services will be obliged to drum up at least three rivals, preferably commercial, to bid for every service.[8]

And in a comment from Cameron reminiscent of Blair's 'scars on his back' from seeking to reform public services, Toynbee and Walker reported:

> Cameron told the Tory spring conference in 2011 he wanted to create a new presumption against the dead hand of the state. Woe betide any civil servant obstructing it: 'If I have to pull those people into my office and get them off the backs of business, then believe me I'll do it'.[9]

In this context of disdain explicitly expressed about those working in the public sector and the civil service, it was the private sector which was to be the favoured resource: not only by providing within a commercial marketplace services which had previously been publicly owned and public sector provided, but also to be at the forefront in creating this marketplace. Ensconced within the government–private sector alliance were the management accountants and consultants based within the big international accountancy firms.

Writing in 2015, Polly Toynbee and David Walker commented:

> Consultants say they are technocrats, offering capacity to stretched [civil service] departments (which were busy cutting posts). This is specious. They carried ideology like a virus; its DNA was pro-market, anti-public sector; they were preferred because their worldview chimed with the government's.[10]

Toynbee and Walker also noted that:

> The Big Four [Deloitte, PricewaterhouseCoopers, Ernst and Young, KPMG] loom large in [the] demonology, the monster accountancy firms that act like a cartel ... How cleverly the Big Four act, helping to draw up contracts for outsourcing public services then bidding themselves or acting for the private bidders.[11]

The concerns expressed by Toynbee and Walker about the role played at the time of Cameron's governments by the accountancy companies in promoting and pursuing privatisation were not new. This had also been a concern, as noted by Anthony Sampson in 2004, at the time of the Blair governments:

> The concentration of the Big Four in Britain now gave them a still more dominating influence. The largest of them PwC, audited forty-three of the Footsie 100 companies in 2002 ... There was a recurring danger of conflicts of interest when they represented two or more big companies – still more so when they represented government departments – and the danger was increased as New Labour extended its private finance initiatives which involved teams of accountants from both sides. In 2002 Unison

found forty-five cases where an accounting firm was both advising a public body *and* [my italic] auditing a member of the consortium which won the PFI contract.[12]

But the creeping tentacles of the accountancy firms were even entangled within government itself, with Sampson commenting that:

> The political influence of the Big Four was becoming a more serious threat to democracy – more pervasive than the Magic Circle of corporate lawyers – as their networks penetrated into Whitehall … The alumni of the Big Four have their own networks spreading between the big corporations and government, and even into St James's Palace, where Prince Charles' private secretary Sir Michael Peat came from one of the founding families of KPMG.[13]

There is a special concern here for social work and social services. Who is it that runs the DfE's Children's Social Care Innovation Programme? (Answer: Deloitte). Who had been engaged in advising the government on the future marketisation of children's social services? (KPMG). Who was awarded the contract for defining the necessary skills of children's social workers and how these social workers should be nationally accredited? (KPMG again). And who chaired PwC's 'Health Industries Oversight Board'? (former Labour Secretary of State for Health Alan Milburn), with the PwC website noting:

> Alan Milburn is Chair of PwC's Health Industries Oversight Board. He is an expert in strategic thinking and health policy. Alan was an MP for 18 years and served for five years in Tony Blair's Cabinet, first as Chief Secretary to the Treasury from 1998 to 1999, and subsequently as Secretary of State for Health until 2003. At the Department of Health, he led a radical reform programme of health and social care services including the creation of a market within the

NHS, autonomous NHS Foundation Trusts, choice for patients and devolution of decision-making.*,[14]

But the international accountancy firms have not been successful and competent even in carrying out their core business as auditors, having been complicit, and indeed conspiring, with the banks in creating the 2008 national and international banking crisis. They apparently were not able to understand the profit-generating high-risk processes and products that the banks had created, and as auditors they failed to spot and stop the financial mess and mayhem which was being produced. They also did not challenge and correct financial accounts which were filed and then published but were subsequently found to have been false.[15, 16, 17] There is an account of more recent concerns about the big accountancy firms in Chapter Eleven.

One of the ways in which the advice and assistance from the consultants would have been useful was in creating what might be seen as the Conservatives' 'mid-way' – but not the 'middle way', as it was never intended as an end position. The mid-way strategy would be to push ahead with public service mutuals as a stepping-stone to full commercialisation and privatisation.

This stepping-stone has been described more fully for children's social work and child protection in Chapter One. But the stepping-stone strategy might not only be deployed for children's social work journey towards privatisation and marketisation. It was a more generally applied strategy, building on the bricks already laid by New Labour and its advisors, among whom, as commented upon earlier, Professor Sir Julian Le Grand had been prominent. As noted by Toynbee and Walker, he, along

---

*   Examples of this intertwining and entangling of the accountancy firms with government include Edwina Currie, a Thatcher Health Minister, who was the wife and sister-in-law of employees of Andersen Consultancy, and Patricia Hewitt, a Blair Secretary of State for Health, who had previously worked for Andersen. After finishing as a government minister in 2007 there was controversy when Hewitt became a non-executive director of a major national pharmaceutical company and a non-executive director of a venture capitalist company which went on to buy 25 hospitals from BUPA (https://www.theguardian.com/politics/2011/may/17/labour-ministers-consultancy-private-sector). She has not been unique or unusual in moving on from being a government minister into relationships with the private sector linked to her ministerial role.

with others, continued his prominence as a government guru and advisor for Cameron's Conservative-led coalition government:

> Professor Julian Le Grand, a former Blair advisor, headed a government panel propagating 'mutuals', viewed by the Tories as merely a precursor to privatisation. Another Labour health professor, Paul Corrigan, joined hardliners at the Reform think tank arguing for maximal competition in the NHS, long after the disaster of the Lansley [the coalition government's Conservative Secretary of State for Health] reforms had been enacted and displayed. We must end 'false loyalty' to equity, he said. Many who might have spoken out were struck dumb. The children's commissioners were hardly audible. The third sector, a hotbed of political naifs, wanted to think the best of ministers. Perhaps they were merely self-interested, despite the patina of saintliness charities liked to paint ... Sir Martin Narey, the former head of Barnardo's, became Michael Gove's advisor on children's social services, where he took it upon himself to defend the private sector's role in child protection. Perhaps that is Narey's sincere belief, but his intervention was conveniently timed from the government's point of view.[18]

So, the privatisation journey initiated by Thatcher has been continued through the subsequent New Labour governments, and the pace has been picked up by the post-2010 Conservative-led governments. But what have been consequences of this journey? These are explored in the following chapters.

Part 3
The impact of privatisation

EIGHT

Privatisation of public services and the undermining of the welfare state

If marketisation, commercialisation and privatisation drove improved performance and generated greater effectiveness, efficiency and economy (and maybe also equity – providing the same opportunities and outcomes for all) the journey would be positive and to be applauded. However, this is not the finding of recent history based on the experience of services which have already been forced or coerced into private ownership and immersed in the contract culture.

In a book on the 'Shadow State', described by Margaret Hodge when chair of the House of Commons Public Accounts Committee as 'Puncturing the myth that the private sector is better at delivering public service', Alan White, a reporter at Buzzfeed News, noted that:

> Supporters of outsourcing will tell you that one thing it brings – which isn't available in the state sector – is competition. If companies don't do their jobs properly – or don't provide value for money while doing it – they'll be replaced by ones that can ... But it just doesn't work like that ... The first reason [that outsourcing does not drive value for money] is the fact that contracts are drawn up in such a way that – disregarding the gigantic fines and reputational damage that companies have occasionally suffered in recent years when things have gone wrong – too often the balance of risk and reward seems unfairly tipped in favour of the firms.[1]

Why might this be so? First, those letting the public service contracts may have experience in contracting but not in the specific field within which they are letting the contract. Secondly, if they buy in contracting advice or capacity it is often (as with central government and its buying in of advice about how to create a statutory children's social services marketplace) from the private sector management consultancy companies which are ingrained and immersed within the ideology of marketisation and privatisation (from which they generate their fees and make their profits). Thirdly, those managing the contracts which have been let may again not know much about the services which have been contracted out, as the public sector quickly loses its own service experience and expertise. Fourthly, it is unlikely that the public sector has retained the capacity to take a failing contract back in house – and certainly not in the short term – so there is a push to not recognise failure, as, fifthly, this also reflects badly on the public sector (such as a local authority or central government) body which has let the contract. And, finally, the public sector contractor is dependent on the company awarded the contract for performance and financial information, and the accuracy and fullness of the presentation of this data is within the control of the company. More likely, if the contract is not working this will first become known to the company, which may seek to pressurise the public body to amend the contract or may just decide to terminate it and walk away from or to sell it on. In essence, the power comes to disproportionately lie with the company receiving the contract rather than with the public body which has drawn up and let the contract.

White gives numerous examples in his book of these processes in play, as does James Meek in *Private Island: Why Britain Now Belongs to Someone Else*.[2] Even more startlingly, Meek notes that despite what was stated as Margaret Thatcher's intention, 'Privatisation failed to turn Britain into a nation of small shareholders',[3] and that much of what were the UK's publicly owned resources and services are now within the ownership of governments in China, France and elsewhere, of venture capitalists in Europe, South-east Asia and the US, or owned and controlled by Russian oligarchs.[4] None are likely to have as a primary concern the welfare of people and communities in the UK. Their intention is to drive a profit out of the contracts they have been awarded and from the public services which they have now turned into money-making businesses.

Even where the privatised former public assets and services might look as though they are still owned in the UK, the companies may be registered in tax havens so that tax on the contracts and contracted-out service incomes is not paid and held within the UK.* Not only profits, but the tax on these profits which should contribute to the government's income and the funding of public services, leak out of the economy and into the increasingly well-filled pockets of those who have captured and corralled what were formerly publicly owned assets.

What is possibly even more startling is that these overseas and offshore tax havens are often 'Crown dependencies' with the protection of the UK government, places such as Jersey, Guernsey, the Isle of Man, Gibraltar and the Cayman Islands, and that there is 'a layered hub–and–spoke array of tax havens centred on the City of London'.[5]

And who advises the companies how to avoid paying taxes by registering within these tax havens and gives advice on the company structures that allow this to happen? It is often the same international accountancy firms who advise the government on how to create a marketplace for what are to be privatised public services (and who are now contracted to define and shape social work and England's social services). As Shaxson notes:

> You may well have heard of the Big Four accountancy firms KPMG, Deloitte, Ernst and Young and PriceWaterhouse Coopers ... These are respectable players among a much larger regiment of smartly dressed accountants, lawyers and banks forming a private global infrastructure which, in league with captured legislatures in the secrecy jurisdictions, makes the whole system work.[6]

---

* This was a cause of concern about David Cameron and his father's business interests and arrangements, with it becoming known that Cameron was a beneficiary of his father's offshore investments (https://www.theguardian.com/politics/2016/apr/09/david-cameron-questions-gift-mother).

And it gets even more concerning when, as recognised by Kerry-Anne Mendoza, a former management consultant who held senior positions in banking:

> A significant number of corporations now have greater financial power than the majority of states, and they have used this to infiltrate and leverage the structural power of states to implement laws and subsidies on their behalf.[7]

Within these corporations are the top executives and the owners, who are already very rich and getting even richer, a process which should be of concern but, as noted by television journalist Robert Peston, is often not acknowledged:

> To admit to concerns about the rise and rise of the billionaire class is not the manifestation of an atavistic socialist prejudice. And if the leaders of the Tory and Labour parties [Peston was writing before Jeremy Corbyn became leader of the Labour Party] were not so thoroughly frightened of being tarnished anti-wealth creation, they would express such concerns. It is really the *sine qua non* of a successful modern economy that there should be no limit on the wealth which any individual can generate and retain. My view, having observed the super-wealthy and pusillanimous politicians at close quarters for twenty years, is that the great new nonsense of our age is that we should take nothing but pride in the proliferation of billionaires and never suggest that they are parasitic. Their charitable giving in the United Kingdom are *de minimis* compared with their peers in the United States. And ... it would be a welcome change if the billionaire class simply paid the same tax as a proportion of income and capital as the rest of us.[8]

Peston was writing in 2008. Nine years later in 2017 it was reported that billionaires had got even richer, owned even more of the total world's wealth, and that they had 'increased their combined global wealth by almost a fifth in the past year to a record $6tn (£4.5tn) – more than twice the GDP of the UK. There are now 1,542 dollar billionaires across the world'.[9]

This is the world and context into which many outsourced public services have been relocated, with the rich getting richer, bigger privatised profits, and tax cuts and tax avoidance for corporations and their owners. It is the world in which social work and social services in England, including statutory children's social services, are now being immersed.

And it is not accidental. Mendoza comments that while the rich thrive, politically chosen austerity targeted at the poor and at public services is an ideological commitment of the Conservative governments of the 1980s and now of the 2010s:

> On arrival in government, the dominant Conservative section of the Coalition government was keen to present Austerity as temporary, necessary and purely practical. Back in 2010, Cameron claimed that he 'didn't come into politics to make cuts', and that Austerity was simply temporary spending restraint based on a necessary effort to cut the deficit, not 'some ideological zeal'. What we can now see is that Austerity is delivering the half-century-long ambition of the Conservative party: to revoke the UK's post-War social contract … This was the social contract the UK public signed up in the aftermath of the Second World War. Why? Because three generations had lived through the horrific consequences of unrestrained capitalism: enormous inequality; widespread poverty and destitution; starving and malnourished children; an entrenched class system; the benefits of the hard work of the many enjoyed by a privileged and undeserving few. David Cameron [and then Prime Minister May, who continued to implement Cameron and Osborne's welfare benefits and public spending cuts] is taking the country back to those dark days. Wearing a white tie, standing at a gilded lectern, speaking to the bankers and brokers of the City of London in late 2013, he stated categorically

that Austerity is ideological and would be permanent under a Tory government.[10]

And here is a comment from Toynbee and Walker in 2017 on politically chosen austerity and cuts which is directly relevant to social workers and others working in local government and in services dependent on grants from local authorities, such as the national and local social welfare charities:

> If Osborne had meant it when he said *we're all in it together* (words that became one of the decade's great clichés), he would have spread austerity fairly and proportionately. Necessary spending cuts would have been transparent and ordered. Instead, ministers tried to disguise them. They 'devolved the axe', pushing cuts on councils, forcing them to take the opprobrium. For example, councils caught the flak for cutting the numbers of meals on wheels delivered in England, which fell from 6.7 million to 3.5 million between 2010–2011 and 2015–2016, despite the fact that over this period the price charged for the services rose by a fifth on average. The Tory-controlled Local Government Association could not or would not put the blame where it lay. They cut according to what they could get away with, not what would cause least pain. Individuals, disconnected, powerless to protest, and regions far from London were easy meat – so it was the families on benefits, children, disabled people and old people at home lacking care who suffered. Ministers have been surprised how far they could go without provoking rebellion.[11]

Cameron and Osborne, and then May and Hammond, repeated the Thatcher-like statements that this was all necessary and that there was no alternative. It is this mantra that is explored and exploded in the final chapter. But it is timely and necessary now to sound alarm bells about what could be the impact of the move to privatise social work and child protection.

Rolling back the welfare state

So how far has the privatisation of public services already gone? In mid–2010s social work and statutory children's services were only reaching their place in the queue to feel the burgeoning brunt of marketisation and commercialisation. It had already overwhelmed and undermined adult social care. Maybe the government had always recognised that privatising the state's responsibilities for the safety and welfare of children was even more radical – and risky – than the outsourcing of other state responsibilities and public services. Maybe the idea of profit being made out of poverty and money out of misery was seen as step too far. But not so, as will be seen in the accounts given in the next chapter of what had already been pursued and pushed forward in dismantling the welfare state and privatising public assets.

The focus in the next chapter is on those very personal needs and services which had been seen as rightly the concern of the state – it does not include accounts of the selling off of former publicly owned manufacturing industries, or public utilities such as electricity, gas and water (and railways, the Post Office and Royal Mail), albeit that these once public utilities are now owned by foreign governments, banks, corporations and venture capitalists, and essential elements of the public infrastructure are now put at risk through fragmentation and through distant ownership and decision-making based on profit, not public good.

What might be termed 'personal services', such as services providing health care, education, housing, social security and public and personal safety, which impact and impinge on the very essence of people's personal lives, have all been exposed to the profit-making market and taken outside the public sector and the state's control and provision.

These service sectors were designed to deal with what Beveridge described as the 'five giants' of *want, ignorance, disease, squalor,* and *idleness,* which he addressed in his 1942 report.[12] They were each addressed by legislation between 1944 and 1948, starting with the 1944 Education Act, and then, amongst others, the 1946 NHS Act, and the 1948 National Assistance Act, 1948 Children's Act, 1948 Employment and Training Act,

1949 Housing Act and 1947 Town and Country Planning Act. These were the building blocks of the welfare state but, over recent years, they have been undermined and the welfare state dismantled.

There are two exceptions – two additions – discussed in the next chapter, which do not feature among Beveridge's five giants. The first might have been termed the sixth giant of *fear and threat*, or what might now be called *community safety*. It is about policing, prisons and probation, which were not issues or services covered by Beveridge. Maybe in the 1940s they were not thought to need addressing and were not controversial or seen to require changes in policies or structures. The state would continue to provide police, courts and prisons as before. But in recent years this assumption no longer holds, as each has been exposed to deep cuts and opened up to non-state provision by commercial, for-profit, organisations.

The other area which was not given much attention in the Beveridge report is what might have been called the seventh giant of *neglect*, which now, in the 21st century, is being addressed through services providing *care*. In the 1940s there were fewer older people and fewer younger disabled people. People died younger, and this was especially so for people who had an impairment or chronic illness. Those who needed help and care largely received it from within their family. Fewer women were in employment outside the home and so women were available to provide care across generations for family members. People also tended to stay local, with much less geographical mobility, so intergenerational extended families would be close to each other, again facilitating care for those who needed it from within the family network. And if families could not – or decided not to – provide this care, there were still the big institutions such as county asylums and large children's homes and cottage home villages, such as Barnardo's at Barkingside and Quarrier's at Bridge-over-Weir, to house and confine (if not care well for) those that needed help. However, there was change as the 1948 National Assistance Act ended the Poor Law and finally formally abolished workhouses, and the 1948 Children Act provided a platform to improve services for children in care – both leading to smaller (but still 25–50 place) residential care homes for children and for older people.

In 1948, Clement Attlee spoke about the universal health and income maintenance legislation which was now being put in place. Attlee said:

> The four Acts which come into force tomorrow [5 July 1948] – National Insurance, National Injuries, National Assistance and the National Health Service – represent the main body of the army of social security … They are comprehensive and available to every citizen. They give security to all members of the family.[13]

It is this comprehensive infrastructure which has been and is being undermined and undone in the mid- and late 2010s by cuts in welfare benefits and by more heavily rationed health care. It is also being challenged by a narrative which has depicted those who at times of difficulty and distress need to use this infrastructure as a drain on society and as feckless failures.

As David Kynaston has reflected on the period of Attlee's Labour government of 1945–51 which created the welfare state:

> It had been an extraordinary hard six years since the end of the war – in some ways even harder than the years of the war itself. The end was in sight of a long, long period of more or less unremitting austerity. Few adults who lived through the 1940s would readily forgo the prospect of a little more ease, a little more comfort. A new world was slowly taking shape, but for most of these adults what mattered far more was the creation and maintenance of a safe, secure home life.[14]

Reviewing the same time period, Peter Hennessy concluded:

> Britain had never – and still hasn't – experienced a progressive phase to match 1945–51. It is largely, though not wholly, the achievement of these years – and the wartime experience, the crucial platform

on which those advances were built – that 1951 Britain, certainly compared to the UK of 1931 or *any* previous decade, was a kinder, gentler and a far, far better place in which to be born, to grow up, to live, love, work and even to die. Such an epitaph cannot be placed with conviction on the plinths of any of the eras to come.[15]

So what has been happening recently to those public services which were built as a part of the welfare state? The next chapter indicates why pursuing the privatisation of statutory children's social services, child protection and social work is fraught with dangers and is a reckless direction of travel.

NINE

The experience and outcomes of privatising public services

When pursuing any policy or service change it is wise to be reflective and to learn from the impact of similar changes elsewhere. There is plenty of scope as statutory children's social services and social work are positioned for privatisation to consider what have been the outcomes of moving other very personal public services into a commercial marketplace. This chapter tracks what has happened to the welfare state public services that were set up following the Beveridge Report[1] in the 1940s and those set up to tackle what in the previous chapter were called the more contemporary concerns: public safety to tackle fear and threat, and care to tackle neglect.

Schools, education and children's centres

First, the Beveridge giant of '*ignorance*'. It was the New Labour government of Tony Blair which provided the platform and process to move publicly funded schools out of the direct control and support of local authorities. Academy schools – like the thrust towards patient choice and creating a market in hospital services – fitted within the public policy initiatives championed by Julian Le Grand to develop 'quasi-markets' in public services[2] where there would be competition between schools and between hospitals.

New Labour's stated intention was that schools which were seen to be poor performers would be moved outside of local authority control, with the local authority itself assumed to be failing, and the school would receive its funding, enhanced by the government, direct from the Department for Education. The school would be given freedoms to design its own curriculum and staffing arrangements and terms and conditions of employment, without the constraint of national requirements, and would be assisted to improve by a sponsor from business or charities.

For New Labour, academy schools were not intended as a mainstream development. They were to be a specific initiative to tackle a specific difficulty – schools which were scoring low on Ofsted inspections and exam performance data and were often located within areas of high deprivation that provided their pupil catchment area. But as with several other New Labour initiatives, it crossed a threshold, broke through a barrier and became a Trojan horse letting in ideologically driven policies of the following Conservative governments. In 2016 the government announced in a White Paper that by 2020 all schools would be removed from the management and oversight of local authorities and would have to become academy schools.[3]

No longer was it expected that schools would be managed and supported by local (education) authorities. No longer would they be within a local authority's remit for strategic planning of schools and school places. No longer would they fall within a national framework of curriculum planning and provision. Essentially a free-for-all, cut-and-thrust, school-against-school, competitive and largely unrestrained marketplace was to be put in place.

And – maybe not surprisingly – there were those who spotted an opportunity to make a profit for themselves out of the publicly funded education of children. These so-called entrepreneurs saw a business opportunity in gathering academy schools together into academy chains through which they could make money by paying themselves high salaries, employing relatives, and charging schools for support services at whatever price was decided by the academy chain.

In December 2017, for example, there were concerns leading to a police investigation about asset-stripping of schools' budgets within the Wakefield City Academies Trust:

> Police have confirmed they are looking at the conduct of a multi-academy trust accused of asset

stripping its schools before collapsing. Wakefield City Academies Trust announced days into the new term in September that it would divest itself of its 21 schools because WCAT could not undertake the 'rapid improvement' they needed. The Department for Education is in the process of arranging for new trusts to take over management of the schools. In October, it was revealed that the trust had transferred millions of pounds of its schools' reserves to centralised accounts before admitting that new sponsors would need to be found for them. Last month, Wakefield city council backed a motion calling for police to investigate the trust's finances and insisted that the DfE ensure 'full restitution' of money transferred from schools into the trust's accounts.[4]

In the same week that this story was making the headlines, the government announced that it was rejecting the recommendation of the Education Select Committee,[5] which had a Conservative chair and majority, that local authorities should be allowed to set up academy school groups. Why? The government stated: 'it is important to maintain the independence of academies'.[6] The government also rejected the Select Committee's recommendation that Ofsted should carry out full inspections of the performance of multi-academy trust chains. The message was that local authorities, although locally embedded and democratically elected, accountable and transparent, were not fit to manage schools, but remote, distant and unaccountable multi-academy chains were, and did not need to be inspected to find out how well they were providing and supporting schools.

The making and taking of profits from schools and education now riddles the system. Here is a 2015 comment from the Institute of Education:

> Both the New Labour and Coalition governments have contributed to a legal and administrative infrastructure which enables profit making. There has been a proliferation of new opportunities for profit-making as schools, colleges, universities, local

authorities and central government award service contracts or buy services from private providers – services that in many cases were previously provided by local authorities or the need for which has been created by policy changes. Most supply teachers are now employed by private agencies. Most school examinations and tests are run by private providers. Since 1992, the work of school inspections has been outsourced to private contractors (though the head of Ofsted, a statutory body, announced in May 2014 that he would bring the management of inspections back in-house).[7]

Is this placing of schools and children's education in a profit-making marketplace just accidental and incidental? Apparently not. James Cusick in *The Independent* in 2013 reported that:

Academies and free schools should become profit-making businesses using hedge funds and venture capitalists to raise money, according to private plans being drawn up by the Education Secretary, Michael Gove. Details of discussions on the proposed redesign of academy regulations were leaked to *The Independent* by Department for Education insiders who are concerned that Mr Gove is going too fast and too far in his ambition to convert all 30,000 schools in England to academies. They are worried that the new setup will divert cash from classrooms, limit the availability of 'expensive' subjects such as music and science and end the public service vocation of teachers. They want to see an end to the secrecy over the proposed reforms, which have not been publicly announced.[8]

The Conservative government's mission to turn all schools into academies has continued beyond Mr Gove's time as Secretary of State for Education, and the profit-making opportunities from academy schools have regularly been reported on as a cause of concern.[9, 10, 11] Taking public money which was meant for children's education as a profit might possibly be argued to be acceptable if the education children received, and the outcomes it generated for them, were positive. However, on this major test – despite the disruption, fragmentation, loss of local influence and community integration, and the higher costs as a consequence of pushing ahead with academy schools – the Royal Society of Arts (RSA) 'Commission' on academy schools noted that 'it is increasingly clear that academy status alone is not a panacea for improvement'.[12] This 'Commission' was chaired for the RSA by Christine Gilbert, who had previously been the Chief Inspector of Schools and head of Ofsted.

A study conducted by Angel Solutions in 2018 found that 'councils beat academy trusts in boosting failing schools' and that 'Researchers looked at how much schools rated inadequate by Ofsted in 2013 had improved by the end of 2017. Those schools that had remained council maintained were more likely to be good or outstanding than those that had become sponsored academies'.[13]

There was particular concern in 2006 about the largest academy chain which ran 67 schools. The BBC reported that:

> Inspectors say that 40% of pupils in primary schools run by AET [the Academies Enterprise Trust] are in 'academies that do not provide a good standard of education'. 'It is even worse in secondary, where 47% of pupils attend academies that are less than good', says Ofsted. The performance of AET's secondary schools is described as 'mediocre' and there has been a lack of progress since Ofsted highlighted weaknesses in the chain's schools two years ago.[14]

The BBC report also noted that 'Ofsted warns that poorer pupils do "particularly badly" in AET schools'.[15] Six months later, in July 2016, the Sutton Trust undertook an analysis across 39 academy chains and concluded that:

> The sponsored academies in this analysis have lower Ofsted inspection grades compared with the national figures for all secondary schools and academies

('mainstream schools').The academies in our analysis group are twice as likely as mainstream schools to be below the floor standard ... The proportion of chains in our analysis group performing above the mainstream average for their disadvantaged pupils has fallen year on year from 2013 to 2015.[16]

This finding led the Conservative leader of Hampshire County Council and chair of the Local Government Association's Children and Young People Board to state:

These figures, and previously published statistics, clearly demonstrate that councils are education improvement partners, rather than barriers to delivering high-quality education that our children deserve.The government should recognise council's role in education improvement, and that imposing structural changes on schools does not guarantee improvement in education.[17]

But despite academy schools being outside of the control of local authorities, and with local authorities having their funding for school support and improvement taken away by the government, Sir Michael Wilshaw, Gilbert's successor as Chief Inspector of Schools, was still calling in September 2016 for local authorities and councillors to take responsibility and to have accountability for improving the academy schools in their area.[18] The lesson here is it that the public body is still in the firing line for criticism and assumed accountability even when its powers have been eroded and withdrawn, and it has little or no leverage over the outsourced services it once provided.

There are particular issues for children's social services raised by the devolved powers and freedoms given to academy schools which are outside of local authority control and influence, and with their only formal public accountability being direct to the Secretary of State for Education.[*]

---

[*] I had an experience of the autonomy of academy schools when in 2013 there was a direction from Michael Gove, the Secretary of State for Education, appointing me

Academy schools had been placed outside of the requirements to be full participants with Local Safeguarding Children Boards. The consequences have been noted by Baginsky and colleagues:

> It is now evident that LSCBs' engagement with schools varies from area to area. In particular, although local authority schools are regularly represented at a senior level on over four-fifths of LSCBs, Academies and independent [private] schools are represented on less than half of all LSCBs, and Academies are represented at a senior level on only one-fifth of Boards.[19]

Baginsky and colleagues also commented that:

> The education sector has been subject to 'marketisation' in recent years, such that schools compete through league tables of assessment criteria and their performance is measured in terms of concrete educational qualifications such as the number of GCSEs children attain at grades A*–C. Teachers are measured also in their success in 'adding value' to their students' predicted performance ... Potentially, there will be an inherent conflict between, on the one hand, pressure on institutions to demonstrate high levels of academic attainment and discipline by pupils in a competitive education 'market' and, on the other hand, the role of the school in recognising and meeting pastoral needs of children who are vulnerable or disadvantaged.[20]

---

to oversee children's services improvement in a local authority area. A large AET secondary school, which was part of a distantly managed academy chain, refused to participate in the training provided by the Local Safeguarding Children Board and also refused to provide data for the Children's Improvement Board which I chaired. There were also concerns about its isolationism, its limited engagement with other agencies, and its response to child protection concerns. The local authority had no levers to pull to get the school to cooperate. The head teacher refused to meet me or to allow me to visit the school. My only recourse was to write to Mr Gove. Civil servants were then active in discussions with the academy chain but with little quick change.

The overwhelming political pressure for schools to compete with each other based on exam result rankings accounts for some of the league table 'game playing' at the expense of pupils, with children not being accepted on schools' rolls, being temporarily suspended during Ofsted inspections, or being officially (and unofficially) permanently excluded.

This has particularly impacted on looked-after children in the care of local authorities, with the *Times Education Supplement* reporting that 'academies appear to be more prepared than maintained schools to delay or challenge [admissions] applications from children in care'.[21] This was a concern raised by Hilary Hibbert-Biles, the Conservative cabinet member within Oxfordshire County Council who was the lead councillor for education, with the council having great difficulty in getting children in care accepted by schools. It was reported by the BBC that:

> Politicians and officials from Oxfordshire are highlighting how more than 30 so called 'looked-after children' in the area have been left without schooling – some for months at a time ... And according to children's services chiefs across England, the problem is not isolated to Oxfordshire ... The main reason for what [Hibbert-Biles] described as a 'completely unacceptable state of affair' is that the council cannot order academy schools, which are independent of the local council, to admit a child in care ... Debbie Barnes, chairman of the Association of Directors of Children's Services [Educational Achievement Policy Committee], said ... 'As schools are getting more anxious about their funding, they are under huge pressures and the pressure of school places. They might think, "How can we meet this child's needs?" because they are likely to have more needs than someone else. If the child is coming into Key Stage 4 GCSE year, they might think, "What results are they going to get?"'.[22]

The Conservative government's focus on the academic outputs of schools (echoing Tony Blair's mantra of the importance of 'education, education, education') in the context of giving schools more freedoms and independence within the competitive marketplace which has been created has generated unintended, but now exposed and understood, outcomes, which remain unrectified. There is a difference of degree between delegation and devolution and disregarding and dismantling previous policy which stated that 'every child matters'.[23]

Beyond the generality of academy schools, one specific group – free schools – has been causing even more unease. The concerns relate to their non-strategic development where free schools are being opened in areas where there is no shortage of school places, and their sustainability and performance is increasingly in doubt. Free schools are also absorbing a disproportionate slice of the government's schools funding. All these concerns were pushed to the margins by the government's ideological commitment to develop more of a competitive market between schools under the mantra of parent choice (albeit that parents were not allowed the chance to choose for their children's schools to remain within the management and support of their local authority).

In April 2017 the House of Commons Public Accounts Committee, with a majority of Conservative MPs, concluded that:

> The system for funding new schools and new places in existing schools is increasingly incoherent and too often poor value for money. The Department for Education (the Department) is spending well over the odds in its bid to create 500 more free schools while other schools are in poor condition ... Add to this that local authorities are legally responsible for ensuring that there are enough school places for all children to attend good schools, even though they have no direct control of free school or academy places or admissions policies. All this made us question how much of a grip the Department really has in providing school places where they are needed. ... The Department indicated that its priority is to meet

the Government's target of creating 500 more free schools by 2020, but we remain to be convinced that this represents the best use of the limited funds available.[24]

The concerns of the Public Accounts Committee in April 2017 about the haphazard and random opening of capital-costly free schools, which may remain high cost if they are not be able to fill all their pupil vacancies, reiterated those expressed in February 2017 in a report by the National Audit Office[25]:

> Ministers are choosing to give billions of pounds to build new free schools while existing schools are crumbling into disrepair, Whitehall's spending watchdog has found … auditors have questioned whether the plans for so many new free schools will be value for money. Some free schools are opening in areas where there are already plenty of places, creating spare capacity that could affect the future financial sustainability of other schools in the area, they said.[26]

Two final comments on academy schools. First, a major academy chain announced in 2016 that it was going to abolish governing bodies for each of its 23 schools.[27] This would remove independent local governance oversight of the schools and would end the role of parent-elected governors. Centralised and commercial interest and control was to replace accountability, participation and transparency within local communities.

Secondly, it is not only children (and parents) who are experiencing the impact of academy schools and multi-academy trusts. Teachers and head teachers are also in the firing line, with one press headline reading 'Disappeared – headteachers are told to clear off and tell no one. In the competitive world of academy trusts school leaders are being ruthlessly fired – and silenced by gagging agreements'.[28] Once upon a time, head teachers (albeit not all) provided continuity, built consistent cultures within schools, and were recognised as leaders within their communities to which they were committed. Now they are agents of multi-academy trusts that determine from a distance their hiring and firing, often at pace and to meet the goals and interests of the trusts and not necessarily the community and its children.

Children's centres

A clear example of passing responsibility from central to local government without giving local authorities the means to fulfil their responsibilities was given by Justine Greening, the Secretary of State for Education, in October 2017. It followed a poll conducted by Action for Children, with a *Children and Young People Now* (CYPNow) report that 'Tory politicians raise concerns over the future of children's centres':

> More than a third of Conservative councillors in local authorities in England are concerned about the future of children's centres, a survey has found. Polling commissioned by Action for Children has found that 38 per cent of 508 Tory councillors questioned believe there is 'a lack of clear direction and funding' from central government for children's centres, family hubs, and family support. Analysis by CYPNow earlier this year revealed that there had been a reduction of more than 1,000 official children's centres in England in the space of seven years, with 2,501 as of February 2017, compared with 3,631 in 2010 ... Action for Children's survey also found that more than half (53 per cent) of Tory councillors agreed that central government funding cuts had made it harder for their council to deliver legally-required responsibilities for children and young people. And nearly three-quarters (72 per cent) agreed that long-term funding for children's services is a major concern for their council.[29]

Two days later Greening appeared before the Education Select Committee, which had a Conservative chair and majority. She was questioned about the closure of Sure Start children's centres. Here is a part of the exchange:

Thelma Walker: "You talk about working more effectively with parents but then we have just referred to the cuts to Sure Start. Having been a head teacher with a Sure Start centre on site, I know that we have very effective partnerships with parents through family outreach workers, through projects like babies into books, which of course links to the oracy and the enjoyment of reading. We had tooth brushing projects, which helped with the dental hygiene, so there was health there as well. There were so many positive projects that if you talked to professionals who were involved in those projects they would say it was working, it was effective. Family outreach workers who would work closely with parents out in the community, bringing parents in to work alongside their children, all of that was effective and that provision has been cut over the last few years."

Justine Greening: "It is a provision that local councils are responsible for. What I am setting out today is our national strategy and councils are able to increase the council tax and manage their own revenue streams if that is what they feel is worthwhile within local communities."[30]

The survey commissioned by Action for Children and this exchange in Parliament raise several points of particular interest for this text on the marketisation and privatisation of social work and social services. First, the survey was commissioned by a major national children's charity which has grown considerably by receiving grants and contracts from local authorities. For Action for Children a significant part of their services has been children's centres built and operated with money from a central government grant specifically allocated to Sure Start and managed by local authorities. The Conservative government withdrew this specific grant and cut the funding. This has had a major impact on the national and local charities who had grown their services based on the government funding. The Sutton Trust reported in 2018 that since 2010 there had been a reduction of 30% in the number of children's centres, with the closure of 1,000 centres in England.[31] In the year 2017/18 alone, Action for Children 'the largest provider of children's centres, in England has been forced to close or downgrade more than half its [children's centre] settings, make nearly 500 staff redundant and work with 69,000 fewer children and families over the past year following "crippling" central government funding cuts', with a reduction over the year of £13.8 million in its income for running children's centres.[32]

Secondly, Justine Greening firmly puts the responsibility on local authorities to raise local taxes to fund children's centres and Sure Start. Maybe this should not be surprising, as the government has abandoned and abdicated from many funding responsibilities. What it ignores, however, is that not only has the government withdrawn the Sure Start specific grant, but it has also cut its general funding to local authorities by 40% over the period since there has been the 30% reduction in the number of children's centres in England.

Greening's funding solution is that local authorities should raise their local council tax to generate the money locally to fund children's centres. Two problems here. First, the local authorities in the most deprived and disadvantaged areas have the greatest need for children's centres to support families experiencing increasingly severe poverty, but it is these local authorities which generate the lowest increase in funding by increasing council tax, and the tax would have to be paid by the disproportionate numbers of poor people in their area, making them even poorer.

There had also been the little local difficulty that the government had not allowed local authorities to increase their council tax by more than 2% without generating a local referendum to seek agreement to the increase. Running a referendum costs money which these local authorities can ill afford, and it may be unlikely that their local populations, already struggling financially as a consequence of government policies, would willingly agree to a higher council tax increase.

Finally, the decimation and decay of the national Sure Start programme shows a lack of evidence-informed policy making and of joined-up government. In the same week that Conservative local councillors and the Conservative-chaired Education Select Committee with a Conservative majority were expressing their concerns about government and Department for Education cuts causing the closure of children's centres, the Ministry of Justice published research[33] which gave rise to a report that 'The Sure Start children's centres network and other early help programmes have been credited as contributing towards a large drop in the number of children becoming involved with the justice system over the past decade'.[34]

The health service and hospitals

The second of Beveridge's giants to be considered is '*disease*'. The National Health Service has been on a similar trajectory to schools, with fragmentation, competition based on league tables, contracting out and outsourcing producing increasing opportunities for money to be made and profits to be taken out of what had been a public service. And as with academy schools, the journey had a significant boost under New Labour.

As noted earlier, it was the 1990 NHS and Community Care Act, based on a report by Sir Roy Griffiths, which established a purchaser–provider separation within the National Health Service. GPs, acting on behalf of patients, were individually and collectively to be the purchasers of other community and hospital health services, but all were still to be within an integrated and locally strategically planned NHS, with health authorities holding all the services together.

It was Alan Milburn as Secretary of State for Health in 2002 who announced the advent of foundation trusts and led on the necessary legislation, which was agreed by Parliament in 2003,[35] and under New Labour and the subsequent Conservative-led governments it had been intended that all NHS providers should become foundation trusts.

Trusts are semi-autonomous within the NHS and were described by the New Labour government in 2005 as being:

at the cutting edge of the Government's commitment to devolution and decentralisation in the public services, and ... at the heart of a patient-led NHS. They are not subject to direction from Whitehall. Instead, local managers and staff working with local people have the freedom to innovate and develop services tailored to the particular needs of their patients and local communities ... NHS Foundation Trusts are there to treat NHS patients, not to make profits or to distribute them. Just like NHS Trusts, most of their income is derived from agreements reached with local NHS Primary Care Trusts to provide locally relevant services for NHS patients at the national tariff rate. Private work is strictly limited.[36]

Foundation trusts were set up as a new legal entities called 'Public Benefit Corporations' but, as with academy schools and education, the initial impetus from New Labour set the health service on a trajectory of competition between providers within a marketplace that was subsequently opened up much more, first by New Labour under the term 'any willing provider' and then extended by Andrew Lansley as Secretary of State for Health in the Conservative-led coalition government, with 'operational guidance' issued in 2011 widening the health services which could be opened up to contractors who were now designated 'any qualified provider':

Since 2010, the Government has been committed to increased choice and personalisation in NHS-funded services. Choice for patients can be about the way care is provided, or the ability to control budgets and self-manage conditions. The government has specifically committed to extending patient choice of Any Qualified Provider for appropriate services. By choice of Any Qualified Provider (AQP) we mean that when patients are referred (usually by their GP) for a particular service, they should be able to choose from a list of qualified providers who meet

NHS service quality requirements, prices and normal contractual obligations. This approach is already in place for routine elective procedures.[37]

In 2015 it was reported that Lansley, now in the House of Lords, 'has taken a job advising corporate clients on healthcare reforms'. Lansley was being employed by Bain & Company:

> Bain & Company, which has its headquarters in the US, has taken a keen interest in the British healthcare system. In 2013 it claimed that the volume of services provided by non-NHS organisations was increasing. A Bain & Company report released that year found that about £5.8bn of NHS work was being advertised to the private sector, up 14% on the previous year.[38]

Lansley was not alone. The *Daily Mirror* in 2014 listed 70 ministers and MPs who had, in various ways, benefited from their relationships and links with private health care and pharmaceutical companies.[39]

The profit being taken out of the NHS by the private sector has grown. From the private–public finance initiative used to build hospitals it is reported that in the six years up to 2017 profits of £831 million were taken out of the NHS,[40] and the British Medical Association reported in 2017 that 'NHS spending on non-NHS and independent sector provision [ISPs] grows each year (there was an increase of £2.6 and £2.1 billion respectively between 2013/14 and 2015/16) [and] the proportion of the total Department of Health budget spent on ISPs is also increasing (from 6.1% in 2013/14 to 7.6% in 2015/16)'.[41]

The track record of the private sector gaining NHS contracts has not been one of outstanding success. In 2006 Serco, the multinational outsourcing company which has increasingly sought to gain contracts for what had been NHS-delivered services, was awarded the contract for the out-of-hours GP services throughout Cornwall. In 2012 *The Guardian* reported that:

When the co-operative of doctors from surgeries across Cornwall that ran the out-of-hours GP service lost its contract with the local primary care trust in 2006, they were not sure why, but suspected money played a large part. The winning bidder was Serco, the private contractor that is a leading provider of services to government and local authorities in many sectors – from defence to prisons and education – but a relative newcomer to health. The terms of the contract are deemed commercially confidential, as is the competitive bidding process, so they are not open to public scrutiny. The former chair of the GP co-operative company, KernowDoc, Dr Gareth Emrys-Jones, said that the service was being run for £7.5m a year until that point. Any private sector bidder would be likely to factor in profits, but the co-operative ran the service as a not-for-profit operation. The PCT was unable to confirm the cost of the previous service when asked by the Guardian, but did say that the first Serco contract was worth £6.1m a year over five years. It was renewed last October for a further five years at a price of £6.4m a year. According to its critics, that dramatic cut and a profitmaking ethos have left the service beset by serious problems and have made it unsafe. A series of claims about its shortcomings are now being investigated by the health regulator, the Care Quality Commission.[42]

A year later in 2013 the House of Commons Public Accounts Committee held hearings about the contracting out of the out-of-hours GP service in Cornwall and about the performance and behaviour of Serco. Their report was damning:

> In early 2012 whistleblowers raised concerns that the out-of-hours service in Cornwall was short staffed and that the contractor, Serco, had lied about its performance by altering data. Serco provides the service under a £32 million five-year contract with the primary care trust, NHS Cornwall and Isles of

Scilly, until 31 March 2013, and since 1 April 2013 with Kernow Clinical Commissioning Group. The primary care trust and the strategic health authority did not demonstrate they had the appropriate skills to negotiate effectively with private providers and hold them to proper account for poor performance. Serco, as a large provider of public services is able to win public sector contracts but has not in this instance proved capable of delivering a good service on the ground. Evidence has confirmed that what the whistleblowers in Cornwall were saying was substantially true. However, Serco appears to have had a bullying culture and management style which inhibited whistleblowers from being open in the patients' interest. The company responded to stories placed in the press by whistleblowers in a heavy handed way, launching internal investigations and searching employees' lockers when issues were raised, and staff were fearful of raising concerns. Serco initially denied the concerns raised by whistleblowers and it was only after reports appeared in the press that it started to accept that things were wrong. Most concerning was the fact that Serco staff altered data on 252 occasions, resulting in Serco overstating the performance it reported to the primary care trust.[43]

Later in 2013 it was reported that:

Serco, the private contractor that falsified its NHS data in Cornwall, is looking to pass on its troubled GP out-of-hours service in the county to a subcontractor … Margaret Hodge, chair of the parliamentary accounts committee (PAC), which held an inquiry into Serco's performance in Cornwall earlier this year, described the move to offload the contract as outrageous. 'It's absurd that the government contracts with one company, which can't cope and misleads us all, and the company then just hands the job over to another. How on earth can you have proper accountability like this?' she said.[44]

In 2015 the Cornwall's Clinical Commissioning Group announced that the out-of-hours GP service for the county would no longer be provided by or through Serco and that it would now be provided by a GP-led, not-for-profit social enterprise.[45]

A second example raises similar concerns and issues about contracting out NHS services to private, for-profit, companies. This time it is about a hospital. Indeed, it is about the first – and to date only – NHS hospital to be passed to the private sector to manage and run. This too was not a successful transfer and transaction. Here is how the 'debacle' was described in 2015, possibly rather surprisingly in the Conservative-supporting *Daily Telegraph*, with reporter Max Pemberton stating:

> As the Public Accounts Committee scrutinises what went wrong at Hinchingbrook, people are still failing to grasp the lessons that need to be learned. Circle took over the running of the hospital in 2012 amid a fanfare. There were grave financial problems and the hospital was facing possible closure when Circle, Europe's largest healthcare partnership, was given the contract to run it in the first ever franchising of an NHS hospital to a private company. It had debts of £39m and a turnover of £73m, but Circle promised to turn this around, bringing the efficiency and leanness of big business to the hospital. This, we were told, was the future of the NHS. It was carefully spun as a John Lewis-style ownership structure. But it was all cynical marketing. Unlike John Lewis, Circle is largely owned by hedge funds; a fact that was repeatedly downplayed when talking about it. Circle went on an all-out PR offensive, courting journalists (myself included) in an attempt to get the maximum positive media coverage. While I declined, many gave unquestioning coverage to the takeover, peddling the line that this was the answer to failing hospitals

and that opening up the NHS to competition had indeed been the solution all along. And then it all went wrong. On January 9, as a highly critical Care Quality Commission report was published, which highlighted major failings in care at the hospital, it was announced that Circle would be terminating its contract. Unsurprisingly, the emails from the PRs have now stopped. Circle claimed it failed because it had not been prepared for rising A&E numbers and reduced charges for operations. I read these reasons and laughed. Welcome to the NHS, Circle. What did you expect it would be like? These are the nightmarish pressures with which every single NHS trust in the country is contending. But, unlike Circle, not every other trust has the luxury of being able to walk away when the going gets tough.[46]

The Hinchingbrooke Hospital experience of being privatised led a former Labour health minister in the 1970s, David Owen, himself a medical doctor, to write:

Advocates of a market-led, partly privatised NHS for England have been saying for years that 'what matters is what works', dismissing those who believe in the 1948 NHS concept as ideological, old-fashioned or plain wrong. Now that their flagship, Hinchingbrooke hospital, the only privately run NHS hospital in the country, is losing its private contractor, Circle, one might have expected the zealots to acknowledge the flawed nature of their policy? Not a bit of it … There should be a fundamental rethink from all those who have identified themselves with this flawed concept, which started to take hold in the debate about foundation hospitals in 2003 and reached its apotheosis in the Cameron/Lansley legislation of 2012 with a full-blown external market for the NHS. The care quality commission (CQC) gave Hinchingbrooke the inspectorate's worst ever rating for 'caring'. The CQC found it 'inadequate' (the worst rating) for safety and leadership, and was so damning overall that Circle threw in the towel hours before the findings were made public.[47]

The House of Commons Public Accounts Committee inquired into the failings of care, and of the outsourcing contract, at the hospital, and its chair, Margaret Hodge, wrote:

> Circle became the first private company to run an NHS hospital when it took operational control of Hinchingbrooke Health Care NHS Trust in February 2012. However, in January 2015, Circle announced that it intended to withdraw from the contract, just three years into the 10-year franchise. Whilst this was an innovative − but ultimately unsuccessful − experiment, we are concerned that none of those involved in the decisions has been properly held to account … Despite our warnings about the risks, oversight of the contract by the various parties who had a role was poor and inadequate and no one has been held accountable for the consequences.[48]

As with the out-of-hours GP privatisation in Cornwall, a private, for-profit, company over-promised and under-delivered on how it would drive down costs as a means of gaining the contract, performance and care got worse, measures introduced to improve performance were not fit for purpose, and those letting the contract were slow to identify and deal with the damning and deleterious situation which was arising. When it all got too difficult the private company withdrew and walked away, leaving the NHS to pick up the pieces.

The two examples examined above about privatisation and the NHS have focused on GP primary care services and hospitals. The third example is focused on the third major arm of NHS provision − community services.* As with Hinchingbrooke

---

* The other major areas of NHS activity are the provision of medicines, with concerns having arisen about the big profits being made by the pharmaceutical companies, and public health, with private commercial companies challenging and resisting

Hospital, it is a story located in Cambridgeshire, and on reviewing the collapse of the community health services contract in Cambridgeshire the National Audit Office commented that:

> The termination of this contract indicates that the health sector may not have learned lessons about assessing and managing risk when working with a private provider, despite the earlier failure of the Hinchingbrooke contract and experience in wider government.[49]

The contract let in 2014 by the clinical commissioning group (CCG) in Cambridgeshire and Peterborough was for the provision of community care for adults over 18 years old, acute emergency care for those over 65 years old, and older people's mental health services. What drove the decision to contract these services outside of the NHS through a process of competitive tendering was the CCG's requirement to cut expenditure on these services as it was facing a combined funding shortfall over five years of £250 million.[50] The savings which had to be made on these services were of such a magnitude (£178 million) that the well-known outsourcing companies, including Serco, Capita and Virgin Care, withdrew from the tendering process as they could not see how to generate the required scale of cost reductions (and with their additional requirement that they make a profit).[51]

An arrangement was made that two local NHS foundation trusts would between them create a private sector limited liability company, UnitingCare Partnership LLP. It then subcontracted with a range of bodies, including the two trusts themselves, other NHS providers and a number of other private sector and voluntary organisations.

What happened next? Soon after the contract was signed UnitingCare quickly concluded that it could not deliver the services within the funding provided by the CCG. This difficulty was compounded by UnitingCare having been set up as a private

---

public health measures such as deterring smoking and reductions in sugar and salt levels in retailed foods.

company outside the NHS. As noted in the National Audit Office report,

> as a separate legal entity, UnitingCare Partnership was not itself an NHS body and was outside NHS VAT arrangements. Therefore NHS subcontractors were no longer able to recover VAT on the services provided to UnitingCare Partnership that had previously been recovered when they provided the same services to the CCG. The partnership had not factored these additional costs into its contract price.[52]

Within eight months of the contract starting in April 2015 it had collapsed, with the BBC's report headed 'Cambridgeshire's £800m NHS outsourcing contract "wasted millions"',[53] and with the House of Commons Public Accounts Committee concluding that 'The termination led to unfunded costs incurred by UnitingCare Partnership totalling at least £16 million, which had to be shared between its two trust partners.'[54]

Meg Hillier, the chair of the Public Accounts Committee, commented:

> It beggars belief that a contract of such vital importance to patients should be handled with such incompetence. The deal went ahead without parties agreeing on what would be provided and at what price – a failure of business acumen that would embarrass a child in a sweet shop, and one with far more serious consequences. Services for patients are likely to suffer and we will be expecting the clinical commissioning group to come clean about precisely how much damage has been done in terms of future service provision and finances. Local MPs have told me that they could not get answers to concerns they raised about this contract, which in turn raises questions about transparency.[55]

But it was not only local health services which were hindered by privatisation. It also impacted on NHS England and its national remit, with the House of Commons Public Accounts Committee finding that:

> NHS England's outsourcing of primary care support services to Capita Business Services Ltd (Capita) was a shambles. Its short-sighted rush to slash by a third the £90 million it cost to provide these services was heedless of the impact it would have on the 39,000 GPs, dentists, opticians and pharmacists affected. Capita recognises that the service it provided was not good enough. Its failures have not only been disruptive to thousands of GPs, dentists, opticians and pharmacists, but potentially have also put patients at risk of serious harm.[56]

A consistent picture of concerns arises from the NHS examples above about privatising health services. First, the contracting-out process carries short-term and continuing costs. Secondly, it adds complexity in accountability and diminishes transparency. Thirdly, there are in-built motivators to bid low to gain contracts, but pressure is then applied back to the NHS to increase the contract value. Fourthly, there may not be openness and honesty about the performance of the contracted-out service and there may be a reluctance and delay by the NHS contractors to recognise that contracts are not delivering what was intended and promised. And, finally, when it all gets too hot to handle, the service is returned to the NHS to retrieve and rescue as, although the services may have been contracted out, the responsibility remains with the commissioners, who are still within the public sector. These are real warning signs about the dangers and difficulties which are likely to arise if crucial services and decision-making to help families and protect children are pushed and placed into a similar commercial privatised market place. As will be seen below, the lessons and warnings do not come only from the examples of health services and schools which have been noted above.

Despite the recent history of privatising health (and social) care being far from reassuring, the contracting out of what had been NHS-provided services to private companies has continued, and indeed has picked up pace, with the BBC reporting in July 2018 that:

> Private firms cash in on over-stretched NHS ... under-pressure NHS services in England are spending over £1bn a year buying care from outside the NHS because they are unable to keep up with demand. The bill is being racked up by hospitals, ambulances and mental health trusts, data obtained by the BBC shows. NHS managers said money was being wasted as often it was done at the last minute, and led to the NHS over-paying.[57]

The British Medical Association (BMA) had expressed concern that as these contracted-out services were still badged as the NHS and displayed the NHS logo, the scale of NHS privatisation may not have been widely recognised.[58]

Criminal justice and community safety

Similarly, it is not always recognised that privatisation has also been rampant within three major arms of the arrangements for criminal justice and community safety – the police, prisons and probation services – and the courts themselves have not been immune from creeping privatisation in the context of cuts. This is the new 'giant' of '*threat and fear*', which was not addressed by Beveridge.

Police

The extent, and even the existence, of private companies getting contracts for what had been public sector police services and responsibilities may be less recognised by the public. This may be because it is partly unseen 'back room' activities which have been taken on by the big outsourcing companies, but it is also a consequence of a gradual drift rather than a dramatic and sudden process, with the police withdrawing and private security firms filling the vacated space. Unlike for the health service and schools there has been no trumpeting that marketisation is the government's policy for the police, justice and security. Yet the scale of the police work outsourced to private security firms is significant and growing. In January 2016 *The Sunday Times* reported that:

> Police [between 2010 and 2014] have spent almost £170m employing investigators, analysts and other staff from G4S and Serco, two private-sector companies that have been investigated for allegedly overcharging the government [for the electronic tagging of offenders]. According to documents obtained under freedom of information laws, forces across the UK have turned to private-sector staff to fill gaps as thousands of officers left or retired after 20% cuts to police budgets.[59]

It was reported, for example, that:

> G4S has been used on sensitive investigations including Operation Yewtree, Scotland Yard's child sex abuse inquiry that has seen several high-profile prosecutions of celebrities collapse; Operation Grange, the long-running hunt for Madelaine McCann; and Operation Withern, the investigation into the London riots in 2011.[60]

The increasing involvement of the private sector in policing was seen to be related to the cuts in police funding and the sizeable reduction in the number of police officers[61] so that at times of high activity the police had to buy in capacity from the security firms, and it was also a consequence of police forces seeking to make savings by contracting out 'back office' functions.

Private security firms have also been one of the UK's leading exports, with their tentacles spreading across the world. In 2016 *The Guardian* reported that:

Britain is the 'mercenary kingpin' of the global private military industry, which has been booming ever since the 'war on terror' began 15 years ago, according to report seen exclusively by The Guardian. The UK multinational G4S is now the world's largest private security company, says the report by the British-based charity War on Want, which adds that no fewer than 14 private military or security companies are based in Hereford, close to the headquarters of the SAS, from whose ranks at least 46 companies higher recruits ... G4S last year [2015] ... signed a five-year £100m contract with the British embassy in Afghanistan ... [and] Foreign Office spending on contracts with private UK security companies rose from £12.6m in 2003 to £48.9m in 2012.[62]

The scale of the cuts-caused crisis in policing was highlighted in 2017 with a police inspectorate report that 'investigations were being shelved'[63] and with concerns about the assessment and supervision of registered sex offenders.[64]

Of particular concern when reflecting on the safety of children, young people and vulnerable adults was the withdrawal of police services from community policing and community intelligence. The cessation of neighbourhood policing teams[65] and the reduction of police community support officers (PCSOs)[66] meant that local knowledge and oversight of 'hot spots' where children might be vulnerable and of networks which might be active in exploiting children and others, would be lost, and this reduction in the 'prevention sphere' was highlighted by senior police officers.[67, 68]

In August 2018 it was reported that:

One in three bobbies on the beat in England and Wales have been axed in just three years as violent crime has surged. A Sunday Times investigation found more than 7,000 traditional neighbourhood police officers, who protect communities and gather intelligence, have been reassigned to other duties or left jobs altogether since March 2015. The number of police community support officers (PCSOs) has also fallen by 18% over the same time period to just over 10,000.[69]

The reality facing police services contending with the cuts was highlighted by the chief constable in the West Midlands:

> The chief constable of England's second largest police force has admitted it sometimes provides a poor service that fails to meet public expectations. Dave Thompson apologised and said budget cuts and fewer officers policing a 'wider spread of crime' had left West Midlands Police at a point where it was not sustainable to tackle everything. He said he was 'drawing the bar higher' as to what would be investigated.[70]

A consequence of cuts leading to police forces 'drawing the bar higher' has been that some communities are turning to private security firms to safeguard their neighbourhoods and communities, with *The Sunday Times* reporting under the headline 'West End elite eye private police force' that 'wealthy landlords are in talks for hundreds of guards to patrol posh areas of central London'.[71] It was not only, however, the rich in London who were looking to 'private police forces'. *The Guardian* published an article in September 2018 about the village of Martock in Somerset where a private security firm was hired by the parish council to patrol the streets after locals were told by Avon and Somerset police that they 'couldn't give us the level of patrolling we thought we needed to deal with [anti-social behaviour]'.[72]

At the same time as the police faced further cuts and retrenchment, the government in 2017 sought to allow powers of arrest to be contracted out to private companies. This was a shock for the *Daily Mail*, which reported:

> Private firms may be given new powers to arrest people in a controversial move that has raised alarm. The proposals would allow, for the first time, staff

from companies such as G4S to arrest members of the public for failing to pay fines imposed by the courts. The plans would see HM Courts and Tribunals Service (HMCTS) privatising part of its compliance and enforcement operations in a deal worth £290 million.[*,73]

This is not, however, something that started in 2017. G4S and Serco have for many years been getting contracts for police, probation, courts and prisons services. *The Guardian* noted in 2013 how these outsourcing companies had already extended into a wide range of public security and justice services:

> [G4S] has a developing business with the police, running custody suites in three forces, providing forensic medical services, including rape reporting centres in 11 forces, and a flagship £229m deal with Lincolnshire police to run its 999 response service, its control room, civilian staff and a police station. The company also runs facilities management services for the courts and employs former police and probation officers to work on temporary contracts to cover staffing gaps in police investigations. The Ministry of Justice contracts together are worth £5.14bn over their lifetime, or about £274m a year. The Home Office contracts are worth a further £301.2m over their lifetime and those with the police £283.8m, making a total of £585m. Together they produce annual revenues of £118m a year. These figures are not insignificant even for a global company like G4S and probably represent about more than half its UK earnings.[74]

The Guardian went on to comment on Serco:

---

*   This is similar to the 2014 changes in statutory regulations which allow statutory children's social work services to be contracted out to profit and non-profit companies and organisations. Both are examples of crucial (and potentially coercive) statutory powers being allowed to be handed over to profit-making outsourcing companies.

205

Serco, an outsourcing specialist, holds the London probation contract, supervising 15,000 offenders carrying out 'community payback' sentences. It also runs six prisons in England and Wales. Two months ago, the group's category-B Thameside prison was the subject of critical report by the chief inspector of prisons, found to be in 'lockdown' after failing to cope with a violent, internal gang culture. It is the single remaining bidder for a contract to run the South Yorkshire cluster of three existing jails but that has been put on hold while the [Ministry of Justice] audit takes place. Overall prison, probation and welfare-to-work contracts in Britain are estimated to account for close to £300m, or 6%, of Serco's £4.9bn global revenues. The two firms [Serco and G4S] are the major private players in criminal justice privatisation and it is hard to see how any further large-scale outsourcing police, probation or prison project can succeed without some sort of involvement by them.[75]

And yet where there have been major public safety contracts given to G4S and Serco, their delivery and performance has been so poor that it has presented risks and dangers to the community, the contracts have had to be terminated, and the cash costs have been considerable. For example, G4S failed to fulfil its government contract to provide security for the 2012 London Olympics, with the BBC reporting that 'Troops were drafted in at the Games after the private company was unable to provide enough security guards. Culture Secretary Jeremy Hunt said it had made him "think again" about the default use of private contractors. And Defence Secretary Philip Hammond said only the state could provide "large-scale" contingency back-up'.[76]

In 2013 G4S, this time with Serco, were again in the news, with the BBC reporting that:

Serco and another company, G4S, allegedly charged the government for electronically monitoring people who were either dead or in jail. The government also uncovered problems with G4S's contract to provide facilities management in courts. The matter has been referred to the Serious Fraud Office (SFO). Both companies have withdrawn from the bidding process to win contracts to supervise offenders on their release from prison. They were stripped of their responsibility for tagging criminals in the UK earlier this month.[77]

Another area of outsourcing within the justice system which has generated concern relates, in particular, to the family courts, with an immediate impact on the decision-making about the lives of children. The concerns here were about the forensic alcohol and drug testing and evidence provided to the family courts by Trimega and Randox Testing. These are two private companies which from 2012 received contracts when the government closed and outsourced its Forensic Science Service:

> The Home Office announced this week [24 November 2017] that 10,000 criminal cases in England and Wales were being reviewed after it emerged that data at a laboratory run by Randox Testing may have been manipulated. The investigation then spread to encompass all child protection proceedings, dating back to 2010, in which drug and alcohol testing had been carried out by the same company. ... 'The problem is that nobody really cares until something like this happens. That's my very strong impression,' said Prof Peter Gill, one of Britain's most distinguished forensic scientists. 'This raises serious questions about ... forensic provision carried out by companies. It shows they can run dubious practice and get away with it for many years.' Gill, who is a professor of forensics at Oslo University, added it was difficult to imagine the scandal having occurred under the Forensic Science Service, where scientists were routinely sent mock cases that were checked as a quality control. 'When you get rid of

that system the quality is quite difficult to maintain,' he said.[78]

Probation

A whole new area for contracts was created for the private sector when the Conservative–Liberal Democrat government, with Chris Grayling as Secretary of State, required that 70% of what had been the Probation Service should be opened up to compulsory competitive tendering. This was greeted at the time with optimism and support from charities and voluntary organisations which were already active in providing rehabilitation services.[79] But while some saw growth opportunities for their charities, others were more cautious and concerned:

> Andrew Neilson, director of campaigns at the Howard League for Penal Reform, feels the entire process is misguided, risky and potentially unworkable. 'The MoJ wants to drive down costs, improve quality and introduce a new system, all at the same time, on a very tight timetable,' he says. 'It's an ambitious political project and they have bitten off more than they can chew.' He predicts that the reforms will end up like the Work Programme: 'We are going to end up worse off – and to make it even worse, we will have missed an opportunity to make it better'.[80]

The government-required and enforced breaking-up of the Probation Service would potentially provide rich picking for the private sector. The 70% of probation responsibilities that were to be outsourced were for offenders deemed to be at lower risk of serious reoffending. The remaining 30% rump of the work, with high-risk serious offenders, would stay with what was left of the Probation Service. In essence, it was the government's plan that most of the high risk was still held within the public sector.

Which organisations got the contracts for the outsourced services? The *Financial Times* reported that:

The government part-privatised its probation service in 2014, awarding £3.7bn of contracts to companies including Sodexo of France, MTCnovo of the US, Ingeus of Australia and Staffline, Interserve and Working Links of the UK to oversee 200,000 medium and low-risk offenders.[81]

Sodexo, in particular, gained a significant number of contracts, for what were now to be known as 'community rehabilitation companies'. They were awarded the contracts for Northumbria, Cumbria, Lancashire, South Yorkshire, Bedfordshire, Northamptonshire, Cambridgeshire, Hertfordshire, Norfolk, Suffolk and Essex. Sodexo was awarded the contracts in partnership with NACRO (the National Association for the Care and Resettlement of Offenders), but where there were partnerships between private companies and voluntary organisations it was primarily the private sector company that was the dominant partner.*

Was the government's breaking-up of the probation service in England and Wales a success? Hardly. Indeed, it has been quite a disaster, and one which was always predictable, as noted in 2014 by witnesses who gave evidence to the House of Commons Justice Select Committee:

> Witnesses in our inquiry, including some supportive of the proposed changes, had significant apprehensions about the scale, architecture, detail and consequences of the reforms—some of which are still to be determined and much of which has not been tested— and the pace at which the Government is seeking to implement them. In particular, our witnesses with professional experience of probation saw potential

---

* Why no probation contracts for G4S and Serco? One might have expected that this would be a significant opportunity for them to capture more public funding and that supervising offenders fitted with their other business interests such as running private prisons and tagging offenders. But *The Guardian* reported that 'G4S and Serco, the private security companies, withdrew their bids after the Serious Fraud Office was called in to investigate overcharging of more than £100m on electronic-tagging contracts involving the two companies' (https://www.theguardian.com/uk-news/2014/oct/29/justice-probation-contracts-private-companies).

risks to the effective management of offenders arising from the Government's decision to split the delivery of probation services between a public National Probation Service dealing with the highest-risk offenders and the new providers who will be dealing with low and medium risk offenders.[82]

Creating fragmentation between workers and agencies supervising offenders, hindering information exchange and making communication more difficult, with offenders passing between organisations and workers as their risk assessment changed, and with no one agency now having the oversight of all offenders within a community to track relationships and networks, was never going to be sensible, and there were accounts in 2015,[83] 2016[84] and 2017[85] of the chaos, complications, costs and confusion which have been created. Added to this the requirement that the contracts being let by the Ministry of Justice were also intended to save significant amounts of money, the shambles which was created was foreseeable.*

It was reported in *The Independent* that problems started to arise very quickly in implementing and delivering the contracts. Within months there was a difficulty with a Sodexo contract:

A privatised part of the Probation Service could be brought back into public hands after the French catering firm chosen to run it in a significant English region failed a Ministry of Justice (MoJ) audit. The South Yorkshire region comes under one of six Community Rehabilitation Companies [CRCs] that Sodexo, previously best known in the UK for feeding school pupils and the military, was chosen to run last December. A document detailing Sodexo's failures in

---

* I had personal professional experience of the complications and difficulties which arose, when overseeing for the government children's services and child protection improvement in three areas of England in 2014–15. Either there was no engagement from the Probation Service and the Community Rehabilitation Company, as both were now stretched too thin with limited management capacity, or both agencies would attend the 'improvement board' meetings I chaired, although neither had a picture and oversight of networks of offenders.

South Yorkshire has been passed to *The Independent* and reinforces fears that privatisation could pose a risk to the public because offenders are not being properly monitored. The document noted 'a lack of contact with offenders, ineffective enforcement and little or no evidence of any offence- or risk-focused work'.[86]

But it was not only Sodexo which was in difficulty delivering the contracts it had been awarded. The difficulties were wide-ranging and largely endemic, with the *Financial Times* reporting in October 2016 that:

> Almost every contract to provide probation services in England and Wales is lossmaking, according to the companies that bid for them two years ago when the system was privatised ... But the companies say the contracts are lossmaking and unsustainable because their bids were based on incorrect assumptions from the Ministry of Justice. The companies complain that the contracts overstated the number of offenders they would manage, suggesting their income would be higher... 'If it is not fixed it will be a disaster,' one provider said. 'It is fine for the big companies with strong balance sheets but some of the smaller players are really struggling.'[87]

These difficulties were covered and confirmed in a report by the National Audit Office,[88] with *The Independent* reporting that:

> Serious failings in the Government's privatisation of the probation services have been exposed in a damning report amid warnings that David Cameron's 'half-baked and reckless' policies have left the criminal justice system in a mess. The report by the independent Parliamentary spending watchdog, the National Audit Office, warns the Government has no way of knowing how well companies responsible for running the country's probation services are performing due to a failure to collect accurate information. It also says

some of the Community Rehabilitation Companies (CRCs) may be manipulating or withholding data from government agencies while others are putting financial profit above public safety by ignoring difficult offenders who require the most help because it costs them too much money to treat them.[89]

But these failings were not primarily teething problems in the early days of new contracts. They were problems which continued into 2016 and beyond.[90, 91]

In July 2018 it was reported in *The Guardian* that 'Private probation companies [are] to have [their] contracts ended early':

> David Gauke, the justice secretary, has announced that eight private firms that run 21 'community rehabilitation companies' (CRCs) in England and Wales are to have their contracts terminated in 2020, two years earlier than agreed ... But despite significant problems identified with the provision of services by the private companies, the government insists that the sector has a role to play and will be putting contracts out to tender for the overhauled framework proposed for 2020 onwards ... The most recent intervention to save the flagging providers will cost the taxpayer £170m. This includes the waiver of £115m in penalties owed by CRCs for failing to meet targets under Grayling's 'payment by results' system, an extra £46m over two years to shore up the 'through the gate' services provided to prisoners on release and a further £9m to correct underpayments. The government has already had to hand over an extra £342m to the CRCs, bringing the total additional cost to the taxpayer to more than £500m.[92]

Prisons

The track record of privatising prisons has been no more successful, and as with the experience of cuts and contracting out in police and probation services, there is an immediate impact on the safety and welfare of children, vulnerable adults and the community.

The UK's recent history on privatising prisons goes back to the Thatcher governments of the 1980s and was continued by New Labour, as noted by the Prison Reform Trust:

> Faced with a rising prison population in the late 1980s the Conservative government turned to the private sector to provide extra prison places. Privatisation was seen as the most cost effective solution to the crisis and was part of the Government's determination to promote private enterprise and extend the free market into public services ... The Labour Party vehemently opposed the Conservatives' policy on private prisons. But within a week of being elected in 1997, it made a dramatic U-turn [and] in a speech to the Prison Officers' Association [in 1998] Mr Straw [Labour's Home Secretary] announced that all new prisons would be privately built and run.[93]

The private companies getting contracts to build and run prisons sought to make their profits by reducing the numbers and the terms and conditions of employment of prison officers.[94] A consequence was increased instability and turnover in the prison officer workforce within the private prisons, with it noted in 2003 that 'low pay is a contributor to the high turnover in many private prisons. Overall, among Prison Custody Officers turnover is 25 per cent – 10 times greater than the 2.5 per cent rate among public sector prison officers'.[95] Not surprisingly in 2003 the House of Commons Public Accounts Committee concluded that 'The performance of the seven PFI prisons against contract has been mixed. All but one have incurred financial deductions for poor performance'.[96]

In 2004 prisons and probation were joined together nationally in what was called the 'National Offender Management Service' (NOMS). This major organisational change was led by Sir Martin Narey (see Chapter Three). Having visited private prisons and the companies that ran them in the US, he was a champion for 'contestability', where public and private providers would be compared and would compete to run prisons, although he denied that this was 'privatisation'.[97] At the time the Prison Reform Trust reported that:

> From 2005 the scope for competition is to be extended under the Government's proposals to introduce 'contestability'. Martin Narey, the Chief Executive of the National Offender Management Service, has said he plans to market test all public sector prisons ... In an interview early last year Martin Narey said, 'Last summer I visited the US and spoke to two viable US private prison providers that are not yet operating in England and Wales. I have started a dialogue with them about the possibility of their bidding for future work'.[98]

In the United States, the Office of the Inspector General of the US Department of Justice reported in 2016 that 'In a majority of the categories we examined, contract prisons incurred more safety and security incidents per capita than comparable [Federal Bureau of Prisons] prisons'[99] and President Obama decided in 2016 that there should be 'No more private federal prisons ... after audit finds they have MORE security breaches than government-run ones'.[100] But in 2017 President Trump reversed this decision and CNN reported that the 'Private prison industry sees boon under Trump administration'.[101]

Has the track record of privatising prisons in England and Wales been any more of a success? In 2012 Chris Poyner of the Public and Commercial Services (PCS) Union wrote in *The Guardian* that:

> It ought to be a national scandal that multimillion-pound global companies are being handed huge amounts of taxpayers' money to profit from locking people up by cutting staff and working conditions. We at the Public and Commercial Services Union (PCS) understand that the going rate for a return is a 7% profit. But all this has happened without any public

debate or discussion, and very little scrutiny. Opened under John Major's government in 1992, HMP Wolds was the first private prison in the UK, prompting the then Labour opposition to condemn the private sector running prisons as 'morally repugnant'.

Performance has been so poor that two were taken back into the public sector and in 2008 it was revealed that 10 of the 11 private prisons in England and Wales were in the bottom quarter of the Ministry of Justice's performance league table.[102]

Maybe it is not surprise that a public sector union should be concerned about prison privatisation but this was not just a concern generated by trade unions. Over the following years there were several scandals involving private prisons, with particular issues about G4S. In 2016 *The Guardian* reported that 'G4S [has been] fined 100 times since 2010 for breaching prison contracts'.[103]

The failings of G4S in running prisons came to a head in summer 2018, with the BBC reporting:

> Birmingham Prison is being taken over by the government from the private firm G4S, after inspectors said it had fallen into a 'state of crisis'. Chief Inspector of Prisons Peter Clarke described it as the worst prison he had ever been to ... There were 1,147 assaults, including fights, recorded at Birmingham in 2017. This was the highest figure for any prison in England and Wales that year, or on record under modern reporting standards. It represented a fivefold increase since 2012, the first full year that it was run by G4S.[104]

There had been particular concern about G4S's Medway Secure Training Centre (STC), where children and young people were assaulted and abused. In January 2016 BBC's Panorama programme exposed through undercover filming the abuse by staff in the centre.[105] A month later the BBC announced that G4S 'is to sell its children's services business including the contract to manage two secure units – one at the centre of abuse claims. The centres are at Oakhill, Buckinghamshire, and Medway, Kent. The sale – as part of a business review – includes its 13 children's homes.'[106]

Three months later, when Medway STC was still being run by G4S, there was a damning report by an Independent Improvement Board appointed by the Secretary of State for Justice which found that 'leadership within the STC has driven a culture that appears to be based on control and contract compliance rather than rehabilitation and safeguarding vulnerable young people. The Board continues to have significant concerns that this culture and the emphasis on contract compliance may be leading to reports of falsification of records'.[107] In May 2016 the Ministry of Justice took over the running of Medway STC,[108] and in February 2017 Medway Local Safeguarding Children Board started a serious case review following criminal convictions of assault and abuse of young people at the STC.[109]

Medway STC was not the first G4S-run service for children and young people to be removed from its running and responsibility. An inspection report in February 2015 about Rainsbrook STC, which accommodated up to 82 children and young people aged 12–18, recorded, among other concerns, that 'there have been serious incidents of gross misconduct by staff, including some who were in positions of leadership. Poor staff behaviour has led to some young people being subject to degrading treatment, racist comments, and being cared for by staff who were under the influence of illegal drugs' and that 'The overall effectiveness of the centre is inadequate'.*,[110]

In September 2016 it was reported that G4S would no longer run Rainsbrook STC and that it was now to be run by MTCnovo.[111] MTCnovo is an American company which also had contracts as a community rehabilitation company. It too

---

* Sir Martin Narey (see Chapter Three) authored an 'independent report' for G4S about Rainsbrook Secure Training Centre for young offenders, which stated that the young people were treated 'overwhelmingly well'. It ran counter to the Ofsted inspection report, which found that G4S staff at Rainsbrook had behaved 'extremely inappropriately' with young people, with Ofsted rating the centre as 'inadequate'. It caused concern when it became known that Sir Martin Narey had previously been paid as a consultant by G4S (https://www.theguardian.com/society/2015/aug/05/g4s-paidmartin-narey-independent-youth-prison-report-consultant).

had been immersed in controversy with Sky News reporting in March 2016 that:

> England's troubled young offender centres could be taken over by an American company accused of managing prisons riddled with violence, corruption and drugs. Two 'Security and Training Centres' (STCs) are being sold by private security firm G4S ... Sky News has learned that one of the frontrunners to succeed G4S is MTC Novo, part of a company currently named in legal action in the US, where inmates claim they were abused. MTC runs the East Mississippi Correctional Facility, a prison described in legal documents as 'an extraordinarily dangerous place'.[112]

In 2017 G4S was again the cause and centre of media and public concern. It followed another BBC Panorama exposé based on under-cover filming, with the BBC reporting that:

> G4S has suspended nine members of staff from an immigration removal centre near Gatwick Airport, following a BBC Panorama undercover investigation. The programme says it has covert footage recorded at Brook House showing officers 'mocking, abusing and assaulting' people being held there. It says it has seen 'widespread self-harm and attempted suicides' in the centre, and that drug use is 'rife'.[113]

The House of Commons Home Affairs Select Committee was so concerned about the evidence of abuse at Brook House that it promptly opened its own inquiry.[114] It held a hearing in September 2017 and it was reported that:

> G4S has been accused of falsifying records to make profits of more than 20 per cent running an immigration detention centre marred by abuse and drugs ... Nathan Ward, who worked as G4S's duty director at Brook House before becoming a vicar, told

the committee the contractor had given inaccurate information to the Home Office on costs.... Rev Ward claimed that G4S had made cost savings but not passed them on to the Government as required, using them instead to drive up profits. He accused the firm of delaying filling vacated posts to save on wages, while demanding money for more staff than were hired. Asked by Yvette Cooper, chair of the committee, whether G4S may have been 'deliberately been giving false information to the Home Office', the former employee replied: 'Categorically, yes.'[115]

The profits being made by G4S from its government contracts to run two immigration removal centres (IRCs) became a topic of interest and debate, with *The Guardian* reporting that:

The security firm G4S appears to have been making more profit than its contract allows from the immigration removal centres (IRCs) it runs for the government, according to an internal document seen by the Guardian. According to an outline of G4S's financial performance at the two IRCs it ran in 2016, the company's margin on its trading profit at Brook House was 20.7%. At Tinsley House, its other IRC, the margin was 41.5%, though that figure may be distorted by the fact that Tinsley House was closed for part of the year.[116]

There is more that can be recounted about G4S and about the dangers to those who are placed in its care, including concerns about the death of Gareth Myatt, aged 15, who died at Rainsbrook STC while being restrained. In 2016 *The Guardian* reported that:

A privately run youth jail where a 15-year-old boy died had the highest number of incidents in which children were caused serious injury by staff attempting to restrain them, according to a government report seen by the Guardian ... The incident is one in a list of restraints-gone-wrong that feature in a Ministry of Justice report. It details incidents where children suffered breathing difficulties or serious injury while being restrained at four STCs and two young offender institutions (YOIs) between April 2014 and March 2015. The worst three institutions were all run by G4S.[117]

Before moving on, here is a summary comment from the BBC which gives a view of the reach and influence of G4S:

> G4S, the security firm that runs the Brook House immigration removal centre where nine members of staff have been suspended, has a chequered history dogged by controversies and accusations of malpractice and mismanagement. The firm operates in around 100 countries worldwide and employs more than 585,000 people. It describes itself as the 'leading global, integrated security company' with a mission to be 'the supply partner of choice in all our markets'. Its website says it is the largest secure outsourcing company in the UK and Ireland, with 34,000 employees and a UK turnover of £1.7bn. Its outsourced operations for the UK government include five private prisons, a secure training centre and two immigration removal centres, as well as accommodation for families awaiting repatriation and secure transportation and electronic monitoring services.[118]

The BBC then listed several of the major concerns which have arisen over recent years about G4S, which included the abuse at Medway STC, the failure to deliver on its contract to provide security at the 2012 London Olympics, its overcharging of the government for its offender tagging contract, and the death of Jimmy Mubenga, who died from a heart attack while he was being restrained by three G4S security guards on a deportation flight bound for Angola.

Despite all of these concerns G4S has continued to get government contracts, including a contract to run the government's equalities helpline, with Mark Serwotka, general secretary of the PCS Union stating that:

> G4S's track record ought to disqualify it from taking on such a sensitive contract. With hate crime and discrimination on the rise in the wake of the Brexit vote, we need good quality support services more than ever. We believe this helpline should be brought back in-house and it is deeply disturbing that the government appears to have dismissed this out of hand.[119]

It was not only G4S that had been a recidivist in failing to deliver government contracts. This had also been the track record of Serco,[120] which had got into difficulty as a consequence of 'a desire to win as much government work as possible, regardless of risk or poor returns'.[121]

Whilst failing to deliver and deceiving about performance on contracts, Serco and G4S continued to get renewed government contracts, including for the accommodation of asylum seekers, with Maurice Wren, the chief executive of the Refugee Council, commenting that 'All too often, people seeking asylum in the UK are forced to live in squalid, unsafe, slum housing conditions, at exorbitant cost to the public purse'.[122]

Social security and employment

But what of Beveridge's giants of '*want*' – which might be called poverty and deprivation – and '*idleness*' – unemployment? As with other areas of outsourcing public services, the privatisation of social security and welfare benefits and their administration goes back to the Thatcher governments of the 1980s[123] and was continued and expanded by New Labour in the late 1990s and 2000s. It was heightened by New Labour's emphasis on assisting and driving those receiving welfare benefits back into employment, and this was to be achieved through contracts awarded to private companies, despite the lessons that could have been learnt from other countries:

> Government plans to 'privatise' the welfare system by paying companies to find jobs for the unemployed are 'fraught with difficulties' and wide open to abuse, a major study finds today. The first international analysis of how similar schemes have worked abroad concludes that while dole queues have been cut and money has been saved, introducing the 'profit motive' into welfare is far from an easy solution. ... Today's report by the centre-Right think tank Policy Exchange will reinforce Left-wing and union opposition by highlighting a history of unscrupulous behaviour by private companies in Australia, the US and elsewhere ... The report uncovered common abuses as companies played the 'payment by results' system to maximise returns rather than further the best interests of unemployed people.[124]

The fears were well founded. In 2012 there was widespread media coverage about the behaviour and performance of a company making big profits out of government contracts to get benefits claimants into employment:

> The company, A4e, which has secured millions of pounds of Government contracts over the past 20 years, was accused of claiming funds despite only placing people in jobs for one day. A4e, which aims to get the unemployed back into work, is headed up by Emma Harrison, who is believed to be worth £70 million. She was named 'back to work tsar' by David Cameron and has run the scheme under Labour and Conservative. Last week, it emerged Mrs Harrison received a dividend of more than £8 million after the company's turnover reached £234 million. A4e has secured millions of pounds of Government contracts over the past 20 years.[125]

In 2015 ten employees of A4e were convicted of fraud having received bonus payments for wrongly claiming that they had got benefits claimants into employment. A4e would also have benefited from being able to claim it was successfully delivering on its government contract.[126]

It seemed, however, that dishonesty and fraud was widespread within A4e and not limited to those employees who were prosecuted, with further examples given by the *Daily Mail*, which stated:

> A series of whistleblowers came forward in 2012 to speak out about a highly-pressurised culture where many employees forged documents to make it look like they were meeting impossible targets. The company would then submit fraudulent claims for payment by the taxpayer based on getting more jobseekers into work than it had actually achieved, the insiders alleged.[127]

There was also profit to be made from the outsourcing of the assessments and administration of social security payments for disabled people, with it reported in 2016 that:

> Two private firms have earned more than £500m in taxpayers' money for carrying out controversial disability benefit assessments. The Department for Work and Pensions (DWP) paid Atos and Capita £507m for personal independence payment (PIP) tests between 2013 and 2016, despite fierce criticism of their services by MPs ... A total of £382m was paid to the IT services firm Atos, a European IT services firm with headquarters in Paris, and £125m to London-based FTSE 100 company Capita.[128]

What is possibly surprising is that despite issues previously raised about the performance of the companies contracted to provide, in particular, disability benefits assessments, concerns about performance and delivery continued at the same time as costs of the contracts were increasing, as was reported in 2011[129] and in 2016.[130] A year later in 2017 MPs were still being told of significant concerns:

> As many as four out of five cases where a claimant has been denied disability benefits are overturned on appeal because of systemic failures in the initial assessment process, MPs have heard. Frontline welfare advisers told the work and pensions select committee that the personal independence payment (PIP) process was 'inherently flawed', resulting in thousands of wrong decisions and causing widespread harm and distress to claimants. In some cases, a decision not to award a PIP was overturned by a tribunal after it had taken account of medical evidence from doctors about the claimant's condition that had been ignored by officials during the initial assessment ... Claimants are assessed by health professionals employed by private firms Atos and Capita.[131]

But it was not only Atos's performance on the benefits assessments contract which was causing long-standing concerns. It was also generating concerns about its performance on other government contracts:

> Atos, the controversial outsourcing company, is facing a government review of all of its major Whitehall contracts, which amount to more than £500m, following another serious IT failure. The Cabinet Office told the Guardian it would undertake a full re-examination of every contract worth more than £10m operated by the French-based firm. Such a review of a single contractor is a rarity in Whitehall and is a reflection of the levels of exasperation both from civil servants and the public accounts committee at the programmes overseen by Atos.[132]

What might be surprising is that recidivist failings to deliver acceptable performance on crucial government contracts, especially to provide services essential to the well-being of disabled people, were tolerated for so long and not urgently addressed. What might also be surprising is that in April 2017 it was reported that Atos and Capita were to receive extra payments of £200 million from the government because the numbers of assessments were beyond those stated in their government contracts. The Labour shadow Work and Pensions Secretary stated that 'it is beyond belief that this Tory government is rewarding failure … The PIP process is in disarray and these companies are receiving huge pay-outs in a time of extreme austerity'.[133]

Housing and homelessness

The one remaining Beveridge giant to consider is *'squalor'*. It was to be tackled through a programme of house building by local authorities. This too has now been largely driven from public provision into an increasingly insecure and expensive profit-generating marketplace which is leaving growing numbers of people homeless and in need of housing. What a change from the intentions and policies of the post-war 1940s, as noted by David Kynaston:

> The belief in 1945 that the public could match the private ran deep. Co-compiling that autumn a Report on Luton for the local council, Richard Titmuss [who as a professor of social administration was to be a shaper of social work in the 1950s and 1960s] ended the section on housing with a clarion call: 'There is evidence that the country is moving towards a wide acceptance of the principle that services provided by the people for themselves through the medium of central and local government, shall compare in standard with those provided by private enterprise. As it is with hospitals and clinics, so it should be with homes and schools. The council house should in the future provide the amenities, space and surroundings which hitherto have been the monopoly of private building'. This was a vision fully shared by Bevan, perversely enough responsible for housing as well

as health, two immensely challenging tasks. His unambiguous policy was severely to restrict private house-building and instead to pour as many resources as he could muster into new local-authority housing. Although there had been significant growth of such housing between the wars, this policy marked the beginning of a fundamental and long-term step-change, so that by the end of the 1970s as much as a third of the national housing stock was in the hands of local authorities.[134]

All of this was to change with a vengeance in the 1980s. The move away from council-provided, affordable rented housing started, as with so much in the privatisation journey tracked in this book, with the policies and practices of the Thatcher governments. It was the 1980 Housing Act, introduced in Thatcher's first year as Prime Minister, which created a statutory right for council tenants to buy, at a subsidy, their council house.[135] As Timmins noted, the move to sell off council-provided public housing gathered pace during the 1980s and 'housing associations were allowed for the first time to find private sector cash to augment public sector grants. This was the first beginnings of private finance for public, or semi-public, projects'.[136]

The changes introduced had a game-changing impact on housing, with 'the intent being, in Thatcher's words, for the state to withdraw "just as far and as fast as possible" from the building, ownership, management and regulation of housing'.[137]

'Tenants Choice' was introduced so that council house tenants could vote to have council houses removed from the control and management of councils and transferred to new landlords – a process which was encouraged by the government's restraints on local authority finances (including restrictions on councils using income from right-to-buy council house sales to replenish the diminishing public housing stock). Local authorities' borrowing was also restricted so that councils struggled to repair and refurbish council housing, with the consequence that tenants found it attractive to have their homes transferred to housing associations whose finances and borrowing capabilities were not so restricted. By 1993 the building of houses by councils had virtually stopped.[138]

If councils were the intended immediate targets of the Thatcher governments' housing policies, the longer-term victims have been those who have been priced out of home ownership and are now forced to rent at a high cost from private landlords, or are homeless. The decimation of public housing provision meant that whilst councils still had a statutory responsibility for homeless people, including families with children, their capacity to respond to increasing homelessness was severely curtailed.[139, 140]

New Labour did invest in housing renovation and improvement through its 'Decent Homes' programme, and had some success in particular in improving the homes provided by housing associations, but the failure to invest in new public housing contributed to the growing shortfall in affordable homes and increasing homelessness, including for families with children and for vulnerable adults.[141, 142]

While housing has been increasingly privatised since the 1980s, albeit with big public subsidies paid through housing benefit, and with privately rented housing replacing council-rented housing, what has been the impact? Toynbee and Walker, writing in 2017, reflected on the position during Cameron's Conservative-led governments in the 2010s:

> Housing is not fairly taxed; house-builders hoard land; 'planning' is passive and restrictive instead of proactive, imaginative and developmental; and dogma prevents the state – local and national – building and letting dwellings. The result is widespread hardship and downright waste of human potential.[143]

Running through the tale and trail of housing, and particularly the disinvestment in and the dismembering of public housing since the 1980s, are two absolutely awful scandals. They each concern neighbouring Conservative-controlled London boroughs.

The first is about Westminster City Council and its leader in the 1980s, Dame Shirley Porter, the daughter of the founder of Tescos. Porter used the sale of council housing as means of turning marginal electoral wards in Westminster into safe Conservative wards and hence securing Conservative control of the council. The process of selling council housing to private developers was intended to bring increased private home ownership into the marginal wards and to move council house tenants, who were assumed to be Labour supporters, out of the wards. It was a process – and an intention – which was found to be illegal and which led to Porter herself being surcharged.[144, 145]

The Westminster City Council scandal showed how the sale of council housing was seen as a strategic opportunity to build and sustain support for a Conservative council, just as nationally the sale of council housing – and other public assets – was anticipated and intended to lead to an increase in Conservative-voting home owners, and owners of shares in the sold-off public utilities.

The second council house scandal, 30 years later in 2017, related to Westminster's neighbour, and another Conservative-controlled local authority, the London Borough of Kensington and Chelsea. It was an even more awful tale of the disregard for council tenants, and the impact and intrusion of the private sector, and this time it led to horrific deaths.

The fire in June 2017 at the Grenfell tower block caused the deaths of 71 people. The tower was managed on behalf of Kensington and Chelsea London Borough Council by Kensington and Chelsea Tenant Management Organisation (KCTMO), the largest tenant management organisation in England, responsible for nearly 10,000 properties in the borough. The properties had previously been managed by Kensington and Chelsea Council, and the tenants of the flats would previously have been council tenants.[146] Although the management of Grenfell Tower had been outsourced by the council, it was the council which still owned the tower block and which in 2012 contracted out its refurbishment to a number of private contractors. Although Kensington and Chelsea is one of the richest boroughs in London it sought to reduce the refurbishment costs by accepting a specification for lower-price cladding for the block rather than more fire-retardant cladding. Residents stated that they had raised concerns for some time about the fire hazards, other safety issues and about building maintenance within the block but that these had largely gone unaddressed by the management organisation and by the council. There was also a concern that government cuts in legal aid had hindered tenants and tenants' associations in seeking to get these matters addressed.

In August 2017 the government set up an inquiry following the fire and deaths which would look at the design, maintenance and refurbishment of Grenfell Tower, the response of emergency services to the fire, and the management of the property and engagement and communication with its residents.[147] What the dreadful Grenfell Tower disaster exposed was the consequences of deregulation, cost-cutting, privatisation and profit-taking, and the opaque and complex accountability that had resulted from outsourcing the management and maintenance of council housing. It also exposed, in one of the richest areas of the country, how those who were poor were marginalised, stranded and left exposed by a council where the boast was of cutting council taxes, with the corollary of cutting public services.

In December 2017, in the week of the memorial service in St Paul's Cathedral for the victims of the Grenfell Tower fire, there was an (interim) report on the review of building regulations which had been ordered by the government. The report was a damning indictment of the privatisation and cost-cutting government policies which led to the context in which the fire occurred:

> A review of building regulations[148] ordered after the Grenfell Tower fire has found the system is 'not fit for purpose' and open to abuse by those trying to save money. Dame Judith Hackitt's interim report into building safety called for an overhaul of the construction industry to put safety above cutting costs. In a foreword, Hackitt said she was shocked by some of the practices she had uncovered. 'The mindset of doing things as cheaply as possible and passing on responsibility for problems and shortcomings of others must stop,' she wrote. Her report highlights concerns about increased privatisation of the building inspection regime leading to safety being

compromised and a reduction in expertise within local authorities.[149]

David Walker, writing on the state of public services in the UK at the end of 2017, commented on the Grenfell Tower tragedy:

> First responders were magnificent and the follow-up, especially with regard to the psychological consequences for residents, showed NHS staff at their best. But Grenfell also exhibited the disjointed, uncommunicative nature of public services and the effects of outsourcing and arms-length management … The Grenfell inquiry won't even begin to ask about the new public management doctrine, which told public bodies 'to steer, not row' and which has pushed much public service delivery to profit-seeking firms or devolved bodies, leaving accountability in tatters and the public befuddled over who does what.[150]

So at Grenfell Tower corners and costs were cut, accountability was made complex and confused, and safety was compromised, all in the context of privatisation. Privatisation, a commitment to largely unrestrained market forces and market dynamics, and deregulation to make the market more attractive and profitable for the private house-building companies (some of which are major financial donors to the Conservative Party[151, 152]), have led to safety being compromised and more costly housing that is unaffordable for many.

With local authorities shunted out of housing provision since the 1980s, housing provision has been derailed, leaving increasing numbers without a home. And the big private house-building companies and their shareholders and senior managers have made big money, including from the taxpayer. In the same week as the Grenfell Tower memorial service it was reported that the chief executive of housebuilders Persimmon was awarded by his board a £100 million bonus and that 'Persimmon is one of the biggest beneficiaries of the government's help-to-buy programme, which has lifted sales and boosted house prices across the UK'.

The bonus 'was attacked by politicians, charities and corporate governance experts, who described it as "obscene", "corporate looting" and a reward based on "taxpayer subsidies"'.*,[153]

---

*   What is of note is that it was a former banker who, as chair of Persimmon's board, had shaped and agreed the payment arrangements for Persimmon's chief executive. £1 million might be seen as a sizeable bonus to be awarded for growing Persimmon's profits from the government's ill-advised 'first time buyers' scheme which – as anticipated by many – put up house prices and benefited the shareholders of house-building companies. If a £1m bonus might be seen as an unearned windfall, £100m is off-the-scale for a largely unearned bonus. BUT playing around with bonuses in the millions and high salaries may not seem so shocking to bankers – like Persimmon's chair.

TEN

The impact to date of the privatisation of social care, social services and social work

This chapter focuses on a more recent 'giant' that was not within Beveridge's original five giants. Alongside want, ignorance, squalor, disease and idleness, and the additional 'giant', identified in the previous chapter, of 'fear and threat' is that of *neglect*.

Since the 1940s, and more so since the 1970s and the creation of local authority social services departments, there has been an increase in publicly funded and public sector provided care services for those who otherwise would be left stranded in a state of neglect. Since before the nineteenth century, there has always been a mixed economy of care services, with charitable and church organisations supplying care alongside state provision. But in the 1980s this balance was to change, as the private sector was promoted by the Thatcher governments and has continued to expand in size and scope.

In the late 2010s the growth of the private sector in what was now often called the 'care industry' can be considered within the context of care services, care organisations, and the care workforce. Each has become territory increasingly captured by commercial companies which are seeking to profit from private and public payments for care.

Care for older people

Since the 1980s care services for older people, and to a lesser extent for younger disabled people, have become primarily provided by private companies. The growth in, and now the dominance of, private sector care homes was noted in a House of Commons Library Briefing Paper:

> The care home market in England is now dominated by private providers ... For over 65 year olds, in 1984 the number of residential care places in local authority-run accommodation for older and physically disabled people peaked at 144,564 (57% of all places), at a time when the private sector provided 66,700 places and the voluntary sector 42,704. However, in 1984, the number of private sector places was approaching double the number in 1980 (37,177), and the rapid expansion of the private sector continued in the following years. By 2017, the number of private sector places had reached 196,600 (76% of all places). Local authority places were just 19,200 (8% of all places), which was under half the number of voluntary sector places (44,400). In terms of nursing care homes, in 2017 the private sector had 179,000 places (86% of all places) compared to 15,200 in the voluntary sector and 10,500 NHS places.[1]

The heavy dominance of and dependence on private care home companies has dramatically reshaped the care home market. As discussed earlier, as a result of government-imposed financial restrictions on local authorities in the 1980s and into the 1990s local authorities closed their ageing care homes which needed modernising and refurbishment or transferred the homes to profit or not-for-profit companies. New homes were primarily built by companies who saw the increasing numbers of older people – and especially people over 80 years of age who were more likely to need care and support – as an expanding market opportunity.

An increasing proportion of older people would also be self-funders as they had income and assets from occupational pensions, home ownership and inherited wealth, providing a flow of funding for the private companies to tap. Those who were not paying for their own care would still be funded by local authorities, which had a statutory requirement to provide care for older people who needed it but could not fund it themselves.

This, therefore, looked like a safe and secure, lucrative and long-lasting expanding market for companies and investors to enter and exploit, despite the experience of local authorities capping the care fees they would pay. The capping of fees did lead to the closure of some homes – often single homes in individual ownership – but it also provided an opportunity for bigger companies to buy up homes and to build their portfolio, even if the company's financial base was not strong, with, as noted by Laing and Buisson, 'the ready availability of sale and leaseback funding [allowing] several large companies with weak balance sheets to embark on a strategy of collecting large care home portfolios'.[2] But more recently the bubble has been bursting:

> Looking back to the turn of the century, risky financial gearing was also responsible for the last spate of financial failures which took place in the early years of the new century as providers which had expanded rapidly with 100% sale and leaseback funding found their narrow margins eliminated by adverse trading conditions brought about by local authority purchasers' unwillingness to increase fee rates by more [than] RPI [Retail Prices Index – a measure of inflation]. As a result, landlords forced several defaulting sale and leaseback operators into receivership.[3]

This statement from LaingBuisson, the health and care sector market analysts, essentially means that the private care companies which grew on the back of selling off care homes (hence securing and banking a financial return for their speculative investors), and then leasing them back to run in the hope of getting a revenue return as well as the capital return, was only a partly successful strategy. They got their capital receipts so made their profit, but they often had weak balance sheets because the investors who took the profit from the care home site sales had actually put in and risked little of their own money. Instead, the companies had borrowed to invest, leaving them with a large continuing debt. The private care companies, many owned by international venture capitalists, had no commitment to the care of older people in the UK. Entering and exploiting the care market was just a way of making money quickly, with the escape route, when needed, of just walking away. The consequence has been a residential care sector for older people which is unstable, and for increasing numbers of care homes unviable. Those who suffer most are older people and their relatives, who are left anxious and with considerable uncertainty about the future, with the threat of having to move on at short notice.

When a care home provider cannot or decides not to continue to trade, where does the buck stop? It is the public sector which has to take the responsibility and come to the rescue – as with the G4S failure to properly prepare for security at the 2012 London Olympics, when the military had to be mobilised by the government. If a care home company withdraws from providing care homes it is local authorities who have to put together a rescue plan and package to provide alternative care for the residents who are now being made homeless. It is the public sector which provides the safety net for older people when private sector investors take high risks to generate high returns. It is a not infrequent occurrence for individual local authorities to have to deal with individual homes withdrawing from providing care, but this has already also happened at scale when major care home companies have imploded because of profit-taking business models. Here are two major examples of older people, in effect, being treated as a commodity to trade on and from which to generate a profit.

Southern Cross grew rapidly in the 2000s to become one of the major private companies in the older people's care home market. In 2001 it had 70 homes. Ten years later, largely through acquisitions, it had 750 care homes, with over 37,000 residents. But, as noted by Peter Scourfield:

This dramatic expansion appeared to be inspired less by the desire to meet the needs of the frail elderly population and more to do with treating care homes as a tradeable commodity and securing profits from asset stripping.[4]

Scourfield described the financial manoeuvres which generated big gains for Southern Cross's investors but which left older people anxious and vulnerable:

A critical point came in 2004 when the private equity company Blackstone bought [Southern Cross] for £162 million. Blackstone also bought another nursing home company, NHP, for £564 million (£1.1 billion including debt). Blackstone then reorganised the companies with Southern Cross providing the care and paying rent to NHP, which now owned most of the properties ... [and in 2006 Blackstone sold NHP to Delta Commercial Properties owned by the Qatar Investment Authority, in a deal which guaranteed rising – and ultimately unaffordable rent payments – to QIA]. In 2007 Blackstone sold their remaining stake in Southern Cross by which time it had made an estimated fourfold return on its investment. In the same year Southern Cross management team left the company, but not before benefitting from 'personal windfalls' totalling £36.6 million, the biggest beneficiary being the then chief executive Philip Scott who made £11.1 million from share sales. Unfortunately, that former investors and managers were profiting so handsomely was not a sign that the company was on a sound financial footing. In fact, the opposite was the case. In June 2008, the company failed to meet a £46 million repayment deadline and was forced into emergency talks with its banks ... By 2011, no longer holding the freehold on most of its properties, Southern Cross was struggling to pay an annual rent bill close to £250,000 owed to its various landlords who now included international financiers, venture capitalists, private equity firms as well as other corporate care providers.[5]

In July 2011 the BBC reported:

> Care home operator Southern Cross is set to shut down after landlords owning all 752 of its care homes said they wanted to leave the group. 'It is currently envisaged that the existing group will cease to be an operator of homes,' the firm said. ... The Darlington-based Southern Cross and its landlords and creditors are a month into a four-month restructuring period, which was agreed in crisis talks in June. The statement said that the details of the restructuring were not yet settled and there was still a possibility of further changes. It had been expected that some of the landlords would leave the group, leaving Southern Cross operating with between 250 and 400 homes, but now it appears that the group is to disappear altogether.[6]

What happened next? The homes were sold on to other corporate companies and in 2014 they were again in the news, with the *Financial Times* reporting:

> Hundreds of former Southern Cross care homes are to be sold to new owners within weeks, two years after Britain's biggest residential care provider collapsed sparking a national debate about care for the elderly. The financial backers of HC-One, which was formed as a management company to run about a third of the estate managed by Southern Cross, has shortlisted five bidders to buy the 241-home portfolio, with a deal in excess of £500m expected by the end of March. ... HC-One is a subsidiary of debt-laden NHP, which owns the freeholds and leaseholds of the properties and is saddled with £1.35bn debt, which its creditors are keen to recoup. The business is

managed by Court Cavendish, led by Dr Chai Patel,
former owner of the Priory rehabilitation clinics. Mr
Patel and his management team are incentivised on
the value of any sale, and could receive between 2
per cent and 6 per cent of the value of an exit, or an
estimated £30m in total.[7]

Tracking and telling the Southern Cross story is complicated
and complex (see above!). But in essence it is a simple tale
which is summed up in *The Guardian* headline 'Southern Cross's
incurably flawed business model let down the vulnerable'.[8] It
was a business model built on seeking quick and big profits for
international venture capitalists and others whilst minimising
their financial risk, and even limiting the amount they had
to personally invest, as compared to borrow, to get their rich
pickings. It was a business model based on asset-stripping. And
it was a business model which left older people exposed and
vulnerable and with local authorities having to work hard and
quickly to put in place alternative care for tens of thousands of
older people who suddenly faced the prospect of being left with
no accommodation and no care.

Is the Southern Cross debacle unique? No. In 2016 and
2017 the story was in many ways replicated by another big
care company conglomerate. In July 2016 the *Evening Standard*
reported that:

> FOUR SEASONS, the stricken care homes operator
> owned by private-equity guru Guy Hands, has
> promised to fix its debt-laden balance sheet by the
> end of the year to help fuel a turnaround. The battered
> group has to pay £55 million a year in interest
> payments following Hands' debt-fuelled acquisition
> of the company in 2012. His firm Terra Firma paid
> £825 million but used £525 million of loans, leaving
> Four Seasons with scores of heavyweight lenders who
> want paying back.[9]

Fifteen months later, after what would have been a lengthy
period of uncertainty for residents, their relatives, and staff of

the Four Seasons care homes, *The Guardian* reported that there
was a respite although still no confirmed solution to the crisis:

> A deal has been agreed to stave off the collapse of
> Four Seasons Health Care, which looks after 17,000
> elderly and vulnerable people, after the company's
> largest creditor agreed to drop several conditions.
> Loss-making Four Seasons had warned it might not
> honour a £26m debt payment due by Friday, raising
> fears the firm could become the largest care home
> operator to fall into administration since Southern
> Cross in 2011.[10]

Nils Pratley summed up the position in a piece headed 'A
shocking way to fund UK care homes':

> Let's not lose sight of the ingredient at the centre of
> the Four Seasons affair. It is debt – too much of it.
> Terra Firma, Guy Hands' private equity firm, over-
> paid for the business in 2012 and loaded up with
> leverage. At heart, this is an old-fashioned tale of
> financial engineering gone wrong. Southern Cross
> came from the same unlovely stable – in that case,
> the financial error was addiction to fancy sale-and-
> leaseback property deals. ... The result, in this case,
> is that control of the biggest care homes operator
> in the land will probably pass from a private equity
> outfit that made a rotten bet on financial leverage to
> an opportunistic US hedge fund that hunts for junk
> bonds to buy at a discount. It's a shocking way to fund
> provision of care homes for the elderly.[11]

It is not only care homes and their residents which have
been pawns in profit-seeking games played by international
hedge funds and venture capitalists. Often on a smaller scale,
private home care providers have also entered, and then left,
the commercial care market – a market which has been made
more difficult by central government cutting funding to local
authorities, which hinders them from paying increased fees for

the services they commission and purchase despite the costs of providing the services increasing, as a consequence, for example, of minimum wage and night payments increasing, and more demanding (and expensive) registration and regulation standards. But the Southern Cross and Four Seasons stories are essentially about seeking and taking big profits to be paid to those who have little interest or commitment to providing care but a lot of interest in making money.

Care for children

The examples above relate to care for older people but children's care provision has also been increasingly privatised, with an example just as alarming as the stories above. This is the story, recounted by Zoe Wood in *The Guardian* in 2007, of Sedgemoor children's homes, owned by a private equity company:

> In the autumn of 2004 the private equity firm ECI made the following boast in its business review: 'Due to the excellent performance of the Sedgemoor business since ECI's initial investment in 2000, an opportunity arose to refinance the business and for ECI to get cash out'. The newsletter flagged the refinancing of three businesses – Sedgemoor, debt management firm Gregory Pennington and restaurant group Tragus, triggering a £20m pay-out to its investors and partners. Fast forward three years, however, and it is a different story. Sedgemoor has gone into administration and is unlikely to be mentioned in despatches. If Sedgemoor was a widget factory, its demise might be described as mere bad luck. But it was one of the UK's largest residential care businesses looking after vulnerable children, and its financial difficulties caused more heartache than just fears about redundancies. The group's demise has renewed concerns among charities and industry professionals about whether the profit-maximising ethos of buyout firms, who tend to operate on three-to five-year investment horizons, is compatible with

the long-term care of the most vulnerable members of society.*,12

And, as with the care homes for older people, it was the residents of the children's homes who were left uncertain and anxious, and local authorities who had to quickly put in place alternative arrangements for care. Who generated an income from the crisis? KPMG:

> More than 50 residential children's homes face an uncertain future after one of the UK's largest providers went into administration. Sedgemoor, which has more than 65 homes and 14 schools throughout the country for children with complex needs, had been involved in talks with potential buyers but was unable to agree. Last week KPMG Restructuring was appointed as administrator and subsequently negotiated the sale of 13 of the company's homes, each of which accommodates one to four children. However, a senior figure in the residential child care sector warned the future is 'uncertain' for the rest of Sedgemoor's homes, schools and staff, adding: 'Local authorities are making contingency plans in case any children have to be moved'.13

The extent of private, for-profit, provision within children's social care may not often be recognised, but it is now significant. Many might think that children's homes are provided by local authorities or by voluntary organisations like Barnardo's, as this is how it used to be. But 72% of children's homes in England (1,538 homes) are now privately owned and operated as for-profit homes, and only 20% (434 homes) are provided by local authorities and 8% (164 homes) by voluntary organisations.14 Many local authorities no longer provide and manage any

---

* I recall that, when a director of social services, along with other social services directors, I had to check at very short notice whether we had any children placed in a Sedgemoor children's home (we didn't!) as all the home's residents had to be moved with less than 48 hours' notice as the company had decided to close the home with little warning.

children's homes but buy all their children's residential care from private providers. Ofsted reported that:

> There were 2,209 children's homes, of all types, on 31 March 2018. This was a net increase of 3% from the same time last year, and follows the patterns of previous years ... At the same time as the number of children's homes rise, the number of local authority (LA)-run children's homes continues to fall ... On 31 March 2018, LAs ran 19% of all children's homes, compared with 23% in 2015. In 2018, more than one in 4 local authorities (44) do not run any children's homes in their area ... Of the 169 new homes opened in 2017–2018, 86% were opened by private organisations ... [and] the 5 largest private organisations owned around 17% of children's homes.[15]

In 2017 it was reported by *Children and Young People Now* magazine that the Independent Children's Homes Association (ICHA) anticipated there might be a legal challenge to local authorities for 'not adhering to public procurement regulation in the way they consult with providers' and that the ICHA wanted a 'dynamic purchasing system [which] could allow approved providers to compete for each individual placement without having to secure a multi-year contract with a local authority'.[16] This looks like a spot-purchasing model whereby any private children's home could bid for a child to be placed within it but where the reality would be that local authorities would be placing children with private providers about whom they had little knowledge and limited continuing relationships.

Private companies are also now significant in providing foster care in England and big profits are being taken from public funding for children social services, as noted by Andy Elvin in 2016:

> Recent research from Corporate Watch shows that in 2014–15, eight commercial fostering agencies made around £41m profit between them from providing

foster placements to local authorities. This is pure profit. It's after allowances for foster carers, staffing costs and support services. Who did this money go to? Well, according to Corporate Watch, one company, Graphite Capital, made £14.4m on shareholder loans from the National Fostering Agency, which it owned, and then sold it on. The Ontario Teachers' Pension Plan accrued £13m from its ownership of Acorn Care and Education. And Sovereign Capital took £1.9m in 2014 alone from company Partnerships in Children's Services, a group that comprises several foster care agencies.[17]

One company Elvin does not mention is Foster Care Associates, a part of the Core Assets Group, and its holding company, Ideapark. Corporate Watch noted that it generated £127.2 million from foster care in 2014 and paid its owners, Jim Cockburn and Janet Rees (after whom the Rees Centre for Research in Fostering and Education at Oxford University is named, having been funded by Core Assets[18]), £9.2 million in 2013, with its highest paid director receiving a salary and benefits of £406,000:*

Founded by carers Jim Cockburn [who was a social worker in Worcestershire] and Janet Rees [a foster carer] in 1994, Foster Care Associates (FCA) has become the biggest foster care company in the

---

* This is a figure comparable with the salary and benefits paid to the Vice-Chancellor of the University of Bath, a large international university with one of the top rankings nationally and in the world. The salary and benefits of the Vice-Chancellor became the subject in 2017 of much media coverage and concern. But big payments to those benefiting from public funding in the private sector receive little comment or criticism, and these are only a fraction of the millions paid individually to senior managers in private sector companies and those in banking and 'financial services' through salaries and bonuses. There is a largely unstated and unexposed hypocrisy from those in the right-wing media who attack public servants for their pay and pensions. It was reported in December 2017, for example, that Paul Dacre, the then editor of the *Daily Mail*, received an annual payment of £2.5 million and has a pension pot that will pay out £708,000 a year (https://www.theguardian.com/media/2017/dec/11/paul-dacre-pay-as-daily-mail-editor-jumps-50-to-almost-25m).

UK, and even has branches in Finland, Australia and Canada. The FCA website assures potential foster carers that it does not have any 'shareholders or private equity interests to serve', but this is only half right. Unlike many of its rivals it is not owned by a private equity firm. But it certainly does have shareholders – principally Jim Cockburn and Janet Rees, through a holding company called Ideapark Ltd. The latest accounts of Core Assets Group Ltd (Foster Care Associates is a trading name) show the company paid out £7m in dividends to Ideapark Ltd in 2014, and £11.6m the year before. Ideapark Ltd's accounts show it only paid out £50,000 to Cockburn and Rees in 2014, but a whopping £9.2m the year before.[19]

The Core Assets Group website described Core Assets as '*industry*-leading experts' [italics added] and as an industry leader Janet Rees was awarded an OBE in 2015 for services to children and families. Core Assets has received Department for Education grants to develop adoption services, was contracted by a number of local authorities, and generated its profits from a range of children's services.[20]

Private companies replacing public service organisations

So, private companies across adult and children's social care services are selling services to public authorities and taking significant profits out of public funding for social care. Private companies are also now being contracted to replace wholesale public authorities in providing social work and social care services. To date this primarily applies to adult social care services with companies such as Virgin Care, for example, having contracts for the majority of community health and adult social services care management and direct provision in several areas of England. In 2017 this included Bath and North East Somerset, where, as reported by *Community Care*, 43 social workers were transferred from the city council to Virgin Care:

The deal struck between Richard Branson's firm, the local authority and NHS commissioners is the first time a profit-making company has taken on responsibility for running a council's core adult social work functions. Under the contract, any profits will be reinvested in services.* Virgin won the tender over a rival bidder from a consortium led by Sirona Care, a community interest company which had previously delivered social care on behalf of the council. The decision met with opposition from anti-privatisation campaigners and trade unions, who questioned Virgin's track-record in social care.[21]

And as commented in *The Guardian*:

The contract, which was approved on Thursday, has sparked new fears about private health firms expanding their role in the provision of publicly funded health services. Virgin Care has been handed the contract by both Bath and North East Somerset NHS clinical commissioning group and Conservative-led Bath and North East Somerset council. It is worth £70m a year for seven years and the contract includes an option to extend it by another three years at the same price. It means that from 1 April Virgin Care will become the prime provider of a wide range of care for adults and children. That will include everything from services for those with diabetes, dementia or who have suffered a stroke, as well as people with

* But money still can be made by Virgin Care by charging for management and facilities costs, and this may be a loss-leader for Virgin Care to get an entry into this marketplace. There should also be a concern that the re-contracting by the NHS and local authority of health and social care services, including adult social work services, in Bath and North East Somerset led to the community interest company which had been providing the services losing out to a profit-driven private company. What lessons can be found here, and what may lie ahead, for statutory children's social work and social services which have been contracted out to community interest companies by councils, in Kingston and Richmond, and elsewhere, when their contracts are re-let by (Conservative) councils – councils which will have lost direct engagement and knowledge, and have less sense of ownership and responsibility, for these crucial core children's services?

mental health conditions. It will also cover care of children with learning disabilities and frail, elderly people who are undergoing rehabilitation to enable them to go back to living at home safely after an operation. NHS campaigners warned that the history of previous privatisations of NHS services in other parts of England may mean the quality of care patients receive drops once Virgin takes over.[22]

Virgin Care are also growing their business by bidding for – and getting – contracts for children's public health services, such as health visiting and school nursing, often bidding against and beating local NHS providers. These contracts are now let by public health departments within local authorities, albeit that the privatisation of these health services for children is causing local and wider concern. For example, it was reported in *The Independent* in December 2017 that 'Campaigners have criticised the "galloping privatisation" of health services after Virgin Care was awarded a £108m contract for providing children's health services in Lancashire' and that 'The decision comes after the NHS made an undisclosed settlement to Virgin Care when it sued a group of NHS bodies in Surrey following its failure to clinch a county-wide children's services contract worth £85m'.[23] So not only are Virgin Care getting contracts for children's services, but there is a history of successfully suing public authority commissioners when they do not get the contract. This is potentially a threatening, intimidating and high-cost liability now on the radar for commissioners and one which may come to distort the contracting process.

Virgin Care has been on the other side of a contract award being challenged and this was when it was the successful contract bidder for the Lancashire contract:

> Last November, Lancashire County Council appointed Virgin to run public health services for 0- to 19-year-olds under a five-year contract worth £104m. The contract covers the delivery of the Healthy Child Programme, health visiting and school nurse services. The Virgin bid was preferred to a rival

one from Lancashire Care NHS Foundation Trust in partnership with Blackpool Teaching Hospitals Foundation Trust, which currently deliver public health services for the council. However, in June, the High Court backed a legal challenge against the decision by the health trusts, who argued the correct procurement process had not been followed. The court found that the council's own records of its moderation process fell short of the standards required to demonstrate how it scored the bidders. The council has now announced that it will re-evaluate the joint health trust bid and that of Virgin, with the scoring and moderation stages re-run with a new independent panel, which will make the decision over awarding the contract.[24]

But what a waste that time, money and attention are being expended on managing the contracting merry-go-rounds rather than keeping the focus on current frontline services and using the resources to maintain these services. And although Virgin Care's Lancashire contract is now to be reviewed it was reported in August 2018 that Virgin Care has enjoyed significant growth built on public funding:

Virgin has been awarded almost £2bn worth of NHS contracts over the past five years as Richard Branson's company has quietly become one of the UK's leading healthcare providers, Guardian analysis has found. In one year alone, the company's health arm, Virgin Care, won deals potentially worth £1bn to provide services around England, making it the biggest winner among private companies bidding for NHS work over the period. The company and its subsidiaries now hold at least 400 contracts across the public sector – ranging from healthcare in prisons to school immunisation programmes and dementia care for the elderly. This aggressive expansion into the public sector means that around a third of the

> turnover for Virgin's UK companies now appear to
> be from government contracts.[25]

And just in case it should be thought that there are some health, care and police services which are too sensitive and personal and too intrusive and intimate to contract out to private, profit-making, companies, G4S and Serco have been awarded contracts in several areas of England to run the examination suites and services for children, women and men who have been sexually assaulted.[26, 27]

The privatisation of the social work workforce

But it is not only by providing profit-generating services that private companies and their owners are achieving big payments. Private companies have also become significant players in, and are profiting from, the recruitment and employment of social workers, who are then working within local authorities.

In autumn 2016 it was reported in *The Guardian* that:

> According to the Department for Education turnover in children's social work was 16% last year and there was an 'unexpected' rise of more than a quarter in vacancy rates, taking them to 17% – but this England-wide figure disguises sharp regional variations, ranging from 7% in Yorkshire and Humber to 29% in outer London. Good news, then, for agencies that supply temporary staff: in adult care, an average 7% of jobs were filled through agencies last year, compared with 3% in 2013, while in children's services the proportion rose by one percentage point to an average 16%, almost 5,000 posts, and as high as 30% in outer London.[28]

The growth of private agencies profiting from supplying agency workers has become a concern through much of the public sector. The chief executive of the NHS, for example, in January 2016 expressed his concerns:

The head of NHS England admitted spending on agency staff is set to hit £4billion this year as he condemned firms who are 'ripping off' taxpayers. Simon Stevens said the soaring bill for temporary workers explained 'the vast majority, if not all' of the record £2billion-plus deficit forecast to be run up by trusts.[29]

The number of agency social workers working within local authority children's social services increased by 14% in one year alone to 5,700 agency workers in September 2015 compared with 4,430 the previous September reflecting a rise in children's social work vacancies to 16%.[30] In inner London a quarter of children's social workers were agency workers and in outer London councils the rate was even higher, at almost a third.[31]

Increasing vacancy levels and the use of agency social workers has also been an issue for adult social services. Skills for Care reported in September 2016 that there was a 13.3% annual turnover rate in adult services social workers, with 6% of the social workers being agency workers.[32] By September 2017 annual turnover had increased to 15.6% and the agency rate to 7%.[33]

The burgeoning cost to local authorities of employing expensive agency social workers, with the costs and impact inflated by the owners of employment agencies taking their profits at a time of cuts in government funding, was noted in 2017 by a BBC Freedom of Information inquiry to councils. It found that the spend on agency social workers had doubled within four years from £180 million in 2012/13 to £355 million in 2016/17.[34]

The biggest agency spend increase during this period was by Northamptonshire County Council, with agency social worker costs rising from £1.7 million to £17.9 million.[35] This may not be unrelated to Northamptonshire voluntarily planning to move all of its children's social services, including its social workers, outside of the council and into a stand-alone company, a controversial intention which may in itself have been destabilising its workforce.

Northamptonshire's council, however, was in the news in 2018 with an even more dramatic concern – it was running out of money, struggling to set a budget, and had put an emergency halt on expenditure.[36] Following a review by an inspector appointed by the government it was recommended that the county council should be abolished and replaced by two unitary authorities. In the meantime, the council leader resigned and commissioners were to be appointed to run the council.[37] Northamptonshire's radical ideological plans to outsource its services had hit the buffers. Outsourcing was no solution to the severe cuts in funding from central government.

In August 2018 Northamptonshire County Council decided to put on hold the outsourcing of its children's services,[38] having already in January 2018 decided to bring adult social care services back within the council because of auditors' concerns about the financial viability and stability of the company created five years before to provide the outsourced services.[39]

Northamptonshire County Council was by no means alone, however, in struggling in 2018 to recruit and retain social workers, with a subsequent high spend on agency workers which was not only leading to an overspend on its children's services budget but was destabilising the council's overall finances. Lewisham, for example, also had high and increasing agency social worker costs which were impacting on the council:

> Lewisham's budget [July 2018] report described the children's services overspend as 'significant'. '[It] is of an order never seen previously in Lewisham,' the report warned. It added that a large increase in agency staff towards the end of the financial year had a 'hugely detrimental' effect on the overall children's services budget, which had been relatively stable until the final quarter … A 'children's social care roadmap', discussed at a select committee meeting in January 2018, had forecasted an overall £7.6 million children's services overspend, £5.7 million of which fell within children's social care. That earlier report predicted that the salaries and wages budget would be overspent by just £1.4 million, as opposed to the

eventual £7.5 million (£6.6 million on agency staff and £0.9 million on wages).[40]

What is possibly surprising is that the two highest–profile councils potentially at risk of imploding were both true-blue Conservative shire councils. Alongside Northamptonshire, Surrey also attracted much media coverage about its financial position,[41] especially about the funding for adult social care, and with further big cuts imminent in 2018/19 for both adult and children's services.[42]

It is within this context that the profits made by employment agencies should be viewed as even more considerable and exceptional, and this is money which might otherwise have been available to invest in and to continue rather than to cut services. Two of the largest social work employment agencies in the UK are Liquid Personnel Limited and Sanctuary Personnel Limited.

Liquid Personnel Ltd was acquired by ICSG Ltd in 2016. ICSG Ltd is a subsidiary of Indigo Parent Ltd. Each of these companies is registered at the same London address and with considerable overlap of company directors. The Liquid Personnel Ltd company accounts for 2016 state that:

> The company operates within the recruitment sector providing niche services to local authorities, charities, NHS trusts and private organisations throughout the United Kingdom. The core business is the provision of temporary and contract social workers and the Board is pleased to note the continuing success of the core business developing substantial and consistent growth … In the 9 month period to 31 December 2016 the company achieved revenue of £71,225,617 in the period and growth of 24% on the previous year pro rata.[44]

The Liquid Personnel company accounts show that it made a pre-tax profit for the nine months to the end of December 2016 of £2,075,309, similar to the full-year profit for the year to the end of March 2016 of £2,893,309. So, in a period of 21 months Liquid Personnel and its owners made a profit of just under

£5 million from the fees and charges paid to the company for the provision of agency workers.

The company accounts for 2016 for Sanctuary Personnel show that it too has been expanding its business:

> This has been the company's ninth consecutive year of turnover growth. This reflects continued growth of the company's renowned Social Work business including an increase in the amount of work undertaken by special project teams. The rate of growth is particularly pleasing given the continued pressures on public finances.[45]

In 2016 Sanctuary Personnel reported a 5% growth in turnover and a 13% gross profit margin and declared an operating profit of £2.2 million, with net assets of almost £3 million. Over the two years of 2015 and 2016 Sanctuary reported its operating profit to have been £6 million.

In addition to the profits accruing to and taken by the owners of these companies, big payments are made to the companies' paid directors. In 2016 one of Sanctuary's directors received £303,120 and the highest-paid director within Liquid Personnel received £292,490.

So just two of the many employment agencies (to which could be added the money made by the interim management and executive search agencies which have also colonised publicly funded social services) in 2015 and 2016 alone made reported profits of almost £11 million, and also made annual payments of over a quarter of a million pounds to individual directors. This is money which has been taken out of social services at a time when services for children, families and disabled and older people are being more heavily rationed and cut.

But it is not only of concern that this is money which had been leaking, and is now flowing, out of personal social services. It is also money which is not well spent, as the growth in interim agency social workers and managers is creating services that are less stable, less secure and less safe, with rapid turnover of workers for service users and no coherent or continuous management oversight and culture-building. In 2018, for example, in

England's Children's Commissioner's annual report on stability for children in care it was noted that 'social worker changes remain significantly more common than placement or school changes. Nearly 19,000 children experienced two or more social worker changes in 2016/17. This works out to around 1 in 4 children in care'.[46]

Why do social workers, albeit still a minority of less than 20%, seek employment and assignments through these profit-making private agencies? *Community Care* reported in 2017 that:

> A survey of 1,351 social workers, undertaken last year, examined how social workers' attitudes to job hunting have changed since a previous survey carried out in 2014. It found that while the majority of social workers preferred permanent work this had dropped from 88% to 84% in line with the subsequent increase in those preferring agency work. Many of those who expressed a preference for locum work cited a better work–life balance, better rates of pay and a greater ability to switch jobs if they feel unhappy with where they are working.[47]

None of these reasons are about service enhancement or about improving service quality. For some it seems to be a lifestyle choice – choosing when to work and how much to work, when to take longer breaks and holidays, and being able to walk away with no notice when workloads build up, secure in the knowledge that they can find similar agency work elsewhere when they want it. It is creating a privatised workforce and a privatised profession providing profits for private companies.

It is not, however, only private, for-profit, employment agencies who are making money out of the social work workforce. The workforce is itself being reshaped by government initiatives led by commercial companies and receiving significant public funding. For example, these companies have received significant payments to design the statement of key skills the government has decided must be met by social workers working in statutory children's services and the government-determined accreditation process for these social workers:

> Private companies have received £8.52 million of
> government funding as part of the implementation
> of social work accreditation ... Responding to
> questions from shadow children's minister Emma
> Lewell-Buck, Goodwill [the children's minister] said
> the government had spent £11.22 million so far on
> the consultation, preparation and introduction of the
> accreditation system and phase one and phase two of
> the implementation. 'This total is split £2.7 million
> for local authorities and £8.52 million for private
> companies', Goodwill said.[48]

One of the companies to benefit by several millions of pounds
from the continuing government funding of the roll-out of the
social worker accreditation process is Mott Macdonald.[49] With
its roots as a global company with big international government
contracts for major engineering projects, its track record and
experience in relation to social work might be seen as quite
limited. However, not only does it now have a major contract
which will reshape the social work profession but it has also been
awarded a government contract to produce a training programme
for social workers on permanence planning for children.[50]

What conclusions to draw about privatisation?

What conclusions might be drawn from the accounts in this
and previous chapters about the outsourcing and privatising of
public services? First, the push to privatise has a history going
back almost 40 years. Initiated by the Thatcher Conservative
governments, it was continued by Blair's New Labour
governments in the 1990s and 2000s. Indeed, it was New Labour
which opened the door for more wide-ranging privatisation
of public services with the introduction of the public–private
finance initiative, NHS Foundation Trusts, academy schools, and
social work practices. The opportunities trailed and created by
New Labour have been seized upon with messianic zeal by the
post-2010 Conservative-led governments, with a mission to go
way beyond what was seen as possible by Margaret Thatcher.
Nothing is now regarded as a step too far in placing public

services into a commercial marketplace. Even the safety and welfare of vulnerable children has now become an opportunity to make a profit.

Secondly, what has been the evidence of the past 40 years from the privatisation of public services? The accounts related above of false reporting, fraud and a focus on gaining a profit from contracts, albeit it in the context of deteriorating services, suggest that there should at least be caution, and at best a rethink and a U-turn, about pushing ahead with further privatisation of public services. To date, privatisation has not delivered on what was promised. It has not led to greater economy, efficiency or effectiveness in services. What it has created is confused accountability, opaqueness rather than transparency about the services which are now within the private sector, and poor performance as a consequence of driving down costs to deliver a profit. When services have then imploded and collapsed – Olympics security, prisons, care homes, privatised national health services – it is residual provision remaining within the public sector that has been called on to rescue and reclaim services withdrawn from or abandoned by the private sector companies who have cut and run.

Thirdly, what is the evidence that lessons have been learnt? Learning seems to have been impeded by politicians and much of the media who have an ideological belief and commitment to a commercialised and privatised marketplace. Most have not worked within public services. Instead, they have experience, and family histories, immersed in making money from marketing, media and management and bonanzas from banking, where it is the financial bottom-line which is the focus, and profit which is the measure of success. Many have used their wealth to buy health care and education from private providers rather than use the public services about which they are often so ignorant and so scathing. Their disdain and couldn't-care-less attitude to public services has resulted in the cuts which have escalated since 2010, and still continue.

If privatisation was ever seen as an answer and salvation from the anticipated consequence of the cuts, the failures of G4S, Serco, Circle Holdings and others to provide the services for which they were contracted with a shrinking pot of money ought to have offered the lesson that privatisation is not so much a solution to cuts but rather compounds problems.

Is the tanker beginning to turn? Is the rose-tinted view taken of those outsourcing companies that now make multi-million profits for their shareholders and directors beginning to fade? Is there an increasing realisation that a self-seeking, profit-focused business taking money out of and away from public services and the public good is actually ripping off the public and the taxpayer (with the wealthy owners and beneficiaries of these companies themselves often immersed in tax avoidance)?

The public's opinion of these companies taking their profits from the public purse is negative and even parts of the right-wing press, quoted above, have turned on the poorly performing privatisation companies.

In 2017 the polling company YouGov, in a report titled 'Nationalisation vs privatisation: the public view', stated that:

> Previous YouGov surveys have always highlighted that state ownership of companies and industries tend to be popular with the public ... The results of our latest research show that there are four services that the public is especially keen to have in public hands: the police (87%), the NHS (84%), the armed forces (83%) and schools (81%) ... While support for nationalisation drops off beyond these services, state ownership is still the preferred option for a majority of people across most of the industries we asked about. In fact, there were only three sectors on the list that the majority of British people wanted to remain in private hands: telephone and internet providers (53% want them run by the private sector), banks (also 53%) and airlines (68%).[51]

With regard to the Royal Mail (65%), railway companies (60%), water companies (59%), the BBC (58%), and energy companies (53%), the majority of the public who were sampled wanted these services to be in public ownership. So, it seems that the public does not favour the privatisation of important and crucial public services.

Parliamentary politicians, as seen in the statements quoted above from House of Commons Select Committees (with Conservative majorities), when confronted with the realities of privatising public services have also been critical and have sought to slow down or pull back from the privatisation process, as noted in these comments from the Public Accounts Committee:

> Government is clearly failing to manage performance across the board, and to achieve the best for citizens out of the contracts into which they have entered. Government needs a far more professional and skilled approach to managing contracts and contractors, and contractors need to demonstrate the high standards of ethics expected in the conduct of public business, and be more transparent about their performance and costs. The public's trust in outsourcing has been undermined recently by the poor performance of G4S in supplying security guards for the Olympics, Capita's failure to deliver court translation services, issues with Atos's work capability assessments, misreporting of out of hours GP services by Serco, and most recently, the astonishing news that G4S and Serco had overcharged for years on electronic tagging contracts: these high profile failures illustrate contractors' failure to live up to standards expected and have exposed serious weaknesses in Government's capability in negotiating and managing private contracts on behalf of the taxpayer ... Some private sector providers have grown significantly in recent years, often through buying up competitors or other organisations in their supply chain–for example, Capita's purchase of the court interpreters' service. But the government has not analysed directly the implications on the operation of the marketplace, and on the delivery of public services. Some public service markets, such as for private prisons, asylum accommodation or the Work Programme are now dominated by a small number of contractors, and the government is exposed to huge delivery and financial

risks should one of these suppliers fail … Contractors have not consistently demonstrated the high ethical standards expected in the conduct of public business. … The Cabinet Office told us that government has a long way to go before it has the skills required to manage contracts properly. This is a concern, given the speed at which some departments–such as the Ministry of Justice–are going ahead with outsourcing, despite a poor track record.[52]

In the 2017 general election Labour, led by Jeremy Corbyn, presented a manifesto which supported public services and committed to halt and start to reverse the tidal wave of privatisation. It led to increased support and votes for Labour and may have started to reset and rebalance the 'public sector bad/private sector good' debate. As John Bew wrote, following the June 2017 election, in a new preface to his biography of Clement Attlee:

The mood of the British people is more receptive to an Attlee-style agenda than at any time for decades. While no one has the authority to deliver upon it [the election led to a hung Parliament, with the Conservatives remaining in government with the support of Northern Ireland's Democratic Unionist Party], it is not beyond the realms of possibility that a new political consensus does begin to emerge over the next decade, with elements of the one that the Attlee government ushered in after the Second World War.[53]

And who do the public trust? Of the occupations listed in the 2016 Ipsos Mori 'Veracity Index' it was public service professionals who were most trusted by the public (nurses 93%; doctors 91%; teachers 88%; judges 81%). Who were least trusted? Politicians generally 15%; government ministers 20%; journalists 24%; estate agents 30%; business leaders 33%.[54]

Turning the tide, however, of the media and political narrative of 'public sector bad/private sector good' will require determination and stamina, as powerful people who are profiting from the national and international commercialisation and globalisation of public services have significant vested interests.

And a warning. As Renwick, in his long view of the antecedents which provided the foundation of the welfare state, concluded:

> The welfare state was never simply a dull system of national insurance that paid benefits out to people who found themselves out of work but an interconnected system of institutions and policies, infused with ideas and values that had been debated and shaped for more than a century. Many of those who had lived through the war and the difficult decades that preceded it greatly appreciated what had come in to being by the end of the 1940s. Yet the generations that followed found it much easier to take for granted something that quickly became central to everyday life in Britain. It is too early to tell if those attitudes will lead to the welfare state unravelling. But as the 150 years before the end of the Second World War show, building something like the welfare is immensely more difficult than allowing it to fall apart.[55]

As Nicholas Timmins has noted in an article headed 'The "welfare state" should be something to be proud of':

> Rather than talk about 'the welfare state' or 'social security', politicians now mainly talk about 'welfare' – and so do the general public. And in this discourse, the meaning of the word has more or less been turned on its head. It has precious little these days to do with faring well; rather, 'welfare' has become almost a term of abuse. To be 'on welfare' is to be on Benefits Street or part of the Great British Benefits Handout: somewhere no one in their right mind wants to be. ... Today the phrase 'the welfare state' has more or less fallen out of the political lexicon,

as indeed has the concept of 'social security'. The language around it has changed, with corrosive effects. ... Does any of this matter? Yes, because with the near disappearance of the language of 'the welfare state' and of 'social security' has gone the sense of inclusion and collectiveness that those phrases imply. It has made 'welfare' a matter of 'them and us': them being the feckless poor, us being the people who pay for them. Even though, as the London School of Economics professor John Hills has so ably demonstrated in his book *Good Times, Bad Times*, we pretty much all benefit from the social security system in particular, and the welfare state in general, over a lifetime.[56]

So much to play for. So much to seek to protect. But so many powerful forces of vested interests seeking to pull it apart. Here is a quote from Clement Attlee from the 1940s:

Capital knows no patriotism and investors look for their return in hard cash not sentiment.[57]

And here is Andrew Mitchell, a Conservative MP and a former minister in Cameron's coalition government, in 2017:

The Paradise Papers [showing widespread offshore tax avoidance by the wealthy in tax havens] show that secrecy is the enemy of good governance, and that powerful people do not go straight because they see the light but because they feel the heat.[58]

The ownership of wealth has changed significantly over the past 30 years, with what had been distributed, owned and shared as public wealth increasingly transferred to the private ownership.[59] In the UK 'the richest 1% control 22% of the country's wealth, up from 15% in 1984. The very richest in the UK have seen a huge increase in their wealth. The top 0.1% – around 50,000 people – have seen their share of the nation's wealth double from 4.5% in 1984 to 9% in 2013.'[60]

What is recounted in much of this book are the self-interested manoeuvres of those who are already rich – in the UK and beyond – as they seek to plunder public services and to reroute public funding to generate greater profit and more and more personal wealth for themselves, enhanced by the avoidance of taxes. And now even those public services which are at the frontline of helping families and protecting children are being opened up to commercial exploitation and profit-taking. But does it have to be this way?

Part 4
Changing course

ELEVEN

No to TINA: an alternative journey for social work and children's social services

Two of Margaret Thatcher's more memorable and often quoted phrases as Prime Minister in the 1980s were that 'there is no alternative' and 'the lady's not for turning'. Thatcher's assertion that 'there is no alternative', in relation to her monetarist policies of public sector cuts while embracing and championing privatisation and the assumed efficiencies of global competitive markets, led to her being known as 'Tina'.[1] The other famous – or infamous – Thatcher phrase was included in the speech she made at the Conservative Party conference in 1980, when she said 'To those waiting with bated breath for that favourite media catchphrase, the 'U' turn, I have only one thing to say. "You turn if you want to. The lady's not for turning".'[2]

Both quotes set the scene for a decade in which Mrs Thatcher launched her crusade to wind back the state, cut public expenditure, and open up what had been publicly owned services provided by the public sector to private companies. It was a crusade which David Cameron continued with renewed vigour within the coalition government which he led from 2010 until 2015, even reprising Mrs Thatcher's slogans, as noted in 2013 in the *Financial Times*:

> David Cameron cast himself in the mould of Margaret Thatcher on Thursday when he insisted the coalition would not be swayed by demands from the left or right to change economic course, declaring: 'There

is no alternative.' Mr Cameron rejected calls from Vince Cable, business secretary, for a relaxation of Plan A to allow more borrowing to fund investment in schools, hospitals and roads, claiming it would unnerve the markets and force up interest rates. 'It's as if they think there's some magic money tree,' Mr Cameron said, mocking those like Mr Cable who believe that extra borrowing for targeted capital spending would boost growth. 'Let me tell you a plain truth: there isn't.' ... He also echoed the heroine of the Tory right by repeating her defiant message from 1980 when she resisted calls for a U-turn on her highly controversial economic policy as Britain plunged into recession. 'This month's Budget will be about sticking to the course,' Mr Cameron said in a speech in Yorkshire. 'There is no alternative that will secure our country's future.'[3]

However, at the beginning of 2018 there was a flurry of concern challenging the statement that there was no alternative to the Conservative government's continuation of politically chosen austerity and reductions in welfare benefits, public sector cuts, and the marketisation and privatisation of public services. What generated this flurry of challenge to the government's policy of privatisation? The answer was: Carillion.

The collapse of Carillion: a turning point in the privatisation journey?

Here is the BBC's description of Carillion:

> Carillion specialises in construction, as well as facilities management and ongoing maintenance. It has worked on big private sector projects such as the Battersea Power station redevelopment and the Anfield Stadium expansion. But it is perhaps best known for being one of the largest suppliers of services to the public sector. Notably, it is part of a consortium that holds a contract to build part of the

forthcoming HS2 high speed railway line, and it is the second largest supplier of maintenance services to Network Rail. It also maintains 50,000 homes for the Ministry of Defence, manages nearly 900 schools and manages highways and prisons.[4]

In essence, Carillion was a construction company which had expanded not only by getting government contracts for major building and engineering projects but also by seeking out other public service contracts, such as providing maintenance, meals and facilities management for schools, hospitals and prisons (it was a company that benefited greatly from the New Labour and Conservative governments' enthusiasm for Public Finance Initiatives). All of these public services were dependent on Carillion to deliver on the contracts to keep their services running.

And, as with other examples discussed earlier in this book about private sector failures, it was the government and the public sector which quickly had to mobilise when Carillion went bust, could not afford to continue to trade, and went into liquidation. This included, for example, the fire service in Oxfordshire being put on standby at very short notice to provide and deliver 18,000 school meals to 90 schools (a private contractor would be likely to state that providing quick and urgent cover was outside the terms of their contract or else would require additional payments to do so).[5]

There were two particular aspects of the Carillion collapse which made it a headline story day after day in the New Year of 2018. The first was the scale and nature of the company and of the contracts it had been awarded, including, for example, for new hospitals in Sandwell and Liverpool, new military barracks in Aldershot and on Salisbury Plain, and schools, as well as for roads and railways. Carillion was also the sponsor of two academy schools. It directly employed 43,000 people and 30,000 small firms were subcontracted by Carillion; and for the direct employees and those working for the subcontracted companies their employment and income was immediately at risk.

This is how Carillion described itself and its financial standing in 2016:

Carillion is one of the UK's leading integrated support services companies, with a substantial portfolio of Public Private Partnership projects, extensive construction capabilities and a sector-leading ability to deliver sustainable solutions ... We have a high-quality order book (including probable orders) worth £16.0 billion, framework contracts that are expected to generate up to £1.5 billion of revenue and a substantial pipeline of specific contract opportunities potentially worth £41.6 billion. In 2016, we won £4.8 billion of new orders and probable orders in our chosen markets, despite tougher conditions in some of our markets, demonstrating our skills in winning work, consistent with our rigorous approach to selecting the contracts for which we bid.[6]

In its 2016 annual report, Carillion reported annual revenue of £5.2 billion, up from £4.6 billion in 2015, and a proposed dividend to shareholders of 18.45p, an increase from 18.25p in 2015. The picture presented was of a company doing well, expanding, and making big payments to its shareholders. But by the end of 2017 Carillion was reporting debts of £1.5 billion.[7]

A second concern about Carillion was that it was still making increasingly big payments to shareholders and directors, even when the company knew that it was in financial difficulty. At the same time that Carillion's workforce was facing the prospect of not being paid and being unemployed, Carillion's senior managers, including some who had already left the company's employment, were still receiving large payments. Roger Barker, the head of corporate governance at the Institute of Directors, was quoted as saying:

There are some worrying signs. The relaxation of clawback conditions for executive bonuses in 2016 appears in retrospect to be highly inappropriate. It does no good to the reputation of UK business when top managers appear to benefit in spite of the collapse of the organisations that they are responsible for.[8]

Mr Barker was also quoted as saying that the collapse of the company 'suggests that effective governance was lacking at Carillion'. He added: 'We must now consider if the board and shareholders have exercised appropriate oversight prior to the collapse.'[9]

It has been suggested that Carillion's board of directors may have been misled by KPMG, Carillion's auditors, with it stated that:

> In the 2016 annual report, KPMG certified that Carillion was on a sound financial footing, and would be so until at least 2019. Its 'viability statement' at the time said: 'We have nothing to report on the disclosures of principal risks ... Based on the knowledge we acquired during our audit, we have nothing material to add or draw attention to in relation to the Directors' viability statement concerning the principal risks, their management, and, based on that, the Directors' assessment and expectations of the Group's continuing in operation over the three years to 2019.' Carillion's board relied on KPMG's certification to insist in the same annual report that the company could survive 'extreme downside scenarios' over the coming three years: 'On the basis of both reasonably probable and more extreme downside scenarios, the Directors believe that they have a reasonable expectation that the Company will be able to continue in operation and meet its liabilities as they fall due over the three-year period of their assessment.'[10]

The role of KPMG, as Carillion's auditors who did not blow the whistle on the financial difficulties which were immersing the company and were soon to lead to its liquidation, itself became a focus of attention in January 2018.[11] The linkages between Carillion and KPMG, its auditors, were long-standing and extensive. KPMG had been Carillion's external auditor for 19 years and had received about £13 million in fees during this period.[12] In 2017 alone KPMG received £1.4 million.[13] Possibly even more surprising and significant, two of Carillion's most recent finance directors had previously worked for KPMG.[14] The UK's Financial Reporting Council decided at the end of January 2018 that it would investigate the role that KPMG had played in relation to Carillion.[15]

The concerns about the actions and possible failings of KPMG are of relevance and interest to those concerned about social work and the personal social services because, as noted earlier, KPMG has been favoured and contracted by the government to lead on the shaping and defining of social work in England.

In January 2018 KPMG, in addition to its part in the Carillion story, was at the centre of two other stories, this time about apparent conflicts of interests in relation to the Grenfell Tower inquiry in London and the development of Hinkley Point nuclear power station in Somerset. In both instances, KPMG was seen as potentially compromised by its previous commercial involvement with private sector contractors whose contracts were now the subject of scrutiny by KPMG!

One of the staggering insensitivities and inappropriate actions within the Grenfell Fire Inquiry was that KPMG was appointed by the government to assist with the Inquiry. It was reported in January 2018 in *The Independent* that:

> Consultancy firm KPMG has been hired by the Government to help plan the inquiry into the Grenfell Tower fire, even though the company has earned millions in auditing fees from three of the bodies being investigated. The multinational corporation based in the Netherlands, has had a lucrative relationship with Rydon, the firm that installed the building's cladding system. Grenfell Tower was encased in panels made up of aluminium sheets with a polyethylene core, which melts and burns at extreme temperatures. These are believed to have contributed to the fire. KPMG reportedly earned £3.5m for services from Rydon. It has also provided £1m worth of auditing to Saint-Gobain Construction Products UK. The firm owns Celotex, which made the synthetic insulation which the panels

were installed on top of. KPMG has also reportedly earned nearly £1m in fees from auditing the Royal Borough of Kensington and Chelsea, which has been heavily criticised for ignoring residents' concerns before and after the deadly fire, which killed 71 people. The Cabinet office has nonetheless hired the firm to provide 'planning and programme management support' [to the Inquiry].[16]

This obvious conflict of interest for KPMG which could have compromised the Inquiry into the fire led to quick and widespread outrage. Three days later KPMG withdrew from advising the government on the Inquiry.

KPMG's conflict of interest in relation to the Grenfell Tower Inquiry, identified in the press, was not unique. In the same month (January 2018), *The Times* reported that:

Consultancy firms working for the government on the Hinkley Point C nuclear power station were advising the project's Chinese investor and its French builder at the same time, an investigation by *The Times* has revealed. KPMG, the professional services group, was paid £4.4 million between 2012 and 2017 as a financial adviser to the energy and business departments, despite telling officials that it was also acting for China General Nuclear Power Corp on the project.[17]

But it was not only KPMG which was exposed in January 2018 as compromised by apparent conflicts of interest. There were also concerns about another of the 'Big Four' accountancy firms, with a report that:

PwC's role in the liquidation process of the collapsed contractor Carillion has come under scrutiny after it emerged that the auditor already has two separate, and apparently conflicting roles, including one advising the defunct company's pension trustees ... Deloitte and KPMG, rival Big Four firms, had been ruled out of the liquidation role because they were already Carillion's internal and external auditors, respectively. This left the government with the choice of PwC; EY, which advised Carillion on restructuring options before its collapse; or one of the smaller accounting firms — highlighting longstanding issues around the Big Four oligopoly and potential conflicts of interest this generates.[18]

At the end of January 2018 there was Parliamentary scrutiny of the 'Big Four' accountancy firms, with the BBC reporting that:

> Frank Field, the chair of the Work and Pensions Committee, asked whether KPMG, PwC, Deloitte and EY should be broken up in the wake of the firm's collapse. Accountancy watchdog head Stephen Haddrill, agreed that the UK's four largest firms needed more competition ... KPMG had handled Carillion's accounts since 1999 and signed off its figures last March, four months before the firm issued its first profit warning.[19]

Carillion was a company with skeletons in its cupboard. It was discovered, for example, in 2009 that it had taken action to deter the employment in the construction industry of those with whom it had been in dispute,[20] with *The Metro* commenting in 2018 that 'The demise of Carillion has been bittersweet for Dave Smith, who was a victim of the construction giant's illegal blacklisting operation. Carillion "ruined his life" after bosses blacklisted him for exposing health and safety dangers'.[21]

Carillion had a history of health and safety concerns and failed and unfilled contracts. In 2013 it was fined £180,000 when a motorcyclist was paralysed after crashing into inadequately signed road works.[22] In the same year it was reported that Clinicenta, a subsidiary of Carillion, had stopped providing a NHS treatment centre in Stevenage following concerns from GPs about the care of patients and a critical report from the Care Quality Commission, but Clinicenta still received £53 million from the NHS to end the contract.[23] In 2015 in Canada Carillion was fined $900,000 for not meeting its contract requirements to clear roads of snow.[24] And in 2016 Nottingham University Hospitals NHS Trust sought to terminate a £200 million five-year facilities and estates management contract with Carillion because of poor performance, and with nurses cleaning wards because of a shortage of Carillion cleaning workers.[25]

Maybe none of this should be too surprising. After all, Carillion is a very big multinational business made up of 326 companies, of which 199 were in the UK, and with 169 directors spread across the Carillion group (including a former chair of Ofsted on its main board).[26] But what is of note is that the failings, faults and unfulfilled contracts noted above are all within public works contracts, which illustrates how widely Carillion had infiltrated and colonised the public sector privatised marketplace.

Setting a new course?

But will the sheer scale of the Carillion scandal turn the tide away from more and more privatisation of public services? It certainly provided a time of reflection, if not retreat from prioritising profit over public good. Here are some comments in January 2018 triggered by the collapse of Carillion.

Simon Jenkins wrote:

> What the Carillion saga demonstrates is the rampant indiscipline in the contracts themselves. The company's demise is attributable to favouritism, cost escalation, excessive risk, obscene remuneration and reckless indebtedness. Carillion and its bankers clearly thought it too big to fail. Whitehall behaved accordingly. It was like a pre-2008 bank. There must now be a review of how privatisation is working.[27]

And Polly Toynbee argued that:

> The era of 'private good, public bad' is drawing to a close. Unshakeable faith in Margaret Thatcher's privatisation creed is being killed off not just by counter-ideology, but by the sheer irrationality,

expense and failure of so many private contracts. Carillion's spectacular collapse makes big headlines, but out of the spotlight local councils, under extreme stress from cuts, are cancelling contracted-out services. Why? Because it saves them money and improves services.[28]

Will Hutton also commented:

> The amount of activity now performed by organisations we all own and whose overriding purpose is public service is minimal. Day-to-day life now depends on private companies with private ambitions ... There is now a sense, growing with every successive scandal, that the privatisation of the everyday has gone too far – a mood captured by startling opinion poll majorities of 80% in favour of renationalising utilities. The opposition leader, Jeremy Corbyn, struck a chord when he said Carillion's failure was a key moment.[29]

A new political agenda was indeed being set, at least by the Labour opposition, with Jeremy Corbyn committing to reverse the trend of privatising public services:

> Labour will call a halt to the 'outsourcing racket' exposed by Carillion's collapse, by tearing up procurement rules to make the public sector the default choice for providing government services, Jeremy Corbyn has revealed. Carillion's collapse has emboldened Corbyn to press home his message that Labour rejects the 'dogma of privatisation'.[30]

Maybe, though, the quotations above should not lead to too much expectation that the privatisation tide is turning. After all, they are all quotes from the left-leaning *Guardian*, and Theresa May's response as Prime Minister was to label Corbyn as being 'anti-business',[31] with a *Guardian* report in June 2018 subheaded

'Government moves to rebuild trust and address criticism following Carillion collapse' noting that:

> In a speech on Monday, David Lidington, the Cabinet Office minister, will reinforce the government's commitment to using the private sector to deliver public services such as running call centres, building railways or providing school meals. About £200bn a year is channelled to private companies providing public services. He will also say that there needs to be a more diverse marketplace of companies bidding for official contracts. The planned measures would encourage and make it easier for small businesses, mutuals, charities, co-operatives and social enterprises to take on government contracts.[32]

So, no change here. The drive to outsource public services and government contracts is planned to continue, albeit in the context of an expanded and potentially more diverse marketplace but one in which there is still no place or space for the public sector.

More surprising, however, is the backtracking and U-turn of George Osborne, who in 2018 was the editor of the *Evening Standard* but was previously Chancellor of the Exchequer in David Cameron's governments. In January 2018 the *Daily Mail* commented:

> Goodness me, how George Osborne has changed his tune! As Chancellor of the Exchequer, he was an ardent advocate of the Private Finance Initiative whereby government projects are contracted out to private firms such as Carillion, which collapsed last week with the potential loss of tens of thousands of jobs. In October 2014, he made Treasury money available to Carillion to help boost its overseas business, saying: 'It's great to see successful companies like Carillion winning contracts around the world.' Today, as editor of the *Evening Standard* after being sacked from the Cabinet by Theresa May, Osborne

takes a different view. 'Why has the State found itself so dependent on a few very large outsourcing firms?' his newspaper thundered. 'The failure to use a variety of smaller mid-sized companies undermines innovation and leaves services hostage when things go wrong'.[33]

Osborne, though, did not see himself as having any responsibility for the Carillion crisis. Instead, in an *Evening Standard* editorial, he blamed civil servants:

> Why has the state found itself so dependent on a few very large outsourcing firms? The failure to use a variety of smaller, mid-size companies undermines innovation and leaves services hostage when things go wrong. Why was Carillion awarded huge contracts by the civil service, with whom rather than ministers almost all procurement decisions lie after they knew it was struggling last year?[34]

Possibly most concerning was the *Metro* report that:

> Mr Osborne earns £650,000 a year from working one day a week for the world's largest fund management company Blackrock, which is thought to have made a £40 million profit by betting on the collapse of Carillion.[35]

It was reported that '18 hedge funds made £80m from the initial [Carillion] share slump, with much more likely to have been banked since then, after further steep falls'.[36] Whilst hedge funds gambled and made their money by betting that Carillion's share price would fall, and Carillion's shareholders received big dividends and directors big payments and protected bonuses, Carillion's workers were to find that Carillion had reduced payments into their pension fund which was in deficit, meaning that future Carillion pensioners would receive reduced pensions.[37]

Further reasons to halt the privatisation journey

The collapse of Carillion in January 2018 was significant but not exceptional or unique in the history of the big outsourcing companies. Carillion had its roots in the construction industry but moved beyond its core competence to hunt out other opportunities – such as in facilities management – to get public service contracts and public funding. Two of the other big outsourcing conglomerates also had expanded beyond their core business focus. Serco had its genesis in bidding for and getting 'blue-collar' public sector contracts for services such as catering and cleaning, but in 2014 its share price tumbled after it announced profit warnings and sought to disinvest itself of its public services business-process contracts.[38] And, following the collapse of Carillion in January 2018, it was quickly reported that Capita, with its foundations in the privatisation of 'white-collar' public services contracts such as IT and business administration, was also reported to be at risk of financial meltdown.[39] Even before the financial vulnerability of these companies had become known, public sector organisations were already ending their contracts with outsourcing companies because of concerns about costs and performance.[40]

In essence, the outsourcing industry seems to be in some disarray as a consequence of expanding beyond the capacity of boards to provide proper governance oversight and with external auditors not spotting – or at least not reporting – danger signals about companies' balance sheets and viability. This is in a context of companies moving beyond their core competencies whilst bidding unrealistically low to gain contracts, and all the while still paying big and escalating salaries and bonuses to senior managers and stripping significant dividends out of the business for shareholders or as profits for venture capitalists.

This is the complicated and complex – and messy, manipulative and murky – morass into which social work and the personal social services are now being immersed. Once upon a time it was so much simpler and more transparent – councils debated and took decisions locally in public for the public, with coverage by the local press and other media, and with council reports and accounts available to all. Now there is much more smoke and mirrors, fuelled by commercial confidentiality, conflicts of interests, and a priority given to generating profit not public benefit.

And if concerns about the business competence of the private companies was not enough to warn against giving them contracts and responsibilities for crucial public services for the welfare and safety of families in difficulty and children and adults who might need help, the behaviour and morality of the leaders of private sector financial and commercial companies might also flag up alerts.

Another media story – at the same time as the stories about Carillion and Capita – running day by day in early 2018 was about an expensive 'men-only' dinner arranged by the 'Presidents Club'. It was attended by what was described as 'leading figures in business, politics and finance',[41] but it was misnamed as a 'men-only' event, as young women were paid to attend and required to the tolerate the sexually exploitative and abusive behaviour of the men who were present.[42]

Among those attending, not for the first time, was Nadhim Zahawi, who had only recently been appointed as the parliamentary under-secretary of state with responsibility for children's social care.[43] His interests on the parliamentary website were listed as 'business and foreign affairs'[44] and he had previously been the European director of a clothing company. The co-chair of The Presidents Club was David Meller, an affluent businessman who had been a donor to the Conservative Party and the founder of a multi-academy schools trust. In 2013 he had been appointed as a non-executive director of the Department for Education's (DfE) board. When the story broke about the scandal of the Presidents Club dinner, Meller resigned from the DfE board.[45]

It may have gone unnoticed that there were no reports of leaders of public sector services or charities attending the event, although one university vice chancellor was listed as attending.[46] It is hardly likely that it would have gone unreported in newspapers such as *The Mail* and the wider press and media if any public sectors leaders had attended. This may suggest that although the public sector is not immune from sexist and abusive behaviour, it does generally possess a different ethic and morality from that exhibited at the Presidents Club dinner.

Is this the end of the rush to privatisation?

It was looking in January 2018 as though the tide may have turned on the trend of outsourcing public services. Jeremy Corbyn and Labour had an agenda to retrieve crucial outsourced services, the public were not in favour of outsourcing, and the big outsourcing companies were known to be unreliable and untrustworthy.

Labour's stated position in Februry 2018 on exiting the European Community included the scope to invest in public services and turn away from privatisation and forced competitive contracting-out, with Corbyn saying:

> Britain will need a bespoke relationship of its own. Labour would negotiate a new and strong relationship with the single market that includes full tariff-free access and a floor under existing rights, standards and protections. That new relationship would need to ensure we can deliver our ambitious economic programme. So we would also seek to negotiate protections, clarifications or exemptions, where necessary, in relation to privatisation and public service competition directives, state aid and procurement rules.[47]

But there had been many false dawns in the past when previous outsourcing failures and scandals had heralded a promised potential halt to public services being raided for private profit, which was then not delivered. Twenty years ago, in 1998 in the year after Labour replaced 17 years of Conservative government, it was thought this could be 'the end of privatisation'.[48] It wasn't.

So, as the Carillion story fades from media coverage and public attention, it may well be a return to business as usual with the big outsourcing corporations getting more public sector contracts, supported by the accountancy firms and the banks and bankers that hardly seem to have been reformed or re-educated since the financial crash they triggered in 2007/08. This is why in relation to social work and statutory social services there remains the requirement to be vigilant and to resist the marketisation and privatisation of these crucial services for people in difficulty and those who may be vulnerable.

A new agenda for social work and the personal social services

The government narrative has been that social work and the personal social services are failing and not fit-for-purpose. In 2012, for example, Michael Gove, as Secretary of State for Education, gave a speech which he headlined 'The failure of child protection and the need for a fresh start'.[49] The solution? Innovation, promoted by specific government grants, with developments led by the private sector and with delivery increasingly taken outside of the public sector and local authorities. This is the script which is writ large and being peddled by politicians in government (and by parts of the press), advised and assisted by civil servants, management accountants and consultants, and others who have little grounded experience or expertise regarding the services which are being opened up to privatisation.

But there is an alternative script, and an alternative future could be created. This draws on the lessons and successes from the past – of which many current government ministers and their advisors will be unaware – whilst moving forward on a journey of continuing improvement. It describes a future which avoids the difficulties and disasters of the contract culture, outsourcing and privatisation.

The contracting-out of social work services has inherent weaknesses which are embedded in the contracting process, with:

- large sums of money now going out of services as profit taken by private companies;
- the downward movement in quality – and qualifications, skills and terms and conditions of workers – as companies seek to cut costs to generate more profit;

- the statutory requirement that companies' first and primary responsibility and accountability is to their owners/shareholders and not to the public or community;
- control by management accountants rather than by professionals experienced in and committed to the services;
- additional costs incurred by central and local government in setting up, letting and managing contracts;
- the increasing complexity and confusion of accountability for services between contractors and contractees;
- the selling on of contracts when companies are taken over or merge and where ownership becomes even more opaque;
- the lack of transparency and openness when services are provided by commercial companies that have no responsibilities for freedom of information and public reporting but can hide behind commercial confidentiality;
- the prevalence of management consultants from the big international accountancy firms acting as government advisors on social work and children's services, whose mission is to generate a market – from which they too will profit – rather than enhance or protect services.

All of these concerns were inherent within the government's strategy of moving statutory children's social work services outside of the direct provision and management by local authorities, as I noted in a *Community Care* article in 2016 headed 'Six reasons to rethink moves to strip councils of children's services: The government's thrust towards trusts could do more harm than good to efforts to improve struggling services'.[50] The six reasons to rethink and reverse the government's strategy were the six 'Ts' of additional costs and complexity:

- **Transition costs**
  It takes at least a year to set up a trust. The set-up process itself consumes the attention of key people in children's services and the wider council. Not only does this cost time, it also costs money (no small consideration at a time of shrinking budgets). In the meantime the focus is not on improving services, which remain trapped in uncertainty.

- **Transaction costs**

  When the new trust is set up and becomes operational there are ongoing added costs. The trust will have to report back on its performance to its own board, the council and the Education Secretary. Generating and delivering data and reports again costs time, attention and cash – with dedicated staff likely to be required to fulfil these activities. At a time when less bureaucracy is needed in children's services, this moves in the opposition direction.

- **Transmission costs**

  One of the early requirements of the new trust is to stabilise a workforce who have had a long period of uncertainty and may still feel uncertain as they are moved without choice into a new organisation. This is made more difficult when the message that has been transmitted, and the news locally and nationally, is that this is a children's service in such disarray that it is no longer to be run by the local authority. Recruitment as well as retention has not been made easier.

- **Transgression costs**

  What if the trust fails to deliver the improvements required? What if – unlike the requirement imposed on other services funded by the council – it goes over budget? What if when Ofsted re-inspects it is still found to be 'inadequate'? This is quite likely if the Ofsted re-inspection comes while the trust, catching up on the improvement delay of the set-up period, has still not had time to generate stability. Are there to be (financial) penalties imposed, as might be expected in a profit-making commercial contract? If so, they will have to be at the expense of the funding of services?

- **Transmutation costs**

  In some areas the stated plan is that after an initial contract period of five years or so, consideration should be given to returning services to the council. But during this time the council will have lost much wisdom, experience and expertise in its corporate, political as well as service leadership for children's services. And if a trust fails should there be an earlier return of services to the council, which still carries the statutory responsibility for the welfare and safety of children in its area? The costs here are in terms of time and cash (unwinding from a contract and setting up another set of new arrangements) and also in the cost of recreating and rebuilding expertise.

- **Transparency costs**
  The greatest concern, however, should not be about financial costs but about the implications of confused and complex accountabilities. The Laming inquiry following the death of Victoria Climbié warned there should be explicit and clear accountability for statutory children's services and child protection. This was enshrined in the 2004 Children Act, with the requirements that there should be a named lead councillor for children's services and the statutory required post of Director of Children's Services. This clear accountability is being made opaque by the transfer of children's services outside the public sector to an independent trust where its relationship with the council is through the management of a contract. As independent, non-public sector organisations, trusts may not be required to comply with freedom of information requests, and indeed may refuse to publish or make available information which they consider to be (commercially) sensitive.

These concerns about contracting statutory children's social work outside of local authorities also apply to adult social work, with the same dynamics and difficulties when social workers are transferred to and managed within companies such as Virgin Care and yet the local authority still holds the statutory responsibility for the welfare and safety of disabled, including older, people.

However, public services, including social work and the personal social services, should not be frozen and immutable and cannot just hold on to the past, especially when the past is recognised as not being good enough for today and the future. Will Hutton, for example, when writing about the Carillion crisis, argued that:

> Britain's nationalised industries suffered from inefficiency and persistent underinvestment. Taking activity back in-house is a strong soundbite, but

no panacea. While some public sector delivery is outstanding, notably in parts of the NHS, the general pattern is more patchy. It is for this reason that governments for decades have been contracting the private sector to deliver goods and services.[53]

But my concern is that there are some responsibilities – for essential community infrastructure such as the provision of energy and safe water supplies, and also for the welfare and protection of children and disabled people – which should be held by the state and should be delivered by the state. They should not be decanted and contracted out to the vagaries of a marketplace where competition is about profit-generation for those who are already wealthy rather than the public good. Markets – increasingly unregulated and unrestrained since the neoliberalism introduced in the 1980s – have not delivered what was promised on the tin. They have been no guarantee of economy, efficiency or effectiveness, and they have certainly not created equity and fairness. What they have generated is greater inequality and greater vulnerability as they have been exploited for personal gain and profit-taking.

The task, therefore, is to determine how to best meet these crucial state responsibilities and provide these essential services, to avoid the vulnerabilities, costs and complexities of contracting them outside of the public sector, and what actions to take if some areas and services are not performing well enough.

So, what makes social work and the provision of the personal social services good? My view increasingly is that what is required is very simple, but difficult to do. It requires:

- the creation and maintenance of a competent and confident stable workforce,
- immersed in a culture which is supportive and performance-focused,
- with senior and top managers who have expertise, calmness and wisdom based on experience of front-line practice and its direct management,
- who stay informed and close to front-line practice,

- who know the strengths and weaknesses of their front-line managers, and
- address concerns when necessary, and where
- they and their colleagues in other agencies stay around for long enough to build trusting relationships and shared agendas, and know their communities and neighbourhoods, and where
- the top managers have the gravitas not to be bullied or bossed around by councillors, council chief executives or central corporate directors who may get too excited by novel central government or corporate agendas, 'innovation' or ideological purity.

Improvement and innovation

A major thread in the government's agenda for social work since 2010, especially in children's services amid politically chosen austerity, has been that struggling services, albeit immersed in funding cuts, would be enhanced by innovation. But innovation is not synonymous with improvement. Indeed, the organisational and worker disruption caused by big restructuring or practice changes may outweigh any (uncertain) gains from the 'innovations' being introduced; even though, as previously noted, one of the government's advisors, Professor Le Grand, sees the 'creative turmoil' and uncertainty being created as itself a positive dynamic,[52] for the social workers and others caught in the uncertainty it may seem more chaotic than constructive.[53]

There are innovations from the recent past which were sensible and desirable but which have already been abandoned. Sure Start, with its area focus on supporting and helping young children and their families, would be a prime example.[54] One of the dangers with the drive for innovation and novelty is that what is already valuable may be lost among the changes in policy and practice, and that the cash and time given to introducing the new changes inevitably create some organisational disruption. This is why, for example, East Sussex has rightly trumpeted its achievements built on creating and maintaining continuity and stability.[55]

This does not mean that innovation should be resisted or placed on the back-burner. Far from it. For example, the evaluation of the first phase of the programmes introduced through the DfE's

Innovation Fund showed positive signs of service improvement.[56] But innovation, if producing positive results, needs to be embedded and sustained to get a real return on the change costs incurred. The danger is that with rapid turnover within the workforce, and especially frequent changes of leadership, there is too much and too frequent change and novelty, with no commitment or ownership of what was only recently introduced by the outgoing senior managers. Change is then experienced as churn, and as disruptive rather than developmental. Managing change also has the danger of taking management attention away from current front-line practice, as was found in 2018 to have happened in Bournemouth, where attention that might have been given to the front line was distracted by a focus on local government reform and council mergers.[57]

Creating stability and continuity, especially in leadership and in the workforce, has been found in Ofsted inspections, as reported in 2018, to generate better performance.[58, 59] Ofsted has also found the corollary to be true – instability undermines performance.[60, 61] This brings into question the short-term, start-stop funding of the Department for Education's Innovation Fund, where new services or models of working are initiated but, in the context of continuing big cuts in mainstream budgets, struggle to be maintained after the short-term funding ends. This became an issue, for example, with the end of government funding for the unit that was supporting the development of Family Drug and Alcohol Courts.[62]

High profile among the government's promoted and funded innovations have been the 'Reclaiming Social Work' model of statutory children's services organisations and the 'Signs of Safety' practice model for child protection. Both have had close relationships with the DfE and its advisors and with significant payments to the creators of the models.

'Reclaiming Social Work'

The 'Reclaiming Social Work' model[63] has generated substantial public funding for Morning Lane Associates (MLA), a company which, as noted in Chapter Three, has one shareholder whom the Chief Social Worker for Children described as 'a close personal friend'. 'Reclaiming Social Work' is an organisational model developed by the Isabelle Trowler, the Chief Social Worker, and Steve Goodman, now the sole shareholder of MLA, when they were previously working together in Hackney. MLA has received payments to roll the model out to other local authorities which have received funding from the 'Innovation Fund'.

It is, however, a model of questionable resilience and sustainability. In a surprising tweet in 2017, referenced in Chapter Three, Steve Goodman stated 'the only people responsible for increased children in care are the ADCS [Association of Directors of Children's Services] – don't blame austerity – adopt the Reclaim Social Work model'.[64] This blatant marketing of a model which generated much of MLA's income led to Twitter exchanges expressing concern that it flew in the face of the evidence about the relationship between the increasing extent and depth of poverty and deprivation for children and families and numbers of child protection investigations, child protection plans, and children in care[65, 66, 67] – evidence which has been confirmed by a study commissioned by the Local Government Association.[68]

The 'Reclaiming Social Work' model is based on small 'pods' consisting of a consultant social worker, maybe two or three social workers, a family therapist, and a unit administrator. The consultant social worker is the manager and supervisor of the 'pod' of workers and is also the named case holder for all the children and families held within the workload of the 'pod'.

The strength of the model was stated to be its emphasis on direct work with children and families using the range of skills within the 'pod', with the workers in the 'pod' practising 'joint working', with discussions and consultation about children and families involving all the workers, all within a practice model prioritising systemic family therapy, and with the ready availability of administrative support.

The roll-out of the 'pure' model created in Hackney has been altered and amended by other councils which have, with the participation of MLA, adopted the model's framework. This is probably inevitable as new practices and policies when more widely rolled out beyond the pioneers rarely if ever stay fully committed or signed up to the model initially owned and championed by its creators. But there are also experiences which highlight the weaknesses of the model.

Between 2010 and 2015 I was appointed by local authorities and the Department for Education to oversee children's services improvement in five areas of England judged by Ofsted to be 'inadequate'. In two of these areas, the Isle of Wight[69] and Devon,[70] the councils had sought to introduce the 'Reclaiming Social Work' model. In each instance the service had imploded and subsequently been rated as 'inadequate' by Ofsted. Major issues had arisen about the management of the extensive organisational change being introduced but also about the role of consultant social workers and about the small size of the work units, especially at a time of increasing child protection workloads, which was the reality throughout England following the media's shaping and telling of 'the Baby P story' in November 2008.[71, 72]

In each authority there had been difficulty in appointing and recruiting experienced social workers as consultant social workers. There was then a difficulty in retaining those who were appointed, as they had the pressure and stress of being the named case holder at any one time for 80-plus cases, for many of which they had not had personal and direct contact before the case was closed. Other cases were in court proceedings where the consultant social worker as the case holder was required to be present at court and to give evidence. There was also a difficulty in identifying and skilling up enough workers for the therapist role in the 'pods'. Social workers in the 'pods' were often without regular management and individual supervision as the consultant social workers were committed to court attendances, and some social workers felt downgraded and disempowered as they were no longer case holders. It may not be too much of a surprise that retention of consultant social workers and social workers became an issue, as did the capacity and continuity of the small 'pods' when there were vacancies, absences because of sickness and annual leave, or a surge in referrals and work to be undertaken.

'Signs of Safety'

The second innovation much supported by the Department for Education's 'Innovation Fund' is the 'Signs of Safety' child protection practice model. It was developed in Australia by Andrew Turnell and Steve Edwards with the participation and assistance of practising social workers. Quite exceptionally for a practice model, in my experience, it has been 'trade mark' protected, which stops people 'stealing or copying' the brand.[73] This seems like a fundamental change. Rather than cooperation and collaboration within a context of professional sharing, the new practice model has been commercialised and has become an income generator for those who have now secured its ownership. In the UK the company which had ownership of the 'Signs of Safety' brand has as its owners Turnell and Edwards, along with Eileen Munro, a professor at the London School of Economics who had been commissioned in 2009 by the government to prepare a report, which was well received by the social work profession, on child protection and children's social work in England.[74] Servelec, an IT and engineering company owned by Scarlet Bidco Ltd which is indirectly owned by Montagu Private Equity,[75] is the 'lead development partner', in the UK for 'Signs of Safety'.[76]

The 'Signs of Safety' model is a strengths-based approach to working with families. It is an asset in giving a framework, structure and tools which can be used when working with families. As with other strengths-based models, such as the NHS 'Mellow Parenting' model which was used as a parent-craft programme with Tracey Connelly, the mother of Peter Connelly ('Baby P'),[77] there is the importance of not getting overly focused on the adults with whom most exchanges might take place and losing sight of the child and their experiences. Some of the 'Signs of Safety' tools help to mitigate this danger.

Losing a focus on and sight of the child is, however, a general difficulty and danger for social workers and others, which has been well researched and recorded by Harry Ferguson.[78] It is still important, therefore, to give attention to the seven 'I's of:

- being Intrigued,
- being Inquisitive,
- being Imaginative,
- being Investigative,
- being Interrogative,
- gathering Information, and
- using intellectual and emotional Intelligence

in trying to understand what is happening within the family and for children when you are not there.

It is why reflective supervision is so important to assist in making sensible judgements, albeit based on what will always be incomplete and untidy knowledge and understanding. The dangers with any practice model is that the model is implemented but the thinking is marginalised.

What is of particular interest for this book about the 'Reclaiming Social Work' and 'Signs of Safety' models, along with the Frontline social work education programme discussed in Chapters One and Three, is how each had received substantial government funding which has then been paid, at least in part, to private companies and consultancies.

The 'Innovation Fund' has sometimes sensibly been used by local authorities to try, however minimally, to offset the bigger reductions in central government funding to local authorities, sometimes with creative twists in re-presenting and reshaping what is being retrieved from previous enforced cuts. For example, the 'Innovation Fund' is used by Hampshire and the Isle of Wight councils[79] to provide personal assistants to work alongside three or four social workers and to take on some of the administrative tasks such as arranging core group meetings with other professionals to review child protection concerns and data inputting and other systems maintenance tasks which otherwise were taking up the time of social workers.

Another positive use of the 'Innovation Fund' is made by Hertfordshire County Council,[80] and also to be found in Hampshire and the Isle of Wight,[81] in integrating adult service workers, such as mental health, drug and alcohol, and domestic violence workers, into front-line children's social services teams.

These positive developments are creative and constructive, but they ought to be able to be made and achieved through the use of mainstream funding rather than the time-consuming, and in itself costly, fragile and fraught, process of having to apply for an (uncertain) grant amid shrinking budgets. The money allocated through the specific 'innovation' grants then gets misleadingly trumpeted by the government and its spokespersons (who often seem to be civil servants – who should remain non-political, unlike government ministers spinning their political interests and agendas) as extra investment in children's services.

The battle over funding

The government has often presented its Children's Services Innovation Fund as new and additional money for children's social services. This is misleading. The short-term, insecure funding made available through the Innovation Fund is a miniscule amount when compared to the much, much bigger cuts the government has made in its funding to local authorities. The Innovation Fund is also by no means the most efficient or effective way of providing money for children's social services. It has high overheads, including the money paid to the private sector companies which it contracts to manage the fund.[82] The Local Government Association (LGA) proposed that it would be more sensible to devolve the Innovation Fund money directly to local authorities, which would, in effect, cut out the private sector intermediaries.[83]

But the window-dressing of the Innovation Fund as additional money for children's social services masks the bigger issue of the cuts and underfunding of the services. The battle and conflict over funding has continued with protagonists for the government matched against, among others, the All-Party Parliamentary Group for Children (APPG Children), the Children's Commissioner in England, the LGA and the Association of Directors of Children's Services (ADCS). Here is how the battle is being fought.

The government's Children's Minister in 2017, Robert Goodwill, and Nadhim Zahawi, the Children's Minister who replaced him in 2018, have presented a consistent line. It was reported that Goodwill's position was that 'Local authorities must prove they are using existing children's services resources efficiently before the Department for Education will approach the Treasury for more money to tackle rising demand' and that 'children's leaders must make better use of existing resources'.[84] In March 2018 when challenged at a meeting of the House of Commons Education Select Committee about the cuts having created severe financial pressures for children's services, Zahawi responded that:

> We want to look at the evidence … We have actually channelled more money into the system including £200m into the innovation programme and a further £20m for those authorities that are struggling. There is very little correlation, at all, between the cost in a local authority for delivering really good childcare, safeguarding and all the other good children's services in a local authority, and the amount of money they spend. Actually, much of the evidence suggests [the importance of] leadership … I think simply focusing on let's just chuck more money at this and it will solve itself – it won't.[85]

So the difficulty according to the ministers is not the impact of the 40% cut in government funding to local councils since 2010. The problem is down to the quality and performance of children's services leaders. Echoes here of the tweet from the director of Morning Lane Associates, Steve Goodman, in October 2017 that 'The only people responsible for increased children in care are the ADCS – don't blame austerity – adopt the Reclaim Social Work model' (see Chapter Three).

This view was challenged by Stuart Gallimore, the ADCS president, in his speech at the 2018 ADCS annual conference, where he stated:

> 'there is not enough money in the system, full stop', and dismissed arguments that current funding is sufficient, but spent disproportionately on care placements. 'There is simply no fat left to trim, instead

authorities up and down the country have found themselves having to cut back on early help services, which makes no financial sense'.[86]

But this is not a view apparently shared by the Chief Social Worker for Children and Families, Isabelle Trowler. In a tweet in June 2018, echoing Goodman's tweet, she wrote 'the ££ is there isn't it? But it's spent disproportionately in the care system rather than support system. The strategy needs to focus on how to switch the balance?'.[87] This tweet from the Chief Social Worker received a Twitter response from Alison Michalska, who had recently finished her term as President of the ADCS, that 'No! The money simply isn't there!! Many good Councils, with excellent preventative services, do not have the money to meet the demand placed on them by rising levels of child poverty and years of austerity'.[88]

However, with the view of ministers being that it still needs to be evidenced that more money is needed for children's services to start to mitigate the year-on-year cuts in funding to local authorities since 2010, and with the view of the Chief Social Worker (and of the director of Morning Lane Associates) being that the money is there but is being wrongly spent, it is hardly surprising that Graham Archer, the senior civil servant for children in the Department of Education, who would be advising ministers alongside the Chief Social Worker, has said it is unlikely children's services will get more money from the government:

> Graham Archer, director of children's social care, improvement and learning at the DfE, told delegates at the Association of Directors of Children's Services (ADCS) annual conference in Manchester that the 'difficult fiscal position' meant it was unlikely 'a lot more money' would be allocated to council children's services at the 2019 spending review … Archer said the sector and the department will need to work together to analyse the factors influencing demand and spend in children's social care and how these related to performance and quality to improve

understanding of whether more money is needed, better commissioning of services or greater roll out of good practice.[89]

So in 2018 it looked as though the concerns about the funding of children's social services were to be kicked into the long grass (rather as has happened with the concerns about the funding for adult social care and care for older people) – apparently more research is needed and, anyway, the immediate issue is about the leadership of children's services.

On the other side of the argument, expressing their fears about the funding gap which has now arisen for children's services, were (in addition to the ADCS, as noted above) the Children's Commissioner in England and the LGA:

> Councils have been warning for some time [said the Children's Commissioner for England] that they are not going to be able to meet their statutory requirements. I can see and hear every day from families and children who simply can't get help ... If you don't help children when the problems aren't at crisis point then the crisis is going to be developing and also it is going to be much more costly when it gets to that point.[90]

> [The LGA] is calling for the services that change children's lives to be properly funded ... By 2020 local government in England will have lost 75 pence out of every pound of core central government funding that it had to spend in 2015. Overall councils are facing a £2 billion funding gap for children's services by 2020. In 2015/16 councils were forced to overspend on their children's services budgets by £605 million across England ... Government funding for the Early Intervention Grant has been cut by almost £500 million since 2013. It is projected to drop by a further £183 million by 2020.[91]

The concerns of the Children's Commissioner and of councillors and senior managers trying to deliver children's services were echoed and emphasised by the MPs and Lords belonging to the APPG for Children in their 2018 report:

> The APPGC received compelling evidence suggesting that thresholds for accessing children's social care are rising. A survey of social workers carried out by the Inquiry found that 70 per cent felt thresholds had risen for qualifying as a 'child in need' under section 17 of the Children Act 1989 and half said the same in relation to making a child subject to a child protection plan. This means that it is getting harder for children and families to access help when they need it ... Evidence received by the Inquiry indicates that funding is influencing, at least implicitly, social workers' decisions about whether to intervene to support a child. These pressures apply more consistently to decisions about early help and preventative services. However, the APPGC was very concerned to hear from social workers and researchers that decisions about whether to take action to safeguard a child – for example taking a child into care or making a child subject to a child protection plan – have also been affected by funding constraints. It is unacceptable that children's safety is potentially being undermined by a lack of sufficient resources. The Inquiry heard evidence that funding pressures are having a disproportionate impact on the most deprived areas. This suggests that in these areas concerns about budgets will loom larger in decisions taken, and access to support for children will be more restricted than in other, wealthier, areas.[92]

Tim Loughton, the Conservative MP and former Children's Minister who has remained an active and committed champion for children and for social work (see Chapter Two), chaired the APPG. It was reported that:

A former Tory children's minister has blamed the government's 'woeful underfunding' of local authorities for a crisis in child protection that is putting the safety of vulnerable young people at risk. The MP Tim Loughton, who served as children's minister in David Cameron's coalition government, said pressure on safeguarding services in some areas was so severe that often the only way to guarantee safety for children was to take them into care ... 'In some places, the pressure on children's services is so acute it is leaving social workers feeling that the only tool available to them to keep a child safe is to remove them from their family,' said Loughton, who is the co-chair of the all-party parliamentary group (APPG) for children. 'As a result, families may look at these skilled and caring professionals with mistrust. But this is wrong. It is the woeful underfunding by government of a proper breadth of social care interventions that is to blame.'[93]

With informed MPs, along with others, expressing their concern about the impact of government cuts on children and families who need assistance from, and sometimes the protection provided by, social workers and children's social services, it really would be timely – indeed urgent – that the government, its ministers and their advisors acknowledged and committed to tackle the crisis in care, a crisis which would be heightened by fragmenting services through marketisation and privatisation, with the consequence of adding costs to and taking a profit out of what has been a shrinking pot of government funding.

A framework for the future

So, what might a positive and constructive alternative future for statutory social work and the personal social services look like? It stands in stark contrast to what is being shaped through the competitive contract culture and the promotion of commercialisation, marketisation and privatisation. The table below shows the contrasts.

Table: A comparison between the current agenda and a positive future agenda for statutory social work and the personal social services

THE CURRENT AGENDA	A POSITIVE FUTURE AGENDA
CONCENTRATING ON FINANCIAL VALUE	CHAMPIONING SOCIAL WORK'S VALUES
ETHICS OF BUSINESS SUCCESS	ETHICS OF PUBLIC SERVICE
FOCUS ON SPREADSHEET BOTTOM-LINE	FOCUS ON FRONT-LINE PRACTICE
EMPHASIS ON COMPETITION	EMPHASIS ON COLLABORATION
FRAGMENTATION	INTEGRATION
FINANCE AND COMMERCIAL FOCUS	FAMILY AND COMMUNITY FOCUS
REMOTE LEADERSHIP AND OWNERSHIP	LOCAL LEADERSHIP AND ACCOUNTABILITY
OPAQENESS	TRANSPARENCY
CREATING MORE COMPLEXITY	SEEKING LESS COMPLEXITY
SHAPED BY MANAGEMENT ACCOUNTANTS	SHAPED BY SERVICE PROFESSIONALS
COMPETITIVE CONTRACT CHANGES	SERVICE CONTINUITY
CHURN	STABILITY
INNOVATION FOCUS	IMPROVEMENT FOCUS
PRIORITISING CUTTING COSTS	PRIORITISING QUALITY
ASSET STRIPPING	INVESTMENT
PROFIT FOCUS	PEOPLE FOCUS

A positive future agenda would reclaim and reset both the style and the context for social work with children and families (and much of this could also apply to social work with adults). Much social work practice has been skewed to focus on risk assessment and risk management, with local authority social workers in particular immersed in the roles of scrutinising and monitoring families. The consequence is that they are sometimes seen as intrusive and threatening rather than helpful and caring. This was, for example, the perception of local authority social workers by parents who were in contact with a Troubled Families programme.[94] This is not a comment on or criticism of the motivation and intentions of the social workers, but it does reflect how their work and roles have been shaped by an overwhelming focus on child (and adult) protection amidst cuts which limit the resources they can mobilise for families and squeeze the time they can give to direct contact and work with the families.

The social workers are also often embedded in centralised offices, as local authorities seek to save money by reducing additional office locations, and departments are structured so that there are frequent handovers of children and families between teams and workers – customer call-centres, and then different teams for referral and initial assessment, early help, children in need, child protection, court proceedings, looked-after children, permanency planning, and leaving care and care leavers. One of the local authorities in difficulty with which I have worked in recent years had eight potential, and sometimes enacted, transfers of teams and social worker for individual children and families, all within a year to 18 months. And this is before any changes of social workers arising from the deployment of short-term interim agency workers or because of other staff turnover. The knowledge and history of families is lost, relationships are aborted or never develop, and children and families never engage or disengage.

There are, however, other local authorities which have maintained or rebuilt a focus on community social work, with social workers based within the areas or localities where they work, and with a knowledge built up over time not only of families but of networks in the community, community resources and of other professionals working across the same patch. Social workers in these authorities are able to see children and families in their social context in and outside the home. They give attention to the deprivation and discrimination impinging on families and are more likely to have the necessary contacts with and access to other agencies and workers to advocate on behalf of the families.

Does it work? The evidence from Ofsted inspection reports is that it does. For example, here are two quotes from Ofsted's inspection report on Kensington and Chelsea (RBKC), a children's service which it rated as 'outstanding':

RBKC uses its well-developed Focus on Practice model of social work, which places a high value on relationship building between children and their social workers, to deliver services that are consistently excellent. Exemplary application of this highly innovative model is also supported by social workers' very low caseloads, social workers remaining with children throughout their journey across all stages of social care intervention, clinicians embedded within social work teams, and the clear and charismatic leadership of RBKC's Director of Family Services (DFS) and its talented senior management team.

Children and families in need of specialist help and support can access social care services directly and quickly through six locality-based and one hospital social care team. Managers report that workers know their locality and the services within it very well, and this enables appropriate services to be swiftly provided.[95]

Leeds is another local authority which has a high positive national profile and where Ofsted rated its children's services as 'good'. Ofsted reported that:

Leeds have successfully integrated local authority, health and third sector services which have evolved into a new early help service, underpinned by the 'Best Start' strategy. Multi-agency, locality 'cluster' arrangements ensure that good and effective use is made of local partnerships – particularly children's centres and learning settings ... A large-scale restructuring of social work services into a locality model, based around 25 multi-agency clusters, is steadily improving the recruitment, retention and professional development of good quality social work staff. A clear career structure and a comprehensive workforce development programme have reduced dependency on agency and temporary staff and raised the status of social work across the city.[96]

The final example is the findings of Ofsted's 2018 inspection of children's services in North Yorkshire, which Ofsted rated as 'outstanding':

> At the heart of the North Yorkshire approach is a belief that stable relationships with workers who know their children and families extremely well is the key to creating and sustaining positive change ... Workers know their children well and manageable caseloads provide them with the conditions to maintain relationships. Children and families do not change worker without good reason, thus facilitating longer term, meaningful relationships. This approach was seen throughout the inspection to be having a significant and positive impact on a number of children and their families.[97]

These leading local authorities have an emphasis on relationship-based and community-located social work. It is a return to what was intended by the Seebohm Committee in the 1960s[98] and what has been a part of social work's history and remit. It is an approach being championed by, for example, Brid Featherstone, Sue White, Kate Morris and Anna Gupta. Their 2014 book *Re-imagining Child Protection: Towards Humane Social Work*[99] and subsequent 2018 book *Protecting Children: A Social Model*[100] challenge much of the basis underlying the context in which social workers are having to practise. They note that:

> A story [of social work] that was rooted in compassion towards the vulnerable in a Keynesian era has morphed into a highly blaming and risk-focused enterprise. Since 2010, and the active policies directed at reducing state support, the focus on the individual family and/or parent has become ethically problematic. In a context of the continued stripping away of many of the key supports necessary to ensure

children and their families flourish (such as decent
incomes, family-friendly working, quality public
transport services, adequate housing and local support
services) an individualised risk-focused practice
culture reinforces rather than ameliorates the struggles
families face. [101]

It is this scenario which Featherstone and her colleagues seek
to change with their focus on community, rights, relationships,
recognising and seeking to address deprivation and discrimination
and its impact, and seeing people's worth and capacity alongside
their troubles. It provides a blueprint which maps out a route
and way forward already being taken by some local authorities
and social workers. It presents an antidote to trends over recent
years (and decades) which have created overly bureaucratised
and risk-focused social work practice.

What to do when performance is not good enough

But what to do when the public sector statutory social work and
the personal social services are not good enough?

The government's thrust, for example, where local authorities
have had their children's social services judged as 'inadequate' by
Ofsted has been to remove the services from direct delivery and
management by the council and outsource them to independent
trusts or other organisations. Indeed, as noted in an earlier
chapter, David Cameron as Prime Minister saw the marketisation
of statutory children's social services as the desired way forward
for all children's social services and across all local authorities.

The difficulties with this recipe for tackling areas where
performance is not good enough are that, as also noted in
Chapter One:

1. it delays and distracts from concentrating on performance
   improvement (note the time taken to set up the independent
   trusts and then to generate improvement in Doncaster and
   Slough[102]);
2. it is costly in terms of cash in the short and longer term.
   The government contributed £2.9 million to set up the
   Doncaster Children's Services Trust, £3.2 million to set

up the Slough Trust and £2.5 million for the Sunderland Community Interest Company. None of this was money to be spent directly on services for children and families.[103] It was money used to fund the move of children's services outside of councils;

3. it is also costly in terms of time. Doncaster received an 'inadequate' rating from Ofsted in 2012. It then took until August 2013 for the Secretary of State to decide that its children's services should be transferred to a trust, and the trust was only in place in September 2014. In November 2015 Doncaster's children's services were re-inspected by Ofsted and still rated as 'inadequate'[104] (although in 2018, over five years on from 2012, Ofsted rated the services as 'good'[105]);

4. it is no guarantee of success despite the considerable investment which will have been made, with Slough Children's Services Trust continuing to be rated by Ofsted as 'inadequate' and with its chief executive stepping down two years after it was formed;[106]

5. it adds complexity and confusion for the accountability and transparency of the services, with, for example, the council still holding the statutory responsibility for the services (for example, the Ofsted reports noted in point (3) above were headed 'Doncaster Metropolitan Borough Council' not 'Doncaster Children's Trust') and having to address the funding, including overspends incurred by trusts, as in Doncaster in 2018;[107] and

6. even where the outsourcing in the first instance is to not-for-profit trusts or community interest companies, this may be a Trojan horse step on the way to the services being placed within private, for-profit, companies when re-contracted. This has happened with NHS community health services being initially contracted out to non-profit community interest companies but then, at the end of the contract, the re-tendered services being transferred to Virgin Care (as in Bath and North East Somerset[108]).

As Jo Miller, the chief executive of Doncaster Council, has noted (and as referred to in Chapter One), other councils such as Rotherham which were allowed by the government to retain direct the management and provision of their children's services despite 'inadequate' judgements by Ofsted have made speedier progress in addressing concerns with assistance from across the council.[109] In relation to Doncaster, 'Miller thinks the improvement was in spite of the trust structure, not because of it. "Yes, services to children have improved since the trust came along," she says. "But so have all the services in the council. Children's services haven't improved any quicker – and the trust costs a lot more money".'[110]

So, what might be an alternative response to poor performance by local authorities? First, it would be wise to understand the reasons for poor performance. Although denied by the government,[111] there is a strong correlation between deprivation, funding and cuts, and Ofsted ratings for services provided by local authorities as 'inadequate', as shown by research undertaken by Hood,[112] Bywaters,[113] Bilson[114] and colleagues. This is not sensibly addressed by adding outsourcing costs to the services in these areas.

Secondly, Ofsted has been a creator of escalating poor performance in areas which were struggling. A review, revamp, realignment and redefinition of the national inspectorate's role was necessary. The inspection culture, process and contribution needed to be reset to focus on service development and improvement rather than on undermining, brutal and damaging one-word judgements and categorisations from a hit-and-run inspectorate which itself has lacked confidence and credibility. A judgement of 'inadequate' has frequently led to a more intense and quickening spiral of increased workloads, greater instability, and a service which is even more battered and overwhelmed, as for example occurred in Tower Hamlets[115] where there was a little irony as its director of children's services was the former head of Ofsted's children's social services inspections.[116]

The changed Ofsted inspection process introduced in 2018 has a positive stronger focus on development, working with local authorities and being proportionate to the local authority's performance record, with Eleanor Schooling, Ofsted's then national director for social care, commenting that: 'In practice this means that Ofsted will have more frequent opportunities to identify any issues of concern, allowing areas to take swifter action to address them. Quite simply, we don't want to wait until the next inspection to find out that practice has deteriorated, we want to be able to 'catch' areas before they fall.'[117]

Thirdly, it is sensible to have and to use comparative information about the performance on key variables between councils (and for the different teams and localities within council's children's services). The data comparisons should be used for benchmarking but not for generating league tables or ratings. The art and science of using performance indicators is about their role in generating reflection, discussion and understanding and then taking action on the basis of the understanding which has been created.

The fallacy is to think that data tells the story. It doesn't. What it should do is trigger where attention should be deployed, and with a considered view then taken about performance based on the benchmarked data. An example: when I was a director of social services we apparently performed poorly on the number of disabled adults aged 18–65 years who received more than 10 hours a week of home care. On the national bar chart tables published by the Department of Health we were way down the league table. But why? It was because we were one of the first authorities to make available and promote direct cash payments to disabled people following the 1996 Community Care (Direct Payments) Act and had a relatively high number of disabled people (across all impairment categories) who had chosen to receive a direct payment. But that would not have been recognised from the bar chart league table. Similarly, we were not one of the higher performers on looked-after children reviews undertaken within timescale. Many councils were recording 97%–100% success. We thought it more important that, whilst mindful of the required timescale set by the government, reviews should be undertaken to fit in with the wishes of the child or young person and the availability of foster or residential key workers and others, even if this meant that the review was a fortnight late, and we were willing to argue this with inspectors from what was then the Social Services Inspectorate, who were rarely less than understanding.

Fourthly, a point not unrelated to point three above, it is sensible to recognise that the expertise about children's social services and social work lies with those who deliver the services and not with firms of management accountants and outsourcing companies. This is why it makes sense to harness the experience and wisdom from within the sector and to make it available to areas which are struggling or failing. This is the approach advocated by Roy Perry, leader of Hampshire County Council, who was also chair of the Local Government Association's children's committee.[118] This view received some acceptance by the government in 2018, with the announcement that it was committing £17 million to promote sector-led improvement. Alison Michalska, the president of the Association of Directors of Children's Services, wrote:

> Funding for sector-led improvement in children's services is to be welcomed – this is the best way to improve the services we provide to children and families. Children's services flourish when corporate and political leadership is well informed and engaged providing effective support and challenge to directors of children's services and their teams. The development of the Partners in Practice programme serves as further recognition from government that the skills, expertise and experience to improve children's services lie in the sector. Whilst we welcome this acknowledgement, ADCS is absolutely clear that all local authorities have something to offer and something to learn, irrespective of their most recent inspection result. We hope Regional Improvement Alliances will bring a greater level of coherence to the ongoing development of sector-led improvement work already happening the regions.[119]

Fifthly, directly injecting the expertise from successful authorities into councils in difficulty is a further stage in the gradation of improvement activities. This might be through the appointment of 'commissioners', in effect performance advisors and scrutineers, or 'improvement partners', who are service leaders and have a strong positive track record from within other local authorities. The commissioners and improvement partners need to have credibility based on their experience, and the gravitas and confidence to give direction without fear or favour. This happened, for example, in Somerset with positive results.[120, 121]

More dramatically, a partnership might be established whereby the senior management team from one council is contracted also to lead and manage the services in another (nearby) council, albeit directly accountable to the councillors in the council where they are now managing the services. This model was first applied, with success, for the Isle of Wight, with senior managers from Hampshire introduced to manage the island's children's services and quickly moving the services on from their 'inadequate' Ofsted rating.[122] In 2018 it is a model also being applied for Torbay, where children's services for the (too small) authority were to be managed by senior managers from Plymouth.[123]

Finally, if all else fails and the local authority is still not delivering its children's services well enough, the Secretary of State should have the power to send in a director or governance and management team to direct the services, and where the council has to accept this direction whilst the service still remains within the council as a locally provided public and accountable service. This is what had happened to some extent in Tower Hamlets, with Alan Wood as one of the commissioners.[124] In 2018 it was the government's remedy for Northamptonshire as it faced financial collapse with two commissioners appointed to manage the council.[125] It is less costly, quicker and less disruptive and complex than outsourcing services.

From TINA to TANIA

As noted above there are new improvement actions (TANIAs!) which can be taken without pushing statutory children's and social work services outside of the transparent and accountable public sector. This may not, however, satisfy those who are on a mission to promote a market for these and other public services. They have wanted to open up the market to David Cameron's 'market insurgents' and to the commercial, private, for-profit, companies which had attended meetings at the DfE and which

LaingBuisson noted had an interest in moving into the children's services 'industry'.

But the marketisation, commercialisation and privatisation of children's social work and child protection is not a sensible response to services collapsing under cuts and politically chosen austerity. The track record of costs and failures of outsourcing and privatisation should sound a loud warning bell that this is not sensible for the care and protection of children or for families who are overwhelmed by increasing poverty.

Will the bell be heard and the warning heeded? Following the debacle of Carillion and the subsequent media coverage, and the resurgence of Labour led by Corbyn, the privatisation script may get less publicity and promotion in the immediate future, but ideological intentions are ingrained and are likely to surface again. Why, for example, during the debates on the 2017 Children and Social Work Act was the government unwilling to review and reverse the 2014 changes in statutory regulation which allow any provider to be contracted to provide statutory children's social work and child protection services? This is what is now allowed, and it is not likely to be a position created by accident or without intention.

It is a part of the privatisation script and journey which, if continued and still pursued, has every danger of leaving children and families, along with social workers, as commodities to be traded in a fragmented, competitive commercial marketplace, adding costs and complexity, and leaking profits out of services, which will undermine children's welfare and safety, and leave families without the assistance they may need to care well for their children.

Notes and references

Introduction

1 Mason, P. (2009) *Meltdown: The End of the Age of Greed*, London, Verso.

2 Tett, G. (2010) *Fool's Gold: How Unrestrained Greed Corrupted a Dream, Shattered Global Markets and Unleashed a Catastrophe*, London, Little Brown.

3 Jones, R. (2014) *The Story of Baby P: Setting the Record Straight*, Bristol: Policy Press.

4 Cardy, S. (2010) '"Care Matters" and the privatisation of looked after children's services in England and Wales: developing a critique of independent "social work practices"', *Critical Social Policy*, 30(3): 430-442.

5 Garrett, P.M. (2008) 'Social work practices: silences and elisions in the plan to "transform" the lives of children "looked after" in England', *Child and Family Social Work*, 13(3): 311-318.

6 Garrett, P.M. (2009) *Transforming Children's Services? Social Work, Neoliberalism and the 'Modern' World*, Maidenhead: McGraw-Hill/Open University Press.

7 Butler, P. (2014) 'Privatise child protection services, Department for Education proposes. Experts sound alarm over proposal from Michael Gove's department to outsource children's services to private firms', 16 May, https://www.theguardian.com/society/2014/may/16/privatise-child-protection-servicesdepartment-for-education-proposes

8 38 Degrees (2016) 'Child protection: we won!', https://home.38degrees.org.uk/2016/11/09/child-protectionwon/

9 Rogowski, S. (2010) *Social Work: The Rise and Fall of a Profession?*, Bristol, Policy Press.

10 Tunstill, J. and Willow, C. (2018) 'Professional social work and the defence of children's and their families' rights in a period of

austerity: a case study', *Social Work & Social Sciences Review*, 19(1): 40-65, DOI: 10.1921/swssr.v19i1.1085

Chapter One

[1] Webb, J. and Bywaters, P. (2018) 'Austerity, rationing and inequity: trends in children's and young peoples' services expenditure in England between 2010 and 2015', *Local Government Studies*, https://www.tandfonline.com/doi/full/10.1080/03003930.2018.1430028?scroll=top&needAccess=true

[2] May, T. (2016) Statement from the new Prime Minister Theresa May, 13 July, https://www.gov.uk/government/speeches/statement-from-the-new-prime-minister-theresa-may

[3] Joseph Rowntree Foundation (2013) 'Poorer areas face £100 per head greater budget cuts compared to rich ones', 28 November, https://www.jrf.org.uk/press/poorer-areas-face-%C2%A3100-head-greater-budget-cuts-compared-rich-ones-%E2%80%93-jrf-report

[4] Elliot, L. (2014) 'If Osborne's plans are followed, public spending will shrink to 1930s levels', https://www.theguardian.com/uk-news/2014/dec/03/osborne-plans-public-spending-shrink-1930s

[5] Child Poverty Action Group (2017) 'Child poverty jumps to 4 million', www.cpag.org.uk/content/child-poverty-jumps-4-million

[6] Jones, R. (2013) 'How to privatise social work in six easy stages', https://www.theguardian.com/society/2013/nov/19/privatise-child-protection-michael-gove-social-workers.

[7] Department for Education (2014a) 'Powers to delegate children's social care functions', https://www.gov.uk/government/uploads/system/uploads/attachment_data/file/304660/Powers_to_Delegate_Con_Doc.pdf

[8] Jones, R. et al (2014) 'Child protection services too important to be privatised', https://www.theguardian.com/society/2014/may/16/child-protection-privatised

[8] Butler, P. (2014a) 'Privatise child protection services, Department for Education proposes', https://www.theguardian.com/society/2014/may/16/privatise-child-protection-services-department-for-education-proposes

[10] Butler (2014a) *op cit.*

[11] BBC (2014) 'Academics warn over child protection privatisation', www.bbc.co.uk/news/education27452457

[12] Department for Education (2014b) 'Consultation on powers to delegate social care functions; Government's response', https://www.gov.uk/government/uploads/system/uploads/attachment_data/file/321863/Extension_regs_consultation_response200614_for_web.pdf.

[13] Department for Education (2014b) *op cit*, p 6.

[14] Department for Education (2014b) *op cit*, p 8.

[15] Butler, P. (2014b) 'Government U-turn over privatising child protection services', 20 June, https://www.theguardian.com/society/2014/jun/20/government-climbdown-privatising-child-protection

[16] Department for Education (2014c) 'Explanatory Memorandum to the Children and Young Persons Act 2008 (Relevant Care Functions) Regulations 2014', www.legislation.gov.uk/uksi/2014/2407/pdfs/uksiem_20142407_en.pdf, p 2.

[17] Department for Education (2014c) *op cit*, p 2.

[18] McCabe, S. (2014) Debate on Draft Children and Young Persons Act 2008 (Relevant Care Functions) (England) Regulations 2014, *Hansard*, 3 September, https://publications.parliament.uk/pa/cm201415/cmgeneral/deleg4/140903/140903s01.htm

[19] Turner, A. (2014) '10 key arguments from the consultation on children's social work outsourcing',www.communitycare.co.uk/2014/06/09/10-key-arguments-consultation-outsourcing-childrens-social-work/

[20] Munn, M. (2014) 'Plans to allow outsourcing of child protection will put young people at risk', www.theguardian.com/society/2014/sep/02/outsource-child-protection-young-people-risk-rotherham

[21] *Hansard* (2014) Debate on Draft Children and Young Persons Act 2008 (Relevant Care Functions) (England) Regulations 2014, 3 September, https://publications.parliament.uk/pa/cm201415/cmgeneral/deleg4/140903/140903s01.htm.

[22] Lewell-Buck, E. (2014) Debate on Draft Children and Young Persons Act 2008 (Relevant Care Functions) (England) Regulations 2014, *Hansard*, 3 September, https://publications.parliament.uk/pa/cm201415/cmgeneral/deleg4/140903/140903s01.htm

23 Owen, J. (2017) 'Top-earning academy bosses revealed', https:// www.tes.com/news/exclusive-top-earning-academy-bosses-revealed

24 Donnelly, L. and Willis, A. (2009) 'Millions spent on NHS management consultants with Labour links', https://www. telegraph.co.uk/news/health/news/6073354/Millions-spent-on-NHS-management-consultants-with-Labour-links.html

25 Warner, N. (2013) 'Why I, a Labour peer, am supporting a regulated market for NHS competition', 23 April, https://www. theguardian.com/commentisfree/2013/apr/23/regulated-market-nhs-competition

26 Butler, P. (2014c) 'Outsourcing: government advisors finesse child protection "sales pitch"', 29 October, https://www. theguardian.com/society/patrick-butler-cuts-blog/2014/oct/29/ governement-advisors-finesse-child-protection-outsourcing-plans-market.

27 Department for Education (2014d) Children's Services Intervention Experts, 2 December, http://www.government-online.net/childrens-services-intervention-experts-department-education/.

28 Jones, R. (2015) 'Plans to privatise child protection are moving at pace', 12 January, https://www.theguardian.com/social-care-network/2015/jan/12/child-protection-privatisation-ray-jones

29 Market Research (2018) Children's Market Research and Industry Analysis, August, https://www.marketresearch.com/Marketing-Market-Research-70/Demographics-c81/Children-c938/

30 Mintel (2018) UK's Children's Social Care Market Report, February, https://store.mintel.com/uk-childrens-social-care-market-report

31 Donaghy, Baroness (2014) Lords Grand Committee debate on Deregulation Bill, Hansard, 18 November, https://www. publications.parliament.uk/pa/ld201415/ldhansrd/text/141118-gc0001.htm, col 116.

32 Donaghy (2014) op cit, cols 116–117.

33 Donaghy (2014) op cit, col 117.

34 Le Grand, J., Wood, A. and Trowler, I. (2014) *Report to the Secretary of State for Education and the Minister for Children and Families on Ways Forward for Children's Social Care Services in Birmingham*, February,

https://www.gov.uk/government/uploads/system/uploads/
attachment_data/file/297748/Birmingham_report _25.03.14.pdf

35 LaingBuisson, Cobic and Cicada (2016) *The Potential for Developing the Capacity and Diversity of Children's Social Care Services in England: Independent Research Report*, December, https://www.gov.uk/government/uploads/system/uploads/attachment_data/file/573035/LaingBuisson_repor t_December_2016.pdf, p 9.

36 Article 39 (2016) 'Secret report on future of children's services finally published', 2 December, http://www.article39.org.uk/news/2016/12/02/secret-report-on-future-of-childrens-services-finallypublished/

37 Department for Education (2016) 'Government response to LaingBuisson report on the potential for delivering the capacity and diversity of children's social care in England', December, https://www.gov.uk/government/uploads/system/uploads/attachment_data/file/574211/Govtresponse_to__LaingBuisson_report_December2016.pdf

38 Le Grand, J., Wood, A., and Gibb, M. (2013) *Report to the Secretary of State for Education on Ways Forward for Children's Services in Doncaster*, May, https://www.gov.uk/government/uploads/system/uploads/attachment_data/file/212598/Ways_forward_for_ children_s_services_in_Doncaster.pdf.

39 Butler, P. (2014d) 'Doncaster launches independent child protection company', 1 October, https://www.theguardian.com/society/2014/oct/01/doncaster-child-protection-company-launched

40 Butler (2014d) *op cit.*

41 Ofsted (2015) *Doncaster Metropolitan Borough Council Inspection of Services for Children in Need of Help and Protection, Children Looked After and Care Leavers, and Review of the Effectiveness of the Local Safeguarding Children Board*, https://reports.ofsted.gov.uk/sites/default/files/documents/local_authority_reports/doncaster/054_Single%20inspection%20of%20LA%20children%27s%20services%20and%20review%20of%20the%20LSCB%20as%20pdf.pdf

42 Ofsted (2106) Letter to Doncaster Council, 2 September, https://reports.ofsted.gov.uk/sites/default/files/documents/local_authority_reports/doncaster/055_Monitori ng%20visit%20of%20LA%20children%27s%20services%20as%20pdf.pdf

[43] Dudman, J. (2016) 'Jo Miller: "Councils can't take more shocks to an already shocked system"', 15 November, https://www. theguardian.com/society/2016/nov/15/jo-miller-doncaster-council-chief-executives-solace

[44] Butler (2014d) *op cit.*

[45] Stevenson, L. (2016) 'Council to outsource children's services to community interest company', 30 September, http://www. communitycare.co.uk/2016/09/30/council-outsource-childrens-services-community-interest-company/

[46] Whitfield, N. (2017), https://www.achievingforchildren.org.uk/about-us/senior-leadership-team/nickwhitfield/

[47] Jones, R. (2016) 'Six reasons to rethink moves to strip councils of children's services', 5 September.

[48] Turner, A. (2017) 'The new service models shaking up children's social work', 19 January, www.communitycare.co.uk/2017/01/19/new-service-models-shaking-childrens-social-work/

[49] Whitehead, M. (2016) 'Sunderland Council to transfer children's services to new company', 23 June, https://www.localgov.co.uk/Sunderland-Council-to-transfer-childrens-services-to-new-company/41113

[50] Rumney, E. (2016) 'Councils trapped by poor Ofsted ratings, say sector leaders', 9 March, www.publicfinance.co.uk/news/2016/03/councils-trapped-poor-ofsted-ratings-say-sector-leaders

[51] Jones, R. (2014) *The Story of Baby P: Setting the Record Straight*, Bristol, Policy Press.

[52] House of Commons Communities and Local Government Select Committee (2015) *Child sexual exploitation in Rotherham: Ofsted and further government issues*, https://publications.parliament.uk/pa/cm201415/cmselect/cmcomloc/1114/1114.pdf

[53] Butler, P. (2015) 'Outsourcing is the future for children's services', 15 December, https://www.theguardian.com/society/2015/dec/15/outsourcing-future-childrens-services

[54] Rumney (2016) *op cit.*

[55] Coughlan, S. (2013) 'Wilshaw's tough message on child protection services', 15 October, www.bbc.co.uk/news/education-24533502

[56] Brindle, D. (2009) 'Child welfare expert defiant over Ofsted criticism', 21 October, https://www.theguardian.com/society/2009/oct/21/ofsted-criticism-rejected

57 Butler, P. (2014e) 'Almost like a PLC: Northamptonshire sees the future of local government now', 18 December, https://www.theguardian.com/society/2014/dec/18/like-plc-northamptonshire-local-governmentfunding-cuts-council

58 Diver, T. (2018) 'Tory authority becomes first UK council in 20 years to impose emergency spending ban', 3 February, https://www.telegraph.co.uk/news/2018/02/03/spending-banned-cuts-force-firstuk-council-emergency-20-years/

59 *The Guardian* (2018) 'The Guardian view on council spending: a crisis unfolding', 4 February, https://www.theguardian.com/commentisfree/2018/feb/04/the-guardian-view-on-council-spending-a-crisis-unfolding

60 Purvis, K. (2018) 'Troubled council says grant released to help pay for adult social care will have "little impact": Adult social care service at Northamptonshire council "on the edge of unsafe", warns its director', 2 March, www.communitycare.co.uk/2018/03/02/troubled-council-says-grant-released-help-pay-adult-social-care-will-little-impact/

61 Gove, M. (2013) Michael Gove's Speech to the NSPCC, 12 November, https://www.gov.uk/government/speeches/getting-it-right-for-children-in-need-speech-to-the-nspcc

62 Randeep, R. (2013) 'Michael Gove on a quest to reform social work training', 12 November, https://www.theguardian.com/society/2013/nov/12/michael-gove-reform-social-work.

63 Gove (2013) *op cit.*

64 Paton, G. (2013) 'Michael Gove: many social workers "not up to the job"', 12 November, www.telegraph.co.uk/news/uknews/10442309/Michael-Gove-many-social-workers-not-up-to-the-job.html

65 Morris, N. (2013) 'Michael Gove: My life was transformed by social workers – but standards must improve', 12 November, www.independent.co.uk/news/uk/politics/michael-gove-my-life-wastransformed-by-social-workers-but-standards-must-improve-8933500.html

66 Cooper, J, (2013) 'Gove Slams Social Work Education', 12 November, www.communitycare.co.uk/2013/11/12/gove-slams-social-work-education/

67 Social Work Action Network (2014) 'In defence of social work: Why Michael Gove is wrong', February, Social Work Action Network pamphlet.

68 Stevenson, L. (2014) '"Social workers will not be sorry to see Gove go": Reactions to Cabinet reshuffle', 16 July, www.communitycare.co.uk/2014/07/16/adoption-frontline-outsourcing-michael-goves-legacy-childrens-social-care/

69 Timpson, E. (2011) 'Improving the adoption system will transform lives', 31 October, www.conservativehome.com/platform/2011/10/edward-timpson-mp-improving-the-adoption-system-will-transform-lives.html

70 Hill, A. (2011) 'Michael Gove relaunches adoption rules with attack on "ridiculous bureaucracy"', 22 February, https://www.theguardian.com/society/2011/feb/22/michael-gove-relaunches-adoption-rules

71 Jones, R. (2017) The Story of Baby P: Setting the Record Straight, updated edition, Bristol, Policy Press.

72 Richardson, H. (2013) 'More child protection takeovers ahead, Gove hints', 12 November, www.bbc.co.uk/news/education-24904031

73 Puffett, N. (2013) 'Reform proposals for social work are "privatisation through the back door"', 26 November, www.cypnow.co.uk/cyp/analysis/1140717/reform-proposals-for-social-work-are-privatisation-through-the-back-door

74 Holehouse, M. (2015) 'David Cameron: social workers must use "common sense" to tackle child abuse', 3 March, www.telegraph.co.uk/news/uknews/law-and-order/11447851/David-Cameron-social-workers-must-use-common-sense-to-tackle-child-abuse.html

75 Department for Education (2015) 'PM: We will not stand by – failing children's services will be taken over', 14 December, https://www.gov.uk/government/news/pm-we-will-not-stand-by-failing-childrens-services-will-be-taken-over

76 Cameron, D. (2015) 'My vision for a smarter state', 11 September, https://www.gov.uk/government/speeches/prime-minister-my-vision-for-a-smarter-state

77 Jones, R. (2015) 'Hedge funds have no place in children's services', 17 September, https://www.theguardian.com/social-

care-network/2015/sep/17/hedge-funds-no-place-childrens-services-market

78   Butler (2015) *op cit.*

79   Elvin, A. (2016a) 'Charities can't just be a critical friend – they should be involved in running children's services', 31 March, www.communitycare.co.uk/2016/03/31/charities-cant-just-critical-friend-involved-running-childrens-services/

80   Elvin, A. (2016b) 'Government opposes profits from child protection – why not from care?', 18 July, http://www.communitycare.co.uk/2016/07/18/government-opposes-profits-child-protection-care/

81   Elvin, A. (2016c) 'Stop treating adoption as the only option for children in care', 1 June, https://www.theguardian.com/social-care-network/2015/jun/01/stop-treating-adoption-as-only-option-for-children-in-care.

82   Elvin, A. (2016d) 'Children in foster care aren't waiting for a loving home – they are already in one', 31 March, https://www.theguardian.com/social-care-network/2016/mar/31/foster-care-nicky-morgan-adoption

83   Elvin, A. (2016e) 'New reforms might just be what social workers and children want – and need', 20 May, www.communitycare.co.uk/2016/05/20/new-reforms-might-just-social-workers-children-want-need/.

84   Elvin, A. (2015) 'Why fear charity involvement in children's social care?', 2 February, https://www.theguardian.com/social-care-network/2015/feb/02/child-protection-privatisation-charities-social-care

85   Virgin Care (2017) 'More than 300 health and social carte services with a difference', http://www.virgincare.co.uk/

86   Department for Education (2016) *Putting Children First: Delivering our vision for excellent children's social care*, July, https://www.gov.uk/government/uploads/system/uploads/attachment_data/file/554573/Putting_children_first_delivering_vision_excellent_childrens_social_care.pdf

87   Stevenson, L. (2016) 'Third of children's services to be "new models" by 2020, government hopes', 5 July, www.communitycare.co.uk/2016/07/05/third-childrens-services-new-models-2020-government-hopes/

88 Butler, P. (2016) 'Labour fears potential privatisation of child protection services', 13 June, https://www.theguardian.com/society/2016/jun/13/labour-fears-potential-privatisation-of-child-protection-services

89 Willow, C. et al (2016) 'Bill puts children's social care at risk', 13 June, https://www.theguardian.com/society/2016/jun/13/bill-puts-childrens-social-care-at-risk

Chapter Two

1 McNicoll, A. and Stevenson, L. (2016) 'Five things social workers need to know about the Children and Social Work Bill', 24 May, www.communitycare.co.uk/2016/05/24/five-things-social-workers-need-know-children-social-work-bill/

2 House of Lords (2017) Debate on Children and Social Work Bill, *Hansard*, 4 April, https://hansard.parliament.uk/lords/2017-0404/debates/B954F5D8-3021-4F93-BA5F-64936118F9FB/ChildrenAndSocialWorkBill

3 Stone, J. (2016) 'Tax credits, disability benefit and nine other U-turns from the first year of a Conservative government', 7 May, www.independent.co.uk/news/uk/politics/tory-conservative-u-turns-policies-david-cameron-benefit-cuts-junior-doctors-academies-a7018276.html

4 LBC (2017) 'As the Chancellor abandons his plan to increase National Insurance Contributions, here is a full list of Theresa May's U-turns during her time at 10 Downing Street', 15 March, http://www.lbc.co.uk/politics/parties/conservatives/theresa-may/theresas-u-turns-key-tory-policy-reversals/

5 Mortimer, C. (2017) 'Child refugees U-turn: Children's Commissioners express "deep concern" over end to Dubs scheme', 15 February, www.independent.co.uk/news/uk/politics/child-refugee-u-turn-dubsamendment-migrant-crisis-alfred-dubs-amendment-a7582711.html

6 Watson, Lord (2016) Children and Social Work Bill, House of Lords Third Reading, *Hansard*, 23 November, https://hansard.parliament.uk/Lords/2016-11-23/debates/BB25F1B0-3E07-446C-97EA-BDFADAD7B300/ChildrenAndSocialWorkBill(HL)

7 Lewell-Buck, E. (2016) Children and Social Work Bill (Lords) First Sitting, *Hansard*, 13 December, https://hansard.parliament.uk/commons/2016-12-13/debates/2fc34fb5-1900-

488f-bb5acb7a94ac25ef/ChildrenAndSocialWorkBill(Lords) (FirstSitting)

8   House of Lords (2016) Children and Social Work Bill (Lords) Third Sitting, *Hansard*, 15 December, https://hansard. parliament.uk/commons/2016-12-15/debates/92b61aa5-249d-4cdc-a26e2e2149c3bdfe/ChildrenAndSocialWorkBill(Lords) (ThirdSitting)

9   House of Lords (2016) Children and Social Work Bill (Lords) First Sitting, *Hansard*, 13 December, https://hansard. parliament.uk/commons/2016-12-13/debates/2fc34fb5-1900-488f-bb5acb7a94ac25ef/ChildrenAndSocialWorkBill(Lords) (FirstSitting)

10 Ramsbotham, Lord (2016) Debate on Children and Social Work Bill, *Hansard*, 8 November, https://hansard.parliament. uk/lords/2016-11-08/debates/5ABC82B8-3486-474C-8A9A9445BBCD382E/ChildrenAndSocialWorkBill(HL)

11 Jones, R. (2016) 'Giving power over social work to a cuts-obsessed government is a mistake', 8 September, https://www.theguardian. com/social-care-network/2016/sep/08/giving-power-over-social-work-to-a-cuts-obsessed-government-is-a-mistake

12 Together for Children (2017), https://togetherforchildren. wordpress.com/

13 Action for Children and the NSPCC (2016) 'Statement on Children and Social Work Bill: Powers to test new ways of working: Second Reading', 5 December 2016, https://www. actionforchildren.org.uk/resources-and-publications/reports/ children-and-social-work-bill/

14 NSPCC (2017) 'Major success in the fight to keep children safe', 14 March, https://www.nspcc.org.uk/whatwe-do/news-opinion/ major-success-fight-keep-children-safe/.

15 Royal College of Paediatrics and Child Health (2017) 'Written evidence submitted by the Royal College of Paediatrics and Child Health (CSWB 06) Children and Social Work Bill [Lords] House of Commons Public Bill Committee', https://www.publications. parliament.uk/pa/cm201617/cmpublic/ChildrenSocialWork/ memo/CSWB06.htm

16 National Children's Bureau (2016) 'Children and Social Work Bill: NCB briefing for the second reading in the House of Commons', 5 December, https://www.ncb.org.uk/sites/default/files/uploads/

Children%20and%20Social%20Work%20Bill%20NCB%20se
cond%20reading%20briefing%20Commons.pdf

17 Willow, C. (and 17 others) (2016) 'Bill puts children's social care
    at risk', 13 June, https://www.theguardian.com/society/2016/
    jun/13/bill-puts-childrens-social-care-at-risk

18 Shennan, G., Allen, R., Featherstone, B., Baron, S., Lavalette, M.,
    Robb, B. and Egan, M. (2016) 'Troubling clauses in children and
    social work bill that should be deleted', Letter, *The Guardian*, 5 July,
    https://www.theguardian.com/society/2016/jul/05/troubling-
    clauses-in-children-and-social-work-bill-that-should-be-deleted

19 Amiss, C., Neale, A., Longstaff, L., Lopez, N. and Sparrow,
    K. (2016) Family support at risk from children's bill, Letter,
    The Guardian, 25 October, https://www.theguardian.com/
    society/2016/oct/25/family-support-at-risk-from-childrens-bill

20 Webb, S. (2017) '"Flexible" arrangements in social work bill may
    endanger children', Letter, *The Guardian*, 11 January, https://www.
    theguardian.com/society/2017/jan/11/flexible-arrangements-in-
    social-work-bill-may-endanger-children

21 Simmonds, J. (2017) 'Children and Social Work Bill could end the
    law as we know it', Letter, *The Guardian*, 10 January, https://www.
    theguardian.com/social-care-network/2017/jan/10/children-
    social-work-bill-end-law

22 Association of Lawyers for Children (2017) 'Child protection',
    Letter, *The Times*, 22 February, http://alc.org.uk/uploads/
    Times_letter_22_Feb_17.pdf

23 38 Degrees (2017) Protect the Rights of Vulnerable Children and
    Care Leavers, https://you.38degrees.org.uk/petitions/protect-
    the-rights-of-vulnerable-children-and-care-leavers

24 Tickle, L. (2016) 'Social workers in fierce row over children's
    bill', 18 October, https://www.theguardian.com/society/2016/
    oct/18/social-workers-fierce-row-childrens-bill.

25 Local Government Association (2017) 'LGA briefing: Children
    and Social Work Bill', http://www.local.gov.uk/briefings-and-
    responses/-/journal_content/56/10180/7858314/ARTICLE

26 McNicoll, A. (2016) 'Scrapping red tape or safeguards? The
    fight for the future of children's services', 13 October, http://
    www.communitycare.co.uk/2016/10/13/scrapping-red-tape-
    safeguards-fight-future-childrens-services/

27 Tickle (2016) *op cit.*

28 Puffett, N. (2017) 'ADCS president speaks out in favour of "exemption clause"', 14 February, https://www.cypnow.co.uk/ cyp/news/2003174/childrens-services-leader-speaks-out-in-favour-of-exemption-clause

29 McNicoll (2016) *op cit.*

30 Elvin, A. (2016) 'Children and Social Work Bill gives workforce a chance to shape services', 18 July, https://www.theguardian.com/ social-care-network/2016/jul/18/children-and-social-work-bill-workforce-services

31 Heyes, D. (2016) 'Government to establish expert panel to vet "exemption clause" bids', 14 October, www.cypnow.co.uk/ print_article/cyp/news/2002595/government-to-establish-expert-panel-to-vetexemption-clause-bids?print=true

32 Jones, R. (2017) 'Submission to the House of Commons Children and Social Work Bill Public Bills Committee', reproduced online at https://togetherforchildren.files.wordpress.com/2016/09/ equal-protection-under-the-law-for-vulnerable-children-and-young-people-9-feb-2017.pdf

33 Stevenson, L. (2017) 'Controversial exemption powers reinstated to social work bill', 10 January, www.communitycare. co.uk/2017/01/10/controversial-exemption-powers-reinstated-social-work-bill/

34 Watson, Lord (2016) Debate on Children and Social Work Bill, *Hansard*, 8 November, https://hansard.parliament. uk/lords/2016-11-08/debates/5ABC82B8-3486-474C-8A9A9445BBCD382E/ChildrenAndSocialWorkBill(HL)

35 Lewell-Buck, E. (2017) Debate on Children and Social Work Bill (Lords) Fifth Sitting, https://hansard.parliament.uk/ commons/2017-01-10/debates/e6e84821-8912-41b2-b4a0-0850e1a4adf1/ChildrenAndSocialWorkBill(Lords)(FifthSitting)

36 Richardson, H. (2017) 'Ministers' U-turn over "bonfire of children's rights"', 2 March, www.bbc.co.uk/news/education-39143396

37 Timpson, E. (2017) 'Oral Answers to questions – Education – in the House of Commons at 1200 am on 20 March 2017', https://www. theyworkforyou.com/debates/?id=2017-03-20a.636.3#g637.6. a.636.3#g637.6https017-03-20a.636.3#g637.6 Questions 12:00 n

38 Laming, Lord (2003) *The Victoria Climbié Inquiry: Report of an inquiry by Lord Laming*, 28 January, https://www.gov.uk/

government/publications/the-victoria-climbie-inquiry-report-of-an-inquiry-by-lord-laming

39   Munro, E. (2011) *Munro Review of Child Protection: Final report – a child-centred system*, 10 May, https://www.gov.uk/government/publications/munro-review-of-child-protection-final-report-a-child-centred-system

40   McNicoll, A. (2017) 'Munro withdraws backing for "dangerous" social care exemptions plan', 10 February, www.communitycare.co.uk/2017/02/10/munro-withdraws-backing-dangerous-social-care-exemption-plan

41   McNicoll, A. (2016) 'Munro backs controversial "innovation" clause in social work bill', 30 June, www.communitycare.co.uk/2016/06/30/munro-backs-controversial-innovation-clause-socialwork-bill/

42   Timpson, E. (2107) Debate on Children and Social Work Bill (Lords) Sixth Sitting, *Hansard*, 10 January, https://hansard.parliament.uk/commons/2017-01-10/debates/501792ec-66bb-4aad-a05f117e43c35b6c/ChildrenAndSocialWorkBill(Lords)(SixthSitting)

43   Reyes, E. (2017) 'Government U-turn on Children's Rights', 6 March, *Law Society Gazette*, http://directories.lawgazette.co.uk/news/government-u-turn-on-childrens-rights/5060825.fullarticle

44   Tunstill, J. and Willow, C. (2018) 'Professional social work and the defence of children's and their families' rights in a period of austerity: A case study', *Social Work & Social Sciences Review* 19(1), https://www.kcl.ac.uk/sspp/policy-institute/scwru/mrc/MRC-News/info/swssr19onetunstillwillow4meeting.pdf

45   Youth Justice Improvement Board (2017) 'Findings and Recommendations of the Youth Custody Improvement Board', www.statewatch.org/news/2017/feb/uk-youth-custody-improvementboard-report-24-2-17.pdf, pp 6-7

46   Youth Justice Improvement Board (2017) *op cit.*

47   Stephenson, J. (2017) 'Inspections: Local Safeguarding Children Boards', April, http://www.cypnow.co.uk/cyp/good-practice/2003504/inspections-local-safeguarding-children-boards

48   Wood, A. (2016) 'Review of the role and functions of Local Safeguarding Children Boards', https://www.gov.uk/government/publications/wood-review-of-local-safeguarding-children-boards, p 7.

49   Puffett, N. (2016) 'Concern over implications of "profound" safeguarding reforms', May, www.cypnow. co.uk/cyp/news/1157496/concern-over-implications-of%E2%80%98profound%E2%80%99-safeguarding-reforms

50   HM Government (2003) *Independent Report: The Victoria Climbié Inquiry: Report of an Inquiry by Lord Laming*, 28 January, Cm 5730, https://assets.publishing.service.gov.uk/government/uploads/system/uploads/attachment_data/file/273183/5730.pdf

51   HM Government (2015) *Working Together to Safeguard Children*, Chapter 3: Local Safeguarding Children Boards, March, /www.workingtogetheronline.co.uk/chapters/chapter_three.html.

52   HM Government (1974) *Report of the Committee of Inquiry into the Care and Supervision provided by Local Authorities and Other Agencies in relation to Maria Colwell and the Co-ordination between them*, London, HMSO.

53   Scorer, R. (2017) 'The government is jeopardising progress on child sexual exploitation', 25 April, https://www.theguardian.com/social-care-network/2017/apr/25/the-government-is-jeopardising-progresson-child-sexual-exploitation

54   Jones, R. (2018) 'The UK child protection system is laudable. Why risk it with reform?', 14 March, https://www.theguardian.com/social-care-network/2018/mar/14/the-uk-child-protection-system-is-laudable-why-risk-it-with-reform

55   Pidd, H. (2013) 'Hamzah Khan: Minister's dismay as report fails to point finger', 13 November, https://www.theguardian.com/society/2013/nov/13/hamzha-khan-ministers-dismay-report

56   Stevenson, L. (2014) 'Serious case reviews "disturbingly variable" in quality, finds expert panel', 31 July, www.communitycare.co.uk/2014/07/31/serious-case-reviews-disturbingly-variable-quality-finds-report/

57   National Panel of Independent Experts on Serious Case Reviews (2014) First Annual Report, July, https://assets.publishing.service.gov.uk/government/uploads/system/uploads/attachment_data/file/474652/First_report_Serious_Case_Review_Panel.pdf

58   Stevenson (2014) *op cit*.

59   Rawlings, A., Paliokosta, P., Maisey, D., Johnson, J., Capstick, J. and Jones, R. (2014) 'Study to investigate the barriers to learning from Serious Case Reviews (SCRs) and identify ways of overcoming these barriers', July, https://www.gov.

uk/government/uploads/system/uploads/attachment_data/
file/331658/RR340.pdf

60 Children and Social Work Act 2017, s 13.

61 Association of Independent LSCB Chairs (2017) 'Written
    Evidence submitted by the Association of Independent LSCB
    Chairs (CSWB 44), Children and Social Work Bill [Lords],
    House of Commons Public Bill Committee', January, https://
    www.publications.parliament.uk/pa/cm201617/cmpublic/
    childrensocialwork/memo/cswb44.htm

62 House of Commons Education Select Committee (2016)
    'Appointment of Her Majesty's Chief Inspector of Education,
    Children's Services and Skills', July, https://www.publications.
    parliament.uk/pa/cm201617/cmselect/cmeduc/170/17004.htm

63 Espinoza, J. (2016) 'Ofsted chairman quits after Isle of Wight
    "inbreeding" comments', August, http://www.telegraph.co.uk/
    education/2016/08/23/ofsted-chairman-quits-after-isle-of-
    wights-inbreedingcomments/

64 Association of Independent LSCB Chairs (2107) *op cit*.

65 Department for Education (2018) 'Members announced for the
    new Child Safeguarding Practice Review Panel', 7 June, https://
    www.gov.uk/government/news/members-announced-for-new-
    child-safeguarding-practice-review-panel

66 Lord Nash (2017) Debate on Children and Social Work
    Bill (HL), *Hansard*, 4 April, https://hansard.parliament.uk/
    lords/2017-04-04/debates/B954F5D8-3021-4F93-BA5F-
    64936118F9FB/ChildrenAndSocialWorkBill

67 McNicoll, A. (2017) 'Government "best placed" to improve
    social work, says minister', 11 April, www.communitycare.
    co.uk/2017/04/11/government-best-placed-improve-social-
    work-says-minister/

68 Social Work Task Force (2009) *Building a Safe and
    Confident Future: The Final Report of the Social Work Task
    Force*, November, http://webarchive.nationalarchives.gov.
    uk/20130321034206/https://www.education.gov.uk/
    publications/eOrderingDownload/01114-2009DOM-EN.pdf

69 Bamford, T. (2015) *A Contemporary History of Social Work*, Bristol,
    Policy Press, p 167.

70 McNicoll, A. (2016) 'Read: The report that triggered College
    of Social Work closure', 15 July, www.communitycare.

co.uk/2016/07/15/read-report-triggered-college-social-work-closure/

71 McNicoll, A. (2015) 'College of Social Work faced £240,000 annual deficit before closure, leaked report reveals', 22 June, www.communitycare.co.uk/2015/06/22/college-social-work-faced-240000-annual-deficit-closure-leaked-report-reveals/

72 Department for Education and Department for Health (2016) Regulating Social Workers Policy Statement, June, http://data.parliament.uk/DepositedPapers/Files/DEP2016-0569/Policy_Statement_Social_Work_Regulation_June_2016.pdf

73 Secretary of State for Health (1998) *Modernising Social Services: Promoting independence, improving protection, raising standards*, November, http://webarchive.nationalarchives.gov.uk/20130107105354/http://www.archive.officialdocuments.co.uk/document/cm41/4169/4169.htm

74 Burt, A. (2016) 'General Social Care Council: Written question – 30718', 10 March, www.parliament.uk/business/publications/written-questions-answers-statements/writtenquestion/Commons/2016-03-10/30718/

75 Romeo, L. and Trowler, I. (2016) 'Chief social workers: Closer link with government will benefit profession: Lyn Romeo and Isabelle Trowler explain why they feel bringing social work regulation closer to government is the right model', June, www.communitycare.co.uk/2016/06/30/chief-social-workers-closer-link-government-will-benefit-profession/

76 McNicoll, A. (2016) 'Trowler: New regulator for social workers "controversial but essential"', 8 July, www.communitycare.co.uk/2016/07/08/trowler-new-regulator-social-workers-controversial-essential/

77 Trowler, I. (2015) 'Social work needs to earn back public trust', 28 July, https://www.theguardian.com/socialcare-network/2015/jul/28/isabelle-trowler-social-work-public-trust-criminal-wilful-neglect

78 Butler, P. (2016) 'Ray Jones: "Social work is under real threat"', 20 July, https://www.theguardian.com/society/2016/jul/20/ray-jones-social-work-threat-childrens-services-privatisation

79 McNicoll, A. (2016) 'Government to regulate social workers from 2018: new social work body will be government executive agency accountable to the education secretary', 29 June, www.

communitycare.co.uk/2016/06/29/government-regulate-social-workers-2018/

80 British Association of Social Workers (2017) 'Children and Social Work Bill: Nine out of ten social workers want an independent regulator for the profession and unequivocal protection of children's rights', January, https://www.basw.co.uk/news/article/?id=1343

81 McNicoll, A. (2016) 'Directors oppose plan for government-controlled social work regulator: Children's services bosses and local government leaders say the new social work body planned by government must be independent', 12 July, www.communitycare.co.uk/2016/07/12/directors-oppose-plan-government-controlled-social-work-regulator/

82 Stevenson, L. (2017) 'Understanding of social work is desirable but not essential for new regulator chief, job ad says', 6 December, www.communitycare.co.uk/2017/12/06/understanding-social-work-desirable-essential-new-regulator-chief/

83 McNicoll, A. (2016) 'Government makes U-turn on plan to control new social work regulator', 20 October, www.communitycare.co.uk/2016/10/20/government-makes-u-turn-plans-control-new-social-work-regulator/

84 Thoburn, J., Featherstone, B. and Morris, K. (2017) 'The future of social work education in universities is under threat', 7 March, www.communitycare.co.uk/2017/03/07/future-social-work-education-universities-threat/

85 Association of Directors of Children's Services (2016) *ADCS Position Statement: The Assessment and Accreditation of Three New Social Work Statuses*, May, http://adcs.org.uk/assets/documentation/ADCS_Position_Statement_The_Assessment_and_Accreditation_of _Three_New_Social_Work_Statuses.pdf

86 Forrester, D. (2016) 'We need to talk about social work education …', 2 August, www.communitycare.co.uk/2016/08/02/need-talk-social-work-education/

87 House of Commons Education Select Committee (2016) *Social Work Reform*, July, https://www.publications.parliament.uk/pa/cm201617/cmselect/cmeduc/201/201.pdf

88 Forrester (2016) *op cit.*

89 White, S., Featherstone, B., Tunstill, J., Gupta, A. and Morris, K. (2013) 'Our concerns over social work training', 15 September,

https://www.theguardian.com/education/2013/sep/15/ concerns-social-work-training.

90   Brindle, D. (2015) 'As fast-track social work training goes north, can it win over its detractors?', 28 October, https://www.theguardian.com/society/2015/oct/28/fast-track-social-work-training-north-east-frontline

91   Smith, A. (2014) 'Teach First or Business First?', in Social Work Action Network, *op cit*, pp 42–43.

92   Cardy, S. (2014) 'Tax avoidance specialists handed teaching role on social work MA course', 7 September, www.socialworkfuture.org/articles-resources/uk-articles/23-tax-avoidance-specialists-teaching-social-workers

93   Frontline (2017) 'Meet Our Team', www.thefrontline.org.uk/about-frontline/meet-our-team

94   Stevenson, L. (2017) 'Union intervenes to try to save social work degrees', 30 May, www.communitycare.co.uk/2017/05/30/union-intervenes-try-save-social-work-degrees/

95   McNicoll, A. (2016) 'Government announces social work bursary allocations', 5 August, www.communitycare.co.uk/2016/08/05/government-announces-social-work-bursary-allocations/

96   McNicoll, A. (2016) 'Government "looking at" scrapping social work bursaries', 25 January, www.communitycare.co.uk/2016/01/25/government-looking-scrapping-social-work-bursaries/

97   McNicoll, A. (2016) 'Social work course closures "alarming"', 21 June, www.communitycare.co.uk/2016/06/21/social-work-course-closures-alarming/

98   Labour Party (2017) *For the Many Not the Few*, www.labour.org.uk/page/-/Images/manifesto2017/Labour%20Manifesto%202017.pdf, p 86.

99   Munro (2011) *op cit*.

100   Munro, E., quoted in Fox, C. (2008) 'A needle in a haystack', 8 December, https://www.localgov.co.uk/Aneedle-in-a-haystack/23796

101   Narey, Sir M. (2014) *Making the Education of Social Workers Consistently Effective: Report of Sir Martin Narey's independent review of the education of children's social workers*, January, https://www.gov.uk/government/uploads/system/uploads/attachment_data/

file/287756/Making_the_education_of_social_workers_
consistently_effective.pdf

102 Croisdale-Appleby, D. (2014) *Re-visioning Social Work Education: An Independent Review*, February, https://www.gov.uk/government/uploads/system/uploads/attachment_data/file/285788/DCA_Accessible.pdf

103 British Association of Social Workers (2014) 'Croisdale-Appleby report combines academic rigour with deep understanding of the social work profession', February, https://www.basw.co.uk/news/article/?id=681

104 Butler, P. (2014) 'Trainee social workers taught too much theory, says report', February, https://www.theguardian.com/society/2014/feb/13/trainee-social-workers-taught-theory

105 McNicoll, A. (2017) 'Frontline graduates face restrictions on practising outside of England', 3 April, www.communitycare.co.uk/2017/04/03/frontline-graduates-face-restrictions-practising-outsideengland/

106 Stevenson, L. (2015) 'It is time to split adults' and children's social work education, says Martin Narey', 10 July, www.communitycare.co.uk/2015/07/10/time-split-adults-childrens-social-work-education-says-martin-narey/

107 Cutmore, M. and Roger, J. (2016) 'Comparing the costs of social work qualification routes', https://www.gov.uk/government/uploads/system/uploads/attachment_data/file/510361/DFE-RR517-Socialwork-qualification-routes-comparing_the_costs.pdf

108 Department for Education (2015) 'Knowledge and skills statements for child and family social work', 19 November, https://www.gov.uk/government/publications/knowledge-and-skills-statements-for-child-and-family-social-work

109 Department for Health (2014) 'Knowledge and skills for social workers in adult services', 10 October, https://consultations.dh.gov.uk/social-care-workforce/knowledge-and-skills-statement-for-social-work-wit/

110 Jones, R. (2015) 'Social work needs a strong independent voice at this time of rapid change', 14 September, *Locum Today*.

111 Morgan, N. (2016) 'Delivering a revolution in children's social care', 14 January, https://www.gov.uk/government/speeches/nicky-morgan-delivering-a-revolution-in-childrens-social-care

112 Silman, J. (2016) 'Children's social workers and compulsory accreditation: what we do and don't know', 19 January, www.communitycare.co.uk/2016/01/19/childrens-social-workers-compulsory-accreditation-know-dont-know/

113 Schraer, R. (2015) 'KPMG and Morning Lane Associates expected to develop pass or fail test for children's social workers', 18 March, www.communitycare.co.uk/2015/03/18/kmpg-morning-lane-associates-expected-develop-pass-fail-test-childrens-social-workers/

114 British Association of Social Workers (2017) 'RiP/RiPfA to be BASW's partner to refresh the Professional Capabilities Framework', 12 May, https://www.basw.co.uk/news/article/?id=1438

115 Policy Communications (2017) 'Transforming Children's Social Care: a national policy conference', 28 April, www.policycommunications.co.uk/events/childsocialcare/programme.html.

116 Department for Education (2016) 'Confidence in practice: child and family social work assessment and accreditation system: Government consultation', 20 December, https://consult.education.gov.uk/social-workreform-unit/naas-consultation/supporting_documents/NAAS_consultation_WEB_FINAL_20170114.pdf

117 McNicoll, A. (2017) '"Flawed" accreditation plans risk social workers quitting', 17 March, www.communitycare.co.uk/2017/03/17/flawed-accreditation-plans-risk-social-workers-quitting/

118 McNicoll, A. (2017) 'Social workers fear being "unfairly penalised" by accreditation tests', 4 April, www.communitycare.co.uk/2017/04/04/social-workers-fear-unfairly-penalised-accreditation-tests/

119 Association of Directors of Children's Services (2016) *ADCS Position Statement: The Assessment and Accreditation of Three New Social Work Statuses*, 9 May, http://adcs.org.uk/assets/documentation/ADCS_Position_Statement_The_Assessment_and_Accreditation_of_Three_New_Social_Work_Statuses.pdf

120 McNicoll, A. (2017) 'Social worker accreditation scheme "poor value", directors warn', 14 March, www.communitycare.co.uk/2017/03/14/social-worker-accreditation-scheme-poor-value-directors-warn/

121 Michalska, A. (2017) 'Change the narrative on social work', *Children and Young People Now*, May, p 29.

122 Carter, R. (2017) 'ADASS president warns against splitting social work into "factions"', 12 May, www.communitycare. co.uk/2017/05/12/adass-president-warns-splitting-social-work-factions/

123 Brown, D. (2016) 'What's it like facing the government's accreditation test? A social worker's story: A social worker speaks about his experience when he sat the accreditation test for children's social workers', 5 May, www.communitycare. co.uk/2016/05/05/like-accredited-social-workers-story/

124 Department for Education (2016) 'Confidence in practice: child and family social work assessment and accreditation system: Equality impact assessment', December, https://consult.education. gov.uk/social-workreform-unit/naas-consultation/supporting_ documents/NAAS_

125 McNicoll, A. (2016) 'One fifth of social workers failed accreditation pilot role play', 7 July, www.communitycare.co.uk/2016/07/07/ one-fifth-social-workers-failed-accreditation-pilot/

126 McNicoll, A. (2016) *op cit*.

127 House of Commons Education Select Committee (2016) *Social Work Reform: Third Report of the Session 2016-2017*, 6 July, https:// www.publications.parliament.uk/pa/cm201617/cmselect/ cmeduc/201/201.pdf

128 House of Commons (2017) Debate on Children and Social Work Bill (Lords) Sixth Sitting, *Hansard*,10 January, https://hansard. parliament.uk/commons/2017-01-10/debates/501792ec-66bb-4aad-a05f117e43c35b6c/ChildrenAndSocialWorkBill(Lords) (SixthSitting)

129 McNicoll, A. (2017) 'Accreditation climb down means just 4% of social workers will be tested by 2020', 17 July, www. communitycare.co.uk/2017/07/17/accreditation-climbdown-means-just-four-per-cent-social-workers-will-tested-2020/

130 Department for Education (2017) 'Confidence in practice: child and family social work assessment and accreditation system', December, https://assets.publishing.service.gov.uk/government/ uploads/system/uploads/attachment_data/file/680351/ Confidence_in_practice_-_Government_consultation_response. pdf

Chapter Three

1 Tickle, L. (2016) 'Social workers in fierce row over Children and Social Work Bill', October, https://www.theguardian.com/society/2016/oct/18/social-workers-fierce-row-childrens-bill

2 McNicoll, A. (2016) 'Government makes U-turn on plan to control new social work regulator', October, www.communitycare.co.uk/2016/10/20/government-makes-u-turn-plans-control-new-social-work-regulator/

3 House of Commons Education Select Committee (2016) *Social Work Reform*, July, para 22, www.publications.parliament.uk/pa/cm201617/cmselect/cmeduc/201/201.pdf

4 Department for Education (2018) *Social work post-qualifying standards: knowledge and skills statements*, https://www.gov.uk/government/uploads/system/uploads/attachment_data/file/338718/140730_Knowledge _and_skills_statement_final_version_AS_RH_Checked.pdf

5 British Association of Social Workers (2018) *Professional Capabilities Framework*, https://www.basw.co.uk/pcf/

6 McNicoll, A. (2015) 'Trowler defends £2 million KPMG contract for social worker accreditation', 21 August, www.communitycare.co.uk/2015/08/21/trowler-defends-2m-kpmg-contract-social-worker-accreditation/

7 McNicoll, A. and Schraer, R. (2015) 'College of Social Work to close due to lack of funds', 18 June, http://www.communitycare.co.uk/2015/06/18/college-social-work-close-due-lack-funds/

8 McNicoll, A. (2016) 'Time to put myths about the College of Social Work closure to bed', 14 July, http://www.communitycare.co.uk/2016/07/14/time-put-myths-college-social-work-closure-bed/

9 @IsabelleTrowler 30 June 2014.

10 Trowler, I. (2015) 'Social work needs to earn back public trust', 28 July, https://www.theguardian.com/social-care-network/2015/jul/28/isabelle-trowler-social-work-public-trust-criminal-wilful-neglect

11 McNicoll, A. (2016) 'Trowler: New regulator for social workers "controversial but essential"', 8 July,, www.communitycare.co.uk/2016/07/08/trowler-new-regulator-social-workers-controversial-essential/

12 Brindle, D. (2013) 'Frontline's founder: "Social work needs life-changing professionals"', 11 September, https://www.theguardian.com/society/2013/sep/11/josh-macalister-social-work-frontline

13 https://twitter.com/isabelletrowler/status/713070175474593792

14 McNicoll, A. (2016) 'Leadership programme re-ignited my passion for social work', 10 November, https://www.communitycare.co.uk/2016/11/10/leadership-training-re-ignited-passion-social-work/

15 Frontline (2018) Mary Jackson, https://thefrontline.org.uk/team-members/mary-jackson/

16 Schraer, R. (2015) 'Sector fears Trowler's agenda undermining reform efforts as Morning Lane set to develop pass/fail test', 26 March, www.communitycare.co.uk/2015/03/26/plans-to-outsource-social-work-accreditation-met-with-concern-from-sector/

17 National Audit Office (2016) 'Investigation: The Department's management of a potential conflict of interest', 26 October, https://www.nao.org.uk/wp-content/uploads/2016/10/11298-001-Conflicts-of-interest-at-DoE.pdf

18 Puffett, N. (2016) 'Trowler firm made £2.9m from DfE contracts, probe finds', 25 October, https://www.cypnow.co.uk/cyp/news/2002664/trowler-firm-made-gbp29m-from-dfe-contracts-probe-finds

19 Department for Education (2015) *Children's Social Care Services Advice, Support and Challenge*, https://www.contractsfinder.service.gov.uk/Notice/9759d127-8539-4ad2-a111-fa68aa97b809

20 Schraer, R. (2015) 'KPMG and Morning Lane Associates expected to develop pass or fail test for social workers', 18 March, www.communitycare.co.uk/2015/03/18/kmpg-morning-lane-associates-expected-develop-pass-fail-test-childrens-social-workers/

21 Morning Lane Associates (2018) Steve Goodman, http://morninglane.org/our-people/

22 Companies House (2017) Morning Lane Associates Limited Unaudited Abbreviated Accounts for Year Ended 30 September 2016.

23 Companies House (2015) Annual return Morning Lane Associates Limited, 6 October

24 Goodman, S. (2017) @Morning_Lane, 5.54 am, 14 October.

25 *The Guardian* (2014) 'Queen's birthday honours list: 2014', 13 June, https://www.theguardian.com/uk-news/2014/jun/13/queensbirthday-honours-obe

26 Government UK (undated) Alan Wood, https://assets.publishing.service.gov.uk/government/uploads/system/uploads/attachment_data/file/424936/Alan_Wood.pdf

27 Lepper, J. (2018) 'Former ADCS president receives knighthood', 2 January, https://www.cypnow.co.uk/cyp/news/2004709/former-adcs-president-receives-knighthood

28 Goodman, S. and Trowler, I. (eds) (2011) *Social Work Reclaimed*, London, Jessica Kingsley.

29 Carter, R. (2014) '"Hackney model" consultants to work in partnership with DfE to reduce bureaucracy: Morning Lane Associates plan to reduce social work bureaucracy in five local authorities by 20%, after securing innovation funding to widen the reach of their "reclaim social work" model', 5 February, www.communitycare.co.uk/2015/02/05/hackney-model-consultants-work-partnership-dfe-reduce-bureaucracy/

30 Jones, R. (2015) 'I've seen the reclaim social work model cause service implosion', 9 April, www.communitycare.co.uk/2015/04/09/ive-seen-local-authorities-reclaiming-social-work-modelcaused-service-implosion/

31 Spring Consortium (2016) *Children's Social Care Innovation Programme Interim Learning Report*, p 13, https://www.innovationunit.org/wp-content/uploads/2017/04/DfE-Innovation-Programme-Interim-Learning-Report.pdf

32 Spring Consortium (2014) Spring Consortium, https://springconsortium.com/.

33 Butler, P. (2014) 'How Alan Wood became the go-to fixer for child protection', 9 July, https://www.theguardian.com/society/2014/jul/09/alan-wood-go-to-fixer-child-protection-hackney-socialwork

34 Butler (2014) *op cit.*

35 Le Grand, J., Wood, A. and Gibb, M. (2013) *Report to the Secretary of State on ways forward for children's services in Doncaster*, May, https://www.gov.uk/government/uploads/system/uploads/attachment_data/file/212598/Ways_forward_for_children_s_services_in_Doncaster.pdf

36 Le Grand, J., Wood, A. and Trowler, I. (2014) *Report to the Secretary of State for Education and the Minister for Children and Families on ways forward for children's services in Birmingham*, February, https://www.gov.uk/government/uploads/system/uploads/attachment_data/file/297748/Birmingham_report_25.03.14.pdf

37 http://csp.sagepub.com/content/early/2015/08/21/0261018315599333

38 Local Government Association (2016) *The Wood Review of the council role in education and children's services*, 29 September, http://lga.moderngov.co.uk/documents/s11173/Wood%20Review%20report%20for%20Sept%202016%20Board%20meeting.pdf

39 Jozwiak, G. (2017) 'Former ADCS president appointed to Youth Justice Board', 24 April, https://www.cypnow.co.uk/cyp/news/2003549/former-adcs-president-appointed-to-youth-justice-board

40 Donovan, T. (2017) 'Former ADCS president takes charge of residential care reforms', 13 November, https://www.cypnow.co.uk/cyp/news/2004498/former-adcs-president-takes-charge-of-residential-care-reforms.

41 Narey, M. (2016) *Residential Care in England: Report of Sir Martin Narey's independent review of children's residential care*, July, https://www.gov.uk/government/uploads/system/uploads/attachment_data/file/534560/Residential-Care-inEngland-Sir-Martin-Narey-July-2016.pdf

42 Donovan, T. (2018) 'Alan Wood to chair £20 m social care evidence centre', 5 July, https://www.cypnow.co.uk/cyp/news/2005516/alan-wood-to-chair-gbp20m-social-care-evidence-centre

43 Gov UK (2014) New Year's Honours 2015, https://www.gov.uk/government/news/new-years-honours-2015

44 Stanley, N., Austerberry, H., Bilson, A., Farrelly, N., Hargreaves, K., Hollingworth, K., Hussein, S., Ingold, C., Larkins, C., Manthorpe, J., Ridley, J. and Strange, V. (2012) *Social Work Practices: Report of the National Evaluation*, https://assets.publishing.service.gov.uk/government/uploads/system/uploads/attachment_data/file/183309/DFE-RR233.pdf

45 Think Ahead (2018) Our Team, http://thinkahead.org/about-us/our-team/

46 Navqui, S. (2016) 'Le Grand Vision', *Professional Social Work*, July-August, http://edition.pagesuite-professional.co.uk/Launch.aspx?EID=1bc0ae46-baef-466b-aa42-6be535f718e9

47 LaingBuisson, *The potential for developing the capacity and diversity of children's social care services in England, Independent research report*, December, https://www.gov.uk/government/uploads/system/uploads/attachment_data/file/573035/LaingBuisson_report_December_2016.pdf

48 Department for Education (2016) *Government response to LaingBuisson's report on the potential for developing the capacity and diversity of children's social care services in England*, https://assets.publishing.service.gov.uk/government/uploads/system/uploads/attachment_data/file/574211/Govt-response_to__LaingBuisson_report_December_2016.pdf

49 McNicoll, A. (2016) 'DfE-commissioned report reveals private sector appetite to run "full range" of children's services', 5 December, http://www.communitycare.co.uk/2016/12/05/dfe-commissioned-report-private-sector-appetite-run-full-range-childrens-services/

50 Puffett, N. (2016) 'DfE report proposes "forced privatisation" of child protection services', 2 December, http://www.cypnow.co.uk/cyp/news/2002841/dfe-report-proposes-forced-privatisation-of-child-protection-services

51 Prison Reform Trust (2005) 'Private Punishment: Who Profits?', January, http://www.prisonreformtrust.org.uk/portals/0/documents/private%20punishment%20who%20profits.pdf

52 Allison, E. and Hattenstone, S. (2015) 'G4S paid author of "independent" youth prison report as consultant', 5 August, https://www.theguardian.com/society/2015/aug/05/g4s-paid-martin-narey-independent-youth-prison-report-consultant

53 Hayes, D. (2014) 'Narey defends private sector role in child protection', 27 May, http://www.cypnow.co.uk/cyp/news/1144301/narey-defends-private-sector-role-in-child-protection

54 Williams, R. (2011) 'Adoption "tsar" Martin Narey in the spotlight', 26 July, https://www.theguardian.com/society/2011/jul/26/adoption-tsar-martin-narey-spotlight

55 Gove, M. (2011) 'Saved by love of strangers: Michael Gove describes how adoption transformed his life', 5 November, http://www.dailymail.co.uk/news/article-2057850/Michael-Gove-describes-adoption-transformed-life.html

56 Rustin, S. (2014) 'Edward Timpson: I wouldn't have been children's minister if my parents hadn't fostered', 29 March, https://www.theguardian.com/lifeandstyle/2014/mar/29/edward-timpson-childrens-minister-parents-fostered

57 Narey, M. (2014) 'Making the education of social workers consistently effective', January, https://assets.publishing.service.gov.uk/government/uploads/system/uploads/attachment_data/file/287756/Making_the_education_of_social_workers_consistently_effective.pdf

58 Croisdale-Appleby, D. (2014) *Re-visionary social work education*, February, https://assets.publishing.service.gov.uk/government/uploads/system/uploads/attachment_data/file/285788/DCA_Accessible.pdf

59 British Association of Social Workers (2014) 'Concern that Narey report would see narrow "checklist" of children's social work skills', February, https://www.basw.co.uk/media/news/2014/feb/concern-narey-report-would-see-narrow-checklist-childrens-social-work-skills

60 Ramesh, R. (2013) 'Michael Gove on a quest to reform social work training', 12 November, https://www.theguardian.com/society/2013/nov/12/michael-gove-reform-social-work

61 Bywaters, P., Brady, G., Bunting, L., Featherstone, B., Jones, C., Morris, K., Scourfield, J., Sparks, T. and Webb, C. (2017) 'Inequalities in English child protection practice under scrutiny: A Universal Challenge?', July, https://onlinelibrary.wiley.com/doi/abs/10.1111/cfs.12383

62 Bilson, A. and Martin, K. (2017) 'Referrals and child protection in England: one in five children referred to children's services and one in nineteen investigated before the age of five', April, https://academic.oup.com/bjsw/article-abstract/47/3/793/2622314

63 Hood, R., Goldacre, A., Grant, R. and Jones, R. (2016) 'Exploring demand and provision in English child protection services', June, https://academic.oup.com/bjsw/article-abstract/46/4/923/2472957

64 Butler, P. (2014) 'Trainee social workers taught too much theory, says report', 13 February, https://www.theguardian.com/society/2014/feb/13/trainee-social-workers-taught-theory

65 Bamford, T. (2015) 'Education – a contested landscape', March, https://www.basw.co.uk/system/files/resources/basw_43830-10_0.pdf

66 Narey, M. (2016) *Residential care in England: Report of Sir Martin Narey's review of children's residential child care*, July, p 32, https://assets.publishing.service.gov.uk/government/uploads/system/uploads/attachment_data/file/534560/Residential-Care-in-England-Sir-Martin-Narey-July-2016.pdf

67 Narey, M. and Owers, M. (2018) *Foster Care in England*, https://www.gov.uk/government/uploads/system/uploads/attachment_data/file/679320/Foster_Care_in_England_Review.pdf

68 Narey and Owers (2018) *op cit*, p 64.

69 Department for Education (2014) Direction for the improvement of children's social care services in Doncaster, September, https://www.gov.uk/government/publications/doncaster-childrens-services-improvement-direction-sept-2014

70 BBC (2013) 'New head for Doncaster children's services', 22 May, www.bbc.co.uk/news/uk-england-south-yorkshire-22629340

71 BBC (2014) 'Eleanor Brazil to head Slough social services', 10 October, www.bbc.co.uk/news/uk-england-berkshire-29559760

72 Sandwell Council (2016) 'Future of children's social care in Sandwell', 6 October, www.sandwell.gov.uk/news/article/3918/future_of_childrens_social_care_in_sandwell

73 McNicoll, A. (2017) 'Social worker who grew up in care recognised in New Year honours', 4 January, www.communitycare.co.uk/2017/01/04/social-worker-grew-care-recognised-new-year-honours/

74 ITV (2017) 'New company takes control of children's services in Sunderland', 31 March, www.itv.com/news/tyne-tees/2017-03-31/new-company-launches-to-improve-childrens-services-in-sunderland-after-inadequate-rating/

75 Mortali, O. (2017) 'Council-owned company to deliver children's services in Reading', 28 July, http://news.reading.gov.uk/childrens-services-company/

76 Achieving for Children (2017) 'Nick Whitfield, Chief Executive, receives CBE in New Year Honours', 30 December, https://www.achievingforchildren.org.uk/news-301217/

77 Puffett, N. (2018) 'Timpson takes up children's commissioner advisory role', 31 January, https://www.cypnow.co.uk/cyp/news/2004845/timpson-takes-up-childrens-commissioner-advisory-role

78 Social Work Task Force (2009) *Building a safe, confident future: The final report of the Social Work Task Force*, December, http://webarchive.nationalarchives.gov.uk/20130403150755/https://www.education.gov.uk/publications/standard/publicationdetail/page1/DCSF-01114-2009

79 Social Work Reform Board (2012) *Building a safe and confident future: Maintaining Momentum: Progress report from the Social Work Reform Board*, June, https://assets.publishing.service.gov.uk/government/uploads/system/uploads/attachment_data/file/175947/SWRB_progress_report_-_June_2012.pdf

80 Department for Education (2014) 'Social Work Reform Board', May, https://www.gov.uk/government/collections/social-work-reform-board

81 House of Commons Education Select Committee (2016) Social Work Reform, 6 July, https://publications.parliament.uk/pa/cm201617/cmselect/cmeduc/201/201.pdf

Chapter Four

1 Beveridge, W. (1942) *Social Insurance and Allied Services*, London: HMSO.

2 Kynaston, D. (2008) *A World to Build*, London, Bloomsbury, p 21.

3 Hennessy, P. (2006) *Never Again: Britain 1945–51*, London, Penguin Books, p 128.

4 Beresford, P. (2016) *All Our Welfare: Towards Participatory Social Policy*, Bristol, Policy Press, pp 31-32.

5 Steadman Jones, D. (2012) *Masters of the Universe: Hayek, Friedman, and the Birth of Neoliberal Politics*, New Jersey, Princeton University Press, pp 28-29.

6 Kynaston, D. (2008) *Smoke in the Valley*, London, Bloomsbury, p 91.

7 Kynaston (2008) *op cit*, p 93.

8   Marwick, A. (1996) *British Society Since 1945*, Harmondsworth, Penguin, p 106.

9   Seebohm, F. (1968) *Report of the Committee on Local Authority and Allied Personal Services*, July 1968, Cmnd 3703, HMSO.

10   Clark, A. (1998) *The Tories: Conservatives and The Nation State 1922–1997*, London, Weidenfeld and Nicolson, p 342.

11   Sandbrook, D. (2011) *State of Emergency: The Way We Were: Britain 1970–1974*, London, Penguin, p 612.

12   Timmins, N. (1996) *The Five Giants: A Biography of the Welfare State*, London, Fontana, p 314.

13   Sandbrook, D. (2013) *Seasons in the Sun: The Battle for Britain 1974–1979*, London, Penguin, p 470.

14   Sandbrook (2013) *op cit*, p 500.

15   Timmins (1996) *op cit*, p 327.

16   Margaret Thatcher Foundation (1979) Remarks on becoming Prime Minister (St Francis's Prayer), 4 May, https://www.margaretthatcher.org/document/104078

17   BBC (2013) 'Ding Dong! The Witch Is Dead enters chart at two', www.bbc.co.uk/news/entertainmentarts-22145306

18   Marwick, A. (1996) *The Tories: Conservatives and the Nation State 1922–1997*, London, Weidenfeld and Nicolson, p 353.

19   McSmith, A. (2011) *No Such Thing as Society: A History of Britain in the 1980s*, London, Constable, p 194.

20   Gilmour, I. and Garnett, M. (1998) *Whatever Happened to the Tories: The Conservatives Since 1945*, London, Fourth Estate, pp 321-322.

21   Gilmour, I. (1992) *Dancing with Dogma: Britain under Thatcherism*, London, Simon and Schuster, p 107.

Chapter Five

1   McSmith, A. (2011) *No Such Thing as Society: A History of Britain in the 1980s*, London, Constable, p 290.

2   Timmins, N. (1996) *The Five Giants: A Biography of the Welfare State*, London, Fontana, p 415.

3   Griffiths, R. (1988) *Community Care: An Agenda for Action*, London, HMSO.

4   Timmins (1996) *op cit*, p 475.

5   Griffiths (1988) *op cit*, p vii.

6   Griffiths (1988) *op cit*, p vi.

7　Challis, D. and Davies, B. (1986) *Case Management in Community Care: An Evaluated Experiment in the Home Care of the Elderly*, Aldershot, Gower.

8　Challis, D., Chessum, R., Chesterman, J., Luckett, R. and Traske, K. (1990) *Case Management in Social and Health Care: The Gateshead Community Care Scheme*, Personal Social Services Research Unit, Canterbury, University of Kent.

9　Challis, D., Darton, R., Johnson, L., Stone, M. and Traske, K. (1995) *Care Management and Health Care of Older People*, Aldershot, Gower.

10　Timmins, N. (1996) *op cit*, pp 472-477.

11　Aitken, J. (2013) *Margaret Thatcher: Power and Personality*, London, Bloomsbury, p 380.

12　Young, H. (1989) *One of Us: A Biography of Margaret Thatcher*, London, Macmillan, p 521.

13　Timmins (1996) *op cit*, p 474.

14　Fowler, N. (1984) 'The Enabling Role of Social Services Departments', Speech to the Joint Social Services Conference, Buxton, September.

15　McCarthy, M. (1989) 'Personal social services', in M. McCarthy (ed) *The New Politics of Welfare: An Agenda for the 1990s?*, Basingstoke, Macmillan, p 43.

16　Seldon, A. and Snowden, P. (2015) *Cameron at 10: The Inside Story 2010–2015*, London, William Collins, pp 147-162.

17　Toynbee, P. and Walker, D. (2017) *Dismembered: How the Attack on the State Harms Us All*, London, Guardian Books, pp 269-270.

18　McSmith (2011) *op cit*, p 5.

19　Timmins (1996) *op cit*, p 474.

20　Young (1989) *op cit*, pp 522-523.

21　Young (1989) *op cit*, p 537.

22　Crewe, I. (1988) 'Has the electorate become more Thatcherite?', in R. Skidelsky (ed) *Thatcherism*, London, Chatto and Windus, pp 35-37.

23　Crewe (1988) *op cit*, pp 44-45.

24　Cockerell, M., Hennessy, P. and Walker, D. (1985) *Sources Close to the Prime Minister: Inside the Hidden World of the News Manipulators*, London, Basingstoke, p 73.

25　Aitken (2013) *op cit*, p 403.

26   Jenkins, S. (2007) *Thatcher and Sons: A Revolution in Three Acts*, London, Penguin Books, p 19.

27   Holman, B. (1993) *A New Deal for Social Welfare*, Oxford, Lion Publishing, p 31.

28   Holman (1993) *op cit*, pp 29–30.

29   Knapp, M. (1989) 'Private and voluntary welfare', in M. McCarthy (ed), *op cit*, pp 235–236.

30   Knapp (1989) *op cit*, p 236.

31   Ibid.

32   Griffiths, R. (1988) *Community Care: Agenda for Action*, London, HMSO, p 1.

33   Campbell, J. and Oliver, M. (1996) *Disability Politics*, London, Routledge, pp 170–171.

34   Beresford, P. (2014) 'Advancing the positives of personalisation/ person-centred support: a multi-perspective view', in C. Needham and J. Glasby (eds) *Debates in Personalisation*, Bristol, Policy Press, pp 155–156.

35   Jones, R. (2008) 'Self-directed support: watching out for the pitfalls', *Journal of Integrated Care*, vol 16, no 1, February, pp 44–47.

Chapter Six

1   Jenkins, S. (2007) *Thatcher and Sons: A Revolution in Three Acts*, London, Penguin Books, p 235.

2   Harris, J. (2003) *The Social Work Business*, Abingdon, Routledge.

3   House of Commons Library Research Briefing (1999) *The Local Government Bill; Best Value and Council Tax Capping*, January, http://researchbriefings.files.parliament.uk/documents/RP99-1/ RP99-1.pdf

4   Blair, T. (2010) *A Journey*, London, Hutchinson, pp 261–262.

5   Barber, M. (2007) *Instruction to Deliver: Fighting to Transform Britain's Public Services*, London, Methuen.

6   Blair (2010) *op cit*, pp 338–339.

7   Blair (2010) *op cit*, pp 480–481.

8   National Audit Office (2018) *PFI and PF2, Report by the Comptroller and Auditor General*, 18 January, https://www.nao.org.uk/wp-content/uploads/2018/01/PFI-and-PF2.pdf, p 15.

9   Sampson, A. (2004) *Who Runs This Place? The Anatomy of Briatin in the 21st Century*, London, John Murray, p 130.

10   Sampson (2004) *op cit*, p 131.

11 Centre for Health and the Public Interest (2017) *PFI: Profiteering from Infirmaries*, https://chpi.org.uk/wpcontent/uploads/2017/08/CHPI-PFI-ProfitingFromInfirmaries.pdf

12 Siddique, H. (2017) 'Private firms poised to make another £1bn from building NHS hospitals', 30 August, https://www.theguardian.com/society/2017/aug/30/private-companies-huge-profits-building-nhs-hospitals.

13 Toynbee, P. (2013) *Hard Work: Life in Low-Pay Britain*, London, Bloomsbury, p 75.

14 Sampson (2004) *op cit*, p 279.

15 Drakeford, M. (2008) 'Going private?', in M. Powell (ed) *Modernising the Welfare State*, Bristol, Policy Press, pp 174-175.

16 Giddens, A. (1998) *The Third Way: The Renewal of Social Democracy*, Cambridge, Polity.

17 Giddens, A. (2007) *Over to You, Mr Brown: How Labour Can Win Again*, Cambridge, Polity Press.

18 Giddens (2007) *op cit*.

19 Seldon, A. (2005) *Blair*, London, Simon and Schuster, p. 175.

20 Le Grand, J. (2003) *Motivation, Agency and Public Policy: Of Knights and Knaves, Pawns and Queens*, Oxford, Oxford University Press, pp 3-4.

21 Le Grand (2003) *op cit*, p 8.

22 Jordan, B. and Jordan, C. (2000) *Social Work and Third Way: Tough Love as Social Policy*, London, Sage, pp 18-19.

23 Jordan, B. (2010) *Why The Third Way Failed: Economics, morality and the origins of the 'Big Society'*, Bristol, Policy Press, pp 1-2.

24 Rawnsley, A. (2010) *The End of the Party: The Rise and Fall of New Labour*, London, Penguin Books, p 7.

25 Toynbee, P. and Walker, D. (2010) *The Verdict: Did Labour Change Britain?*, London, Granta, p 302.

26 Toynbee and Walker (2010) *op cit*, pp 266-267.

27 Sainsbury, D. (2013) *Progressive Capitalism: How to Achieve Growth, Liberty and Social Justice*, London, Biteback Publishing, p 21.

28 Mason, P. (2009) *Meltdown: The End of the Age of Greed*, London, Verso, p 111.

29 Tett, G. (2009) *Fool's Gold: How unrestrained greed corrupted a dream, shattered global markets and unleashed a catastrophe*, London, Little, Brown.

30 Tett (2009) *op cit*, p 83.

31 Luyendijk, J. (2015) *Swimming with Sharks: My journey into the world of the bankers*, London, Guardian Books.

32 Cable, V. (2009) *The Storm: The world economic crisis and what it means*, London, Atlantic Books, p 1.

33 Peston, R. (2007) *Who Runs Britain? How the super-rich are changing our lives*, London, Hodder and Stoughton, pp 347-348.

34 Toynbee, P. and Walker, D. (2008) *Unjust Rewards: Ending the Greed that is Bankrupting Britain*, London, Granta, p 54.

Chapter Seven

1 Darling, A. (2011) *Back from the Brink: 1,000 Days at Number 11*, London, Atlantic Books, pp 308-309.

2 Jones, O. (2014) *The Establishment and How They Got Away With It*, London, Allen Lane, p 241.

3 Darling (2011) *op cit*, p 310.

4 Quoted in Milne, S. (2012) *The Revenge of History: The Battle for the 21st Century*, London, Verso, pp 228-229.

5 Klein, N. (2007) *The Shock Doctrine*, London, Penguin Books, p 288.

6 Klein, N. (2017) *No Is Not Enough: Defeating the New Shock Politics*, London, Allen Lane, pp 1 and 138–139.

7 Shipman, T. (2016) *All Out War: The Full Story of How Brexit Sank Britain's Political Class*, London, William Collins, p 603.

8 Toynbee, P. and Walker, D. (2012) *Dogma and Disarray: Cameron at Half-Time*, London, Granta, pp 81-82.

9 Toynbee and Walker (2012) *op cit*, p 82.

10 Toynbee, P. and Walker, D. (2015) *Cameron's Coup: How the Tories Took Britain to the Brink*, London, Guardian Books, p 262.

11 Toynbee and Walker (2015) *op cit*, pp 97-98.

12 Sampson, A. (2004) *Who Runs This Place? The Anatomy of Britain in the 21st Century*, London, John Murray, p 318.

13 Sampson (2004) *op cit*, p 319.

14 PwC (2017) 'Health Industries Oversight Board Chair', www.pwc.co.uk/contacts/a/alan-milburn.html.

15 Mathiason, N. (2009) 'Auditors face being called to account for their role in the global financial crisis: "Cosy cabal" of accountants to be grilled by politicians over self-regulation and apparent conflicts of interest', 25 October, https://www.theguardian.com/business/2009/oct/25/auditors-role-financial-crisis

16 Ahmed, K. (2011) 'Lords inquiry to damn Big Four auditors' role in financial crisis', 26 March, www.telegraph.co.uk/finance/newsbysector/supportservices/8408593/Lords-inquiry-to-damn-BigFour-auditors-role-in-financial-crisis.html

17 Economic Affairs Committee (2011) 'Auditors: Market concentration and their role', https://publications.parliament.uk/pa/ld201011/ldselect/ldeconaf/119/11909.htm.

18 Toynbee and Walker (2015) *op cit*, p 277.

Chapter Eight

1 White, A. (2016) *Shadow State: Inside the Secret Companies that Run Britain*, London, Oneworld Publications, p 204.

2 Meek, J. (2014) *Private Island: Why Britain Now Belongs to Someone Else*, London, Verso.

3 Meek (2014) *op cit*, p 15.

4 Meek (2014) *op cit*, p 23.

5 Shaxson, N. (2011) *Treasure Islands: Tax Havens and the Men Who Stole the World*, London, Bodley Head, p 15.

6 Shaxson (2011) *op cit*, p 22.

7 Mendoza, K-A. (2015) *Austerity: The Demolition of the Welfare State and the Rise of the Zombie Economy*, Oxford, New Internationalists Publications.

8 Peston, R. (2008) *Who Runs Britain? How the Super-Rich are Changing Our Lives*, London, Hodder and Stoughton, p 347.

9 Neate, R. (2017) 'World's witnessing a new Gilded Age as billionaires' wealth swells to $6tn: Not since the time of the Carnegies, Rockefellers and Vanderbilts at the turn of the 20th century was so much owned by so few', www.theguardian.com/business/2017/oct/26/worlds-witnessing-a-new-gilded-age-as-billionaires-wealth-swells-to-6tn

10 Mendoza (2015) *op cit*, pp 78-79.

11 Toynbee, P. and Walker, D. (2017) *Dismembered: How the Attack on the State Harms Us All*, London, Guardian Books, pp 65-66.

12 Beveridge, W. (1942) *Social Insurance and Allied Services*, London: HMSO.

13 Attlee, C., quoted in J. Bew (2017) *Citizen Clem: A Biography of Attlee*, London, Riverrun, p 467.

14 Kynaston, D. (2007) *Austerity Britain 1945–1951*, London, Bloomsbury, p 633.

15 Hennessy, P. (2006) *Never Again: Britain 1945–51*, London, Penguin Books, p 454.

Chapter Nine

1   Beveridge, W. (1942) *Social Insurance and Allied Services*, London, HMSO.

2   Le Grand, J. (undated) *Delivering Britain's Public Services through 'Quasi-markets': What we have Achieved so far*, Centre for Market and Public Organisation Research in Public Policy, www.bristol. ac.uk/medialibrary/sites/cmpo/migrated/documents/legrand.pdf

3   Department for Education (2016) *Educational Excellence Everywhere*, March, Cm 9230, https://www.gov.uk/government/uploads/ system/uploads/attachment_data/file/508447/Educational_ Excellence_Everywhere.pdf

4   Perraudin, F. (2017) 'Police investigate multi-academy trust accused of asset stripping: West Yorkshire police receive information about Wakefield City Academies Trust, which is divesting itself of 21 schools', 7 December, https://www.theguardian.com/ education/2017/dec/06/wakefield-city-academies-trustwest-yorkshire-police

5   Donovan, T. (2017) 'Government rejects call to hand councils academy powers', 1 December, https://www.cypnow.co.uk/ cyp/news/2004595/government-rejects-call-to-hand-councils-academy-powers

6   House of Commons Education Select Committee (2017) 'Multi-Academy Trusts', Seventh Report of the Session 2016-2017, 22 February, https://publications.parliament.uk/pa/cm201617/ cmselect/cmeduc/204/204.pdf

7   Ball, S. (2015) 'Why should we be worried about profit-making in schools?', https://ioelondonblog.wordpress.com/2015/05/07/ why-should-we-be-worried-about-profit-making-in-schools/

8   Cusick, J. (2013) 'Cash for classrooms: Michael Gove plans to let firms run schools for profit: Exclusive: Details leaked by Department for Education insiders concerned that he is going too fast and too far', http://www.independent.co.uk/news/uk/ politics/cash-for-classrooms-michael-gove-plans-to-let-firms-run-schools-for-profit-8682395.html

9   Boffey, D. and Warwick, M. (2016) 'Are England's academies becoming a cash cow for business? Special investigation: how not-

for-profit academies have been thrown open to entrepreneurial interests in an unprecedented fashion', https://www.theguardian.com/education/2016/jun/12/academy-schools-cash-cowbusiness

10 Perraudin, F. (2017) 'Labour urges ministers to "come clean" over collapsed academy trust', https://www.theguardian.com/education/2017/oct/24/labour-urges-ministers-to-come-clean-over-collapsed-academy-trust

11 Munro, B. (2018) 'Academy chain accused of misusing public funds', 10 September, https://www.bbc.co.uk/news/education-45472189

12 Royal Society of Arts (2013) *Unleashing greatness: Getting the best from an academised system: The Report of the Academies Commission*, https://www.thersa.org/discover/publications-and-articles/reports/unleashingagreatness-getting-the-best-from-an-academised-system, p 4.

13 Burns, J. (2018) 'Councils beat academy trusts in boosting failing schools', 5 July, https://www.bbc.co.uk/news/education-44698272

14 Coughlan, S. (2016) England's largest academy chain 'failing too many pupils', 4 February, www.bbc.co.uk/news/education-35492433

15 Coughlan, S. (2016) *op cit*.

16 The Sutton Trust (2016) Chain Effects 2016, 7 July, https://www.suttontrust.com/researchpaper/chaineffects2016/

17 Perry, R. (2016), quoted in J. Brown (2016) 'Academies fail disadvantaged children, finds charity', 7 July, https://www.cypnow.co.uk/cyp/news/1158113/academies-fail-disadvantaged-children-finds-charity

18 Brown, J. (2016) 'Wilshaw urges councils to "shoulder responsibility" for school improvement', https://www.cypnow.co.uk/cyp/news/2002361/wilshaw-urges-councils-to-shoulder-responsibility-for-school-improvement

19 Baginsky, M., Driscoll, J. and Manthoroe, J. (2015) 'Thinking aloud: decentralisation and safeguarding in English schools', *Journal of Integrated Care*, 23(6): 357.

20 Baginsky et al (2015) *op cit*, p 358.

21 Santry, C. (2018) 'Children in care turned away in their hour of need', *TES* (*Times Education Supplement*), 23 February, p 13.

22 Richardson, H. (2015) 'The children in care left without a school place', 23 October, www.bbc.co.uk/news/education-41664460

23 HM Government (2003) *Every Child Matters*, Cm 5860, https://www.education.gov.uk/consultations/downloadableDocs/EveryChildMatters.pdf

24 House of Commons Public Accounts Committee (2017) 'Capital funding for schools', Fifty-seventh Report of Session 2016–17, https://publications.parliament.uk/pa/cm201617/cmselect/cmpubacc/961/961.pdf

25 National Audit Office (2017) 'Capital funding for schools', 21 February, https://www.nao.org.uk/wpcontent/uploads/2017/02/Capital-funding-for-schools.pdf

26 Syal, R. (2017) 'Billions spent on free schools while existing schools decay', 22 February, https://www.theguardian.com/education/2017/feb/22/government-spending-billions-on-free-schools-while-existing-schools-crumble

27 Coughlan, S. (2017) 'Academy chain to scrap governing bodies', 19 January, www.bbc.co.uk/news/education-35347602

28 Tickle, L. (2017) 'Disappared – headtachers told to clear off and tell no one', 24 October, https://www.theguardian.com/education/2017/oct/24/disappeared-headteacher-sacked-academy-dismissal

29 Puffett, N. (2017) 'Tory politicians raise concerns over future of children's centres', 23 October, https://www.cypnow.co.uk/cyp/news/2004377/tory-politicians-raise-concerns-over-future-of-childrenscentres

30 House of Commons Education Committee (2017) Oral evidence: Accountability Hearings, HC 341, 25 October, Question 14, http://data.parliament.uk/writtenevidence/committeeevidence.svc/evidencedocument/educationcommittee/accountability-hearings/oral/72035.pdf

31 Smith, G., Sylva, P., Sammons, P., Smith, T. and Omonigho, A. (2018) *Start Stop*, Sutton Trust, 5 April, https://www.suttontrust.com/research-author/with-aghogho-omonigho/

32 Donovan, T. (2018) 'Charity sees children's centre income fall by £14m', 14 August, https://www.cypnow.co.uk/cyp/news/2005653/council-spending-cuts-slashes-charitys-childrens-centre-income-by-nearly-gbp14m

33 Sutherland, A., Disley, E., Cattell, J. and Bauchowitz, S. (2017) 'An analysis of trends in first time entrants to the youth justice system', RAND Europe and Get the Data, https://www.gov.uk/government/uploads/system/uploads/attachment_data/file/653182/trends-in-fte-to-the-youth-justice-system.pdf

34 Puffett, N. (2017) 'Children's centres credited with role in youth justice progress', 24 October, https://www.cypnow.co.uk/cyp/news/2004383/childrens-centres-credited-with-role-in-youth-justiceprogress

35 Health and Social Care (Community Health and Standards) Act 2003.

36 Department of Health (2005) *A Short Guide to NHS Foundation Trusts,* https://www.cmft.nhs.uk/published/UserUpload/file/A%20Short%20Guide%20to%20Foundation%20Trusts.pdf, pp 2-3

37 Department of Health (2011) 'Operational Guidance to the NHS Extending Patient Choice of Provider', https://www.gov.uk/government/publications/operational-guidance-to-the-nhs-extending-patient-choice-of-provider

38 Syal, R. and Hughes, S. (2015) 'Ex-health secretary Andrew Lansley to advise firms on healthcare reforms', 20 October, https://www.theguardian.com/politics/2015/oct/20/andrew-lansley-advise-firms-healthcarereforms

39 Blanchard, J. (2014) '"Selling off NHS for profit": Full list of MPs with links to private healthcare firms', www.mirror.co.uk/news/uk-news/selling-nhs-profit-full-list-4646154

40 Pickard, J. and Tetlow, G. (2017) 'Private companies make £831 million profits from NHS contracts', 30 August, https://www.ft.com/content/71201382-8cd6-11e7-9084-d0c17942ba93

41 British Medical Association (2017) 'Hidden Figures: Private Care in the NHS', p 1, https://www.bma.org.uk/collective-voice/influence/key-negotiations/nhs-funding/privatisation-report

42 Lawrence, F. (2012) 'Cornish complaints raise questions about drive to outsource NHS care: Allegations in Cornwall are still being investigated as health service go out to tender in line with new policies', https://www.theguardian.com/society/2012/may/25/questions-outsource-nhs-care

43 House of Commons Public Accounts Committee (2013) 'The provision of the out-of-hours GP service in Cornwall', 11 July,

https://publications.parliament.uk/pa/cm201314/cmselect/cmpubacc/471/47103.htm

44   Lawrence, F. (2013) 'Serco condemned over move to offload troubled GP service in Cornwall: Private contractor in talks with NHS to pass on out-of-hours service to not-for-profit enterprise', 11 October, https://www.theguardian.com/business/2013/oct/11/serco-gp-service-cornwall

45   NHS Kernow (2015) 'New GP out of hours service for Cornwall', https://www.kernowccg.nhs.uk/news/2015/02/new-gp-out-of-hours-service-for-cornwall/

46   Pemberton, M. (2015) 'Hinchingbrooke: what else did they expect? The NHS is now picking up the pieces at Hinchingbrooke Hospital after the private company Circle terminated its contract after failings in care. Is that really a surprise?', 9 February, www.telegraph.co.uk/lifestyle/11392213/Hinchingbrooke-what-else-did-they-expect.html

47   Owen, D. (2015) 'Lesson one from the Hinchingbrooke hospital scandal: beware the "mutual": Supporters of the flagship hospital said its structure was a blueprint for the future. In fact it was privatisation by another name', 19 January, https://www.theguardian.com/commentisfree/2015/jan/19/hinchingbrooke-hospital-scandal-mutual-privately-run

48   Hodge, M. (2015) Circle's withdrawal from Hinchingbrooke Hospital update report published, 18 March, https://www.parliament.uk/business/committees/committees-a-z/commons-select/public-accounts-committee/news/report-circle-withdrawal-from-hinchingbrooke-hospital/.

49   National Audit Office (2016a) 'Investigation into the collapse of the UnitingCare Partnership contract in Cambridgeshire and Peterborough', July, https://www.nao.org.uk/report/investigation-into-the-collapse-of-the-unitingcare-partnership-contract-in-cambridgeshire-and-peterborough/

50   National Audit Office (2016b) 'Investigation into the collapse of the UnitingCare Partnership contract in Cambridgeshire and Peterborough', HC 512 Session 2016-17, 14 July 2016, https://www.nao.org.uk/wpcontent/uploads/2016/07/The-collapse-of-the-UnitingCare-Partnership-contract-in-Cambridgeshire-and-Peterborough.pdf, p 5.

51   National Audit Office (2016b) *op cit*, p 7.

52 National Audit Office (2016b) *op cit*, p 6.

53 BBC (2016) 'Cambridgeshire's £800m NHS outsourcing contract "wasted millions"', 14 July, www.bbc.co.uk/news/uk-england-cambridgeshire-36792483

54 House of Commons Public Accounts Select Committee (2016) '"Grossly irresponsible" rush into contract led to catastrophic failure', November, https://www.parliament.uk/business/committees/committees-a-z/commons-select/public-accounts-committee/news-parliament-2015/unitingcare-partnership-contract-report-published16-17/

55 House of Commons Public Accounts Select Committee (2016) *op cit*.

56 House of Commons Public Accounts Select Committee (2018) 'Supporting Primary Care Services: NHS England's contract with Capita', 25 July, https://www.parliament.uk/business/committees/committees-a-z/commons-select/public-accounts-committee/news-parliament-2017/nhs-contract-capita-report-published-17-19/

57 Triggle, N. (2018) 'Private firms cash in on over-stretched NHS', 19 July, https://www.bbc.co.uk/news/health-44874238

58 British Medical Association (2017) *op cit*, p 2.

59 Harper, T. and Greenwood, G. (2016) 'Security firms are paid £170m to do police job', 3 January, https://www.thetimes.co.uk/article/police-pay-firms-pound170m-to-plug-gaps-j3lbchzrm9s

60 Kandhola, T. (2016) 'Scotland Yard used ex-police from private firm G4S to help hunt for missing Madeleine McCann', 3 January, www.mirror.co.uk/news/uk-news/scotland-yard-used-ex-police-7112764

61 Harper and Greenwood (2016) *op cit*.

62 Norton-Taylor, R. (2016) 'Britain is mercenary kingpin of private security, says charity', 4 February, https://www.theguardian.com/business/2016/feb/03/britain-g4s-at-centre-of-global-mercenary-industry-says-charity

63 Grierson, J. (2017) 'Watchdog says police cuts have left forces in "perilous state"', 2 March, https://www.theguardian.com/uk-news/2017/mar/02/inspectorate-police-engaging-dangerous-practices-austerity-cuts-diane-abbott

64 Grierson, J. (2017) *op cit*.

65   Dodd, V. (2017) 'Cuts "threaten disaster" for policing terror', 11 November, https://www.theguardian.com/uknews/2017/nov/10/police-cutbacks-threaten-national-security-warns-counter-terrorism-head-neil-basu

66   Dodd, V. (2017) 'Norfolk police plan to axe all community support officers', 20 October, https://www.theguardian.com/uk-news/2017/oct/19/norfolk-police-plan-to-axe-all-community-support-officers

67   Dodd, V. (2017) 'Met police chief warns further cuts will make it harder to fight crime', 31 October, https://www.theguardian.com/uk-news/2017/oct/31/met-police-chief-warns-further-cuts-will-make-it-harder-to-fight-crime

68   Dodd, V. (2017), 11 November, *op cit.*

69   Shveda, K., Harper, T. and Thomas, J. (2018) 'Bobbies on beat slashed by a third', 26 August, https://www.thetimes.co.uk/edition/news/bobbies-onbeat-slashed-by-a-third-2gtg28f3f

70   Kotecha, S. (2018) 'West Midlands Police chief says force offers "poor service"', 28 July, https://www.bbc.co.uk/news/uk-england-birmingham-44941173

71   Gilligan, A. (2018) 'West End elite eye private police force', 26 August, https://www.thetimes.co.uk/article/west-end-elite-eye-private-police-force-5n7dgpl2m

72   Harris, J. (2018) 'The growth of private policing is eroding justice for all', 10 September, https://www.theguardian.com/commentisfree/2018/sep/10/growth-private-policing-eroding-justice-for-all

73   Drury, I. (2017) 'Private firms may be given powers to arrest people: Companies would be able to hold individuals who fail to pay fines imposed by courts', 28 September, www.dailymail.co.uk/news/article4927688/Private-firms-given-powers-arrest-people.html

74   Travis, A. and Bowers, S. (2013) 'G4S and Serco: key players in criminal justice privatisation', 11 July, https://www.theguardian.com/politics/2013/jul/11/g4s-serco-criminal-justice-privatisation

75   Travis, A. and Bowers, S. (2013) *op cit.*

76   BBC (2012) 'G4S Olympic failure prompts ministers to "think again" over outsourcing', 14 August, www.bbc.co.uk/news/uk-19251772

77 BBC (2013) 'Serco agrees to repay £68.5m after tagging scandal', 19 December, http://www.bbc.co.uk/news/uk-25448944

78 Devlin, H. (2017) 'Fears over lack of regulation for forensic testing in family courts', 24 November, https://www.theguardian.com/politics/2017/nov/23/regulator-calls-for-better-scrutiny-of-drug-testing-infamily-courts

79 Ainsworth, D. (2013) 'Analysis: "A step in the right direction" on probation service contracts', 25 June, www.thirdsector.co.uk/analysis-a-step-right-direction-probation-servicecontracts/management/article/1187238

80 Ainsworth, D. (2013) *op cit.*

81 Plimmer, G. (2016) 'UK probation deals are failing, say providers', 12 October, https://www.ft.com/content/c2fde9ba-8c71-11e6-8aa5-f79f5696c731

82 House of Commons Justice Select Committee (2014) 'Crime reduction policies: a co-ordinated approach?', Interim report on the Government's Transforming Rehabilitation programme, 22 January, https://publications.parliament.uk/pa/cm201314/cmselect/cmjust/1004/100403.htm

83 Rutter, T. (2015) 'Probation service split: "staff are staring into the abyss"', 9 April, https://www.theguardian.com/public-leaders-network/2015/apr/09/probation-service-split-staff-demoralised-divided-private-services

84 Rutter, T. (2016) 'Privatised probation staff: stressed, deskilled and facing job cuts', 23 February, https://www.theguardian.com/public-leaders-network/2016/feb/23/privatisation-probation-service-stressed-job-cuts

85 Brewer, K. (2017) 'Why are privatised probation services using public libraries to see clients?', 1 November, https://www.theguardian.com/society/2017/nov/01/privatised-probation-services-libraries-ex-offenders

86 Leftly, M. (2015) 'Probation Services in South Yorkshire could be renationalised after firm fails Ministry of Justice audit', 20 December, www.independent.co.uk/news/uk/crime/probation-services-in-southyorkshire-could-be-renationalised-after-firm-fails-ministry-of-justice-a6780881.html

87 Plimmer, G. (2016) 'UK probation deals are failing, say providers: Companies say they were given misleading figures when bidding

for £3.7bn contracts', 12 October, https://www.ft.com/content/c2fde9ba-8c71-11e68aa5-f79f5696c731

88 National Audit Office (2016) *Transforming Rehabilitation*, 28 April, https://www.nao.org.uk/wpcontent/uploads/2016/04/Transforming-rehabilitation.pdf

89 Fenton, S. (2016) 'Watchdog criticises Government's privatisation of probation services', 2 May, http://www.independent.co.uk/news/uk/politics/national-audit-office-watchdog-savages-governments-disastrous-privatisation-of-probation-services-a7010496.html

90 *The Guardian* (2016) 'The Guardian view on probation: another Grayling casualty', Editorial, 15 December, https://www.theguardian.com/commentisfree/2016/dec/15/the-guardian-view-on-probation-another-grayling-casualty

91 Plimmer, G. (2016) 'Outsourced London probation services "putting people at risk": Damning inspectorate report could see US firm MTCNovo lose contract', 15 December, https://www.ft.com/content/aab6a7d2-c21a11e6-9bca-2b93a6856354

92 Grierson, J. (2018) 'Private probation companies to have contracts ended early', 27 July, https://www.theguardian.com/society/2018/jul/27/private-probation-companies-contracts-ended-early-justice?CMP=Share_iOSApp_Other

93 Prison Reform Trust (2005) 'Private Punishment: Who Profits?', January, www.prisonreformtrust.org.uk/Portals/0/Documents/private%20punishment%20who%20profits.pdf

94 Prison Reform Trust (2005) *op cit.*

95 Prison Reform Trust (2005) *op cit.*

96 House of Commons Public Accounts Committee (2003) 'Public Accounts – Forty-Ninth Report', https://publications.parliament.uk/pa/cm200203/cmselect/cmpubacc/904/90406.htm .

97 Travis, A. (2004) 'Taking no prisoners', 17 November, https://www.theguardian.com/society/2004/nov/17/guardiansocietysupplement.crime

98 Prison Reform Trust (2005) *op cit.*

99 Office of the Inspector General of the US Department of Justice (2016) *Review of the Federal Bureau of Prisons' Monitoring of Contract Prisons*, August, https://oig.justice.gov/reports/2016/e1606.pdf

100 *Daily Mail* (2016) 'No more private federal prisons Obama rules after audit finds they have MORE security breaches than

government-run ones', 18 August, www.dailymail.co.uk/news/article3747479/Obama-administration-end-use-private-prisons.html

101 Watkins, E. and Tatum, S. (2017) 'Private prison industry sees boon under Trump administration', 18 August, http://edition.cnn.com/2017/08/18/politics/private-prison-department-of-justice/index.html

102 Poyner, C. (2012) 'Prison privatisation should be a national scandal', 8 November, https://www.theguardian.com/commentisfree/2012/nov/08/prison-privatisation-g4s-wolds

103 Mason, R. (2016) 'G4S fined 100 times since 2010 for breaching prison contracts', 15 April, https://www.theguardian.com/society/2016/apr/15/g4s-fined-100-times-since-2010-prison-contracts

104 Shaw, D. (2018) 'Birmingham Prison: Government takes over from G4S', 20 August, https://www.bbc.co.uk/news/uk-england-birmingham-45240742

105 BBC Panorama (2016) 'Teenage Prison Abuse Exposed', 20 January, www.bbc.co.uk/programmes/b06ymzly

106 BBC (2016) 'G4S Medway unit: Security firm to sell children's services', 26 February, www.bbc.co.uk/news/uk-england-35671385

107 Medway Improvement Board (2016) 'Final Report of the Board's Advice to Secretary of State for Justice', 30 March, https://www.gov.uk/government/uploads/system/uploads/attachment_data/file/523167/medway-report.pdf

108 Plimmer, G. (2016) 'Ministry takes over youth custody centre from private operator', 5 May, https://www.ft.com/content/dea0b368-12b0-11e6-91da-096d89bd2173

109 BBC (2017) 'G4S Medway unit: Serious case review launched', 13 February, www.bbc.co.uk/news/uk-england-kent-38956281

110 Care Quality Commission, HM Inspector of Prisons, and Ofsted (2016) 'Inspection of Rainsbrook Secure Training Centre', February, p 8, https://reports.ofsted.gov.uk/sites/default/files/documents/secure-training-centre-reports/rainsbrook/Rainsbrook%20STC%20Ofsted%20report%20February%202015%20%28PDF%29.pdf

111 *The Guardian* (2015) 'G4S loses contract to run Rainsbrook young offender facility', 4 September, https://www.theguardian.com/

uk-news/2015/sep/04/g4s-loses-contract-to-run-rainsbrook-young-offender-facility

112 Hirsch, A. (2016) 'US firm could take over Young Offender Centres: An American company accused of managing prisons riddled with violence, corruption and drugs could soon be running two UK centres', 27 March, https://news.sky.com/story/us-firm-could-take-over-young-offender-centres-10220549

113 BBC (2017) 'Detainees "mocked and abused" at immigration centre', 1 September, www.bbc.co.uk/news/uk-41121692

114 House of Commons Home Affairs Committee (2017) *Brook House Immigration Removal Centre Inquiry*, 14 September, https://www.parliament.uk/business/committees/committees-a-z/commons-select/home-affairs-committee/inquiries/parliament-2017/inquiry/publications/

115 Dearden, L. (2017) 'G4S lied to Government so it could make big profit on scandal-hit immigration detention centre, MPs told', 14 September, www.independent.co.uk/news/uk/home-news/g4s-immigration-profits-detention-centre-brook-house-abuse-scandal-gatwick-inmates-panorama-a7946776.html

116 Allinson, E. and Hattenstone, S. (2017) 'G4S may make more profit than allowed from removal centres, figures suggest', 13 September, https://www.theguardian.com/business/2017/sep/13/g4s-may-make-more-profit-than-allowed-from-removal-centres-figures-suggest

117 Allison, E. and Grierson, J. (2016) 'Restraint injuries persist at youth jail where boy died 12 years ago MoJ report says there were 65 incidents across six facilities in 2014-15', the highest number at G4s-run Rainsbrook, 5 May, https://www.theguardian.com/society/2016/may/05/restraint-injuries-youth-jailsrainsbrook-gareth-myatt

118 BBC (2017) 'A global security giant with a chequered record', 1 September, https://www.bbc.co.uk/news/uk-41123840

119 White, A. (2016) 'G4S to take over running of government discrimination helpline, 26 July, https://www.buzzfeed.com/alanwhite/exclusive-g4s-to-take-over-vital-government-discrimination-s

120 Maidment, N. (2014) 'Serco chastened by costly lesson in outsourcing risk', 14 November, http://uk.reuters.com/

article/uk-britain-serco/serco-chastened-by-costly-lesson-in-outsourcing-riskidUKKCN0IY0VL20141114

121 Maidment (2014) *op cit.*

122 Perraudin, F. (2017) 'UK asylum seekers living in "squalid, unsafe slum conditions"', 27 October, https://www.theguardian.com/uk-news/2017/oct/27/uk-asylum-seekers-living-in-squalid-unsafe-slum-conditions

123 Edmiston, D. (2014) 'Social security privatisation in the UK: a means to whose end?', *People, Place and Policy*, 8(2): 113-128.

124 Helm, T. (2008) 'Privatised welfare system plan "open to abuse"', 14 April, www.telegraph.co.uk/news/uknews/1585112/Privatised-welfare-system-plan-open-to-abuse.html

125 Bowater, D. (2012) 'Fraud probe into "back to work" programme: a Government-backed work scheme is facing a police investigation over allegations of fraud dating back to 2010', 20 February, www.telegraph.co.uk/news/uknews/crime/9092308/Fraud-probe-into-back-to-work-programme.html

126 Marsden, S. and Mullin, G. (2015) 'Government back-to-work contractors who forged signatures to con taxpayers out of £300,000 jailed for total of 15 years', 1 April, http://www.dailymail.co.uk/news/article3020303/Government-work-contractors-forged-signatures-taxpayers-300-000-jailed-total-15-years.html

127 Marsden and Mullin (2015) *op cit.*

128 Walker, J. (2016) 'Private firms earn £500m from disability benefit assessments', 26 December, https://www.theguardian.com/society/2016/dec/27/private-firms-500m-governments-fit-to-work-scheme

129 House of Commons Work and Pensions Select Committee (2011) 'The role of incapacity benefit reassessment in helping claimants into employment', Sixth Report of Session 2010–12, Volume I: Report, together with formal minutes, oral and written evidence, Summary, 13 July, https://publications.parliament.uk/pa/cm201012/cmselect/cmworpen/1015/1015.pdf

130 House of Commons Committee of Public Accounts Committee (2016) 'Contracted out health and disability assessments', Thirty-third Report of Session 2015–16, 17 March, https://publications.parliament.uk/pa/cm201516/cmselect/cmpubacc/727/727.pdf

131 Butler, P. (2017) 'Disability benefits process is "inherently flawed", MPs told', 6 March, https://www.theguardian.com/

society/2017/mar/06/disability-benefits-process-is-inherently-flawed-mps-told

132 Syal, R. (2016) 'Government to review £500m-worth of Atos contracts after IT failure: Cabinet Office to examine Whitehall contracts worth £10m in move suggesting lack of confidence in outsourcing company', 6 March, https://www.theguardian.com/society/2016/mar/06/government-to-review500m-worth-of-atos-contracts-after-it-failure

133 BBC (2017) 'Disability benefits: PIPs assessment firms "to get extra £200m"', 14 April, www.bbc.co.uk/news/uk-39599331

134 Kynaston, D. (2007) *Austerity Britain 1945–1951*, London, Bloomsbury, pp 154-155.

135 Disney, R. and Luo, G. (2014) 'The Right to Buy Public Housing in Britain: A Welfare Analysis', December, IFS Working Paper W15/05, London, Institute of Fiscal Studies, p 4.

136 Timmins, N. (1996) *The Five Giants: A Biography of the Welfare State*, London, Fontana Press, pp 434-435.

137 Timmins (1996) *op cit*, p 435.

138 Timmins (1996) *op cit*, pp 435-436.

139 Meek, J. (2014) *Private Island: Why Britain Now Belongs to Someone Else*, London, Verso, pp 193-194.

140 Toynbee and Walker (2010) *op cit*, p 141.

141 Butler, P. (2017) 'Families with stable jobs at risk of homelessness in England, report finds: Nurses are among those ending up with nowhere to live after being evicted by private-sector landlords, says watchdog', 15 December, https://www.theguardian.com/society/2017/dec/15/homelessness-report-workingfamilies-stable-jobs-local-government-ombudsman

142 House of Commons Public Accounts Committee (2017) 'Homeless Households': Eleventh Report of Session 2017–2019, HC462, 20 December, https://publications.parliament.uk/pa/cm201719/cmselect/cmpubacc/462/462.pdf

143 Toynbee, P. and Walker, D. (2017) *Dismembered: How the Attack on the State Harms Us All*, London, Guardian Books, pp 74–75.

144 Doughty, S. (2001) 'Law Lords order Dame Shirley to pay £27 million', www.dailymail.co.uk/news/article-89909/Law-Lords-order-Dame-Shirley-pay-27-million.html

145 BBC (2004) 'Porter pays £12m to Westminster', 5 July, http://news.bbc.co.uk/1/hi/uk_politics/3867387.stm

146 BBC (2017) 'London fire: What happened at Grenfell Tower?', 19 July, www.bbc.co.uk/news/ukengland-london-40272168

147 Grenfell Tower Inquiry (2017) https://www.grenfelltowerinquiry.org.uk/

148 Hackitt, J. (2017) *Building a Safer Future: Independent Review of Building Regulations and Fire Safety: Interim Report*, December, Cm 9551, https://www.gov.uk/government/uploads/system/uploads/attachment_data/file/668831/Independent_Review_of_Building_Regulations_and_Fire_Safety_web_accessible.pdf

149 Weaver, M. (2017) 'Building regulations unfit for purpose, Grenfell review finds: Interim report says system to ensure homes are built to be safe is open to abuse and there are concerns about privatisation', 18 December, https://www.theguardian.com/uk-news/2017/dec/18/put-safety-ahead-of-costcutting-urges-grenfell-tower-building-report

150 Walker, D. (2017) 'So 2017 ends as it began, with urgent questions about UK public services', 20 December, https://www.theguardian.com/public-leaders-network/2017/dec/20/2017-review-uk-public-services-local-government

151 Blake, H. (2011) 'Conservatives given millions by property developers', 9 September, www.telegraph.co.uk/news/earth/hands-off-our-land/8754027/Conservatives-given-millions-byproperty-developers.html

152 Branson, A. (2017) 'Property provides 37% of Tory corporate donations', 2 June, https://www.propertyweek.com/news/property-provides-37-of-tory-corporate-donations/5089611.article

153 Neate, R. (2017) 'Persimmon chair quits over failure to rein in CEO's "obscene" £100m+ bonus', 15 December, https://www.theguardian.com/business/2017/dec/15/persimmon-chair-resigns-chief-executive-obscene-bonus

Chapter Ten

1 Jarrett, T. (2018) 'Social care: care home market – structure, issues, and cross-subsidisation (England)', House of Commons Library Briefing Paper No 8003, 13 February, https://researchbriefings.parliament.uk/ResearchBriefing/Summary/CBP-8003

2 Laing and Buisson (2010) *Care of Elderly People UK Market Survey 2010–2011*, London, Laing and Buisson, p 79.

3   LaingBuisson (2016) *Care of Older People: UK Market Report*, 27th edn, London, LaingBuisson, p 114.

4   Scourfield, P. (2011) 'Caretelization revisited and the lessons of Southern Cross', *Critical Social Policy*, 32(1): 140.

5   Scourfield (2011) *op cit*, pp. 140-141.

6   BBC (2011) 'Southern Cross set to shut down and stop running homes', 11 July, www.bbc.co.uk/news/business-14102750

7   Plimmer, G. (2014) 'Former Southern Cross Care homes set for sell off', 2 March, https://www.ft.com/content/8a72fac0-9fb8-11e3-b6c7-00144feab7de

8   Wachman, R. (2011) 'Southern Cross's incurably flawed business model let down the vulnerable', 16 July, https://www.theguardian.com/business/2011/jul/16/southern-cross-incurable-sick-business-model

9   Bow, M. (2016) 'Four Seasons plans restructure to slash its mountain of debt', 23 August, https://www.standard.co.uk/business/four-seasons-plans-restructure-to-slash-its-mountain-of-debta3327521.html

10 Davies, R. (2017) 'Four Seasons Health Care earns reprieve after deal with creditors: Uncertainty for 17,000 care home residents ended temporarily after troubled firm strikes debt holiday deal with private equity investors', 14 December, https://www.theguardian.com/society/2017/dec/14/fourseasons-health-care-saved-from-collapse-after-deal-with-creditors

11 Pratley, N. (2017) 'A shocking way to fund UK care homes', 12 December, https://www.theguardian.com/business/nils-pratley-on-finance/2017/dec/12/a-shocking-way-to-fund-ukcare-homes

12 Wood, Z. (2007) 'Should profit come before children? Sedgemoor's demise has fuelled fears about firms looking after vulnerable youngsters', 21 October, https://www.theguardian.com/business/2007/oct/21/observerbusiness.businessandmedia13.

13 Meghji, S. (2007) 'Children's homes in limbo', *Children and Young People Now*, 2 October, https://www.cypnow.co.uk/cyp/news/1054683/childrens-homes-left-in-limbo

14 Ofsted (2017) 'Children's Social Care Data in England 2017: Main findings', 31 August, https://www.gov.uk/government/publications/childrens-social-care-data-in-england-2017/childrens-social-care-data-in-england-2017-main-findings

15   Bradbury, J. (2018) 'The changing picture in the children's home sector', 22 August, Ofsted, https://socialcareinspection.blog.gov.uk/2018/08/22/the-changing-picture-in-the-childrens-homes-sector/

16   Donovan, T. (2017) 'Children's home commissioning must change or risk legal action, warns ICHA', 11 December, https://www.cypnow.co.uk/cyp/news/2004627/childrens-home-commissioning-must-change-or-risk-legal-action-warns-icha

17   Elvin, A. (2106) 'Why do we let fostering agencies profit from caring for vulnerable children?', 11 July, https://www.theguardian.com/social-care-network/2016/jan/11/why-let-fostering-agencies-profit-caring-children

18   University of Oxford (2017) Rees Centre for Research in Fostering and Education, http://reescentre.education.ox.ac.uk/

19   Corporate Watch (2015) 'The Foster Care Business', 15 December, https://corporatewatch.org/the-fostercare-business/

20   Core Assets (2016) Impact Report, https://www.coreassets.com/mediacentre/wpcontent/uploads/2017/04/Core-Assets-Childrens-Services-Impact-Report-2016.pdf

21   Turner, A. (2017) 'Social workers transferred to Virgin Care under landmark deal', 26 April, http://www.communitycare.co.uk/2017/04/26/social-workers-transferred-virgin-care-landmark-deal/

22   Campbell, D. (2016) 'Virgin Care wins £700m contract to run 200 NHS and social care services', 11 November, https://www.theguardian.com/society/2016/nov/11/virgin-care-700m-contract-200-nhs-social-care-services-bath-somerset

23   Matthews-King, A. (2017) 'Virgin's £100m children's health services contract signals 'galloping privatisation' of NHS, warn MPs', 12 December, www.independent.co.uk/news/health/virgin-children-health-service-contract-nhs-privatisation-mps-warn-drugs-healthcare-lancashire-a8105606.html

24   Hayes, D. (2018) 'Council to reassess bids to run children's health services', 15 August, https://www.cypnow.co.uk/cyp/news/2005659/council-to-reassess-bids-to-run-childrens-health-services

25   Osborne, H. (2018) 'Virgin awarded almost £2bn of health contracts in past five years: Richard Branson's company now one of UK's leading healthcare providers, analysis reveals', 5

August, https://www.theguardian.com/society/2018/aug/05/virgin-awarded-almost-2bn-of-nhs-contracts-in-the-past-five-years?CMP=Share_iOSApp_Other

26   Travis, A. (2013) 'G4S contract to run sexual assault referral centres damned: Campaigners criticise "sell-off" of sensitive services to private company that bungled Olympics security contract', https://www.theguardian.com/business/2013/may/24/g4s-contract-sexual-assault-referral-centres

27   Serco (2013) *Contract News Update 16*, May, https://www.serco.com/media/676/676.original.pdf?1473336847

28   Brindle, D. (2016) 'How can social work find a sustainable solution to its recruitment crisis?', 6 September, https://www.theguardian.com/social-care-network/2016/sep/06/social-work-sustainable-solution-recruitment-crisis

29   Tapsfield, J. (2016) 'Health chief: Agency staff "rip-off" will cost us £4bn', 19 January, *The Metro*, p 2.

30   Puffett, N. (2016) 'Unexpected rise in children's social worker vacancies', 25 February, https://www.cypnow.co.uk/cyp/news/1156125/unexpected-rise-in-children%E2%80%99s-social-worker-vacancies

31   Donovan, T. (2016) 'Children's social work vacancies soared 27% in past year, government reports', 26 February, http://www.communitycare.co.uk/2016/02/26/childrens-social-work-vacancies-soared-27-past-year-government-reports/

32   Skills for Care (2016) *The state of the adult social care sector and workforce in England September 2016*, https://www.nmds-sc-online.org.uk/Get.aspx?id=980099

33   Skills for Care (2016) *The state of the adult social care sector and workforce in England September 2017*, p 26, www.skillsforcare.org.uk/Documents/NMDS-SC-and-intelligence/NMDS-SC/Analysis-pages/State-of17/State-of-the-adult-social-care-sector-and-workforce-2017.pdf, p 26

34   Holt, A. and Greenwood, G. (2017) 'Councils spend doubles on social workers hired from agencies', 1 November, https://www.bbc.co.uk/news/education-39659252

35   BASW (2017) 'Spending on agency staff has doubled', *Professional Social Worker Magazine*, December 2017/January 2018, p 7.

36 BBC News (2018) 'Struggling Northamptonshire County Council bans spending', 2 February, www.bbc.co.uk/news/uk-england-northamptonshire-42920716

37 BBC News (2018) 'Northamptonshire County Council "should be scrapped"', 15 March, www.bbc.co.uk/news/uk-england-northamptonshire-40610349

38 Lepper, J. (2018) 'Troubled council shelves plan to outsource children's services', 24 August, https://www.cypnow.co.uk/cyp/news/2005680/troubled-council-puts-plans-to-outsource-childrens-services-on-hold

39 Donovan, T. (2018) 'Council takes adult social care services back in house after viability concerns', 18 January, www.communitycare.co.uk/2018/01/18/council-takes-adult-social-care-services-back-house-viability-concerns/

40 Turner, A. (2018) '£6.6m agency staff overspend "hugely detrimental" to council's children's services', 30 July, https://www.communitycare.co.uk/2018/07/30/agency-staff-overspend-lewisham-childrens-services/

41 Zeffman, H. (2018) 'Surrey county council raises pay despite funding crisis', 9 February, https://www.thetimes.co.uk/article/surrey-county-council-raises-pay-despite-funding-crisis-88znnsvmb.

42 Davies, G. (2018) 'Is Surrey the next council in crisis?', 7 February, https://www.thebureauinvestigates.com/stories/2018-02-07/is-surrey-the-next-council-in-crisis

43 Sleator, L. (2018) 'Council under financial strain', 7 September, https://www.bbc.co.uk/news/uk-politics-45435368

44 Liquid Personnel Ltd (2016) Annual Report and Financial Statements for the period ended 31 December 2016.

45 Sanctuary Personnel Ltd (2016) Director's Report and Financial Statements for the Year Ended 31 October 2016.

46 Children's Commissioner (2018) Stability Index 2018, June, https://www.childrenscommissioner.gov.uk/wp-content/uploads/2018/05/Childrens-Commissioners-2018-Stability-Index-Overview.pdf

47 Donovan, T. (2017) 'Number of social workers who prefer locum work on the increase: Community Care research shows the majority of social workers still prefer permanent work but this is beginning to change', 22 February, www.communitycare.

co.uk/2017/02/22/number-social-workers-prefer-locum-work-increase/

48   Stevenson, L. (2017) '£8.5 million given to private companies to develop social worker accreditation, government reveals', 22 December, www.communitycare.co.uk/2017/12/22/8-5-million-given-privatecompanies-develop-social-worker-accreditation-government-reveals/

49   Stevenson, L. (2018) 'International consultancy firm handed £3.6 million social work accreditation contract', 7 February, www.communitycare.co.uk/2018/02/07/international-consultancy-firm-handed-3-6-million-social-work-accreditation-contract/

50   Mott Macdonald (2017) 'Development of a CPD programme on permanence for children and family social workers', https://www.mottmac.com/article/35830/development-of-a-cpd-programme-on-permanence-for-child-and-family-social-workers

51   Smith, M. (2017) 'Nationalisation vs privatisation: the public view', 19 May, https://yougov.co.uk/news/2017/05/19/nationalisation-vs-privatisation-public-view/

52   House of Commons Committee of Public Accounts (2014) 'Contracting out public services to the private sector', Forty-seventh Report of Session 2013–14, 26 February, p 3, https://publications.parliament.uk/pa/cm201314/cmselect/cmpubacc/777/777.pdf

53   Bew, J. (2017) *Citizen Clem: A Biography of Attlee*, London, Riverrun, p xxiii.

54   Skinner, G. and Clemence, M. (2016) Veracity Index 2016, Ipsos MORI, https://www.ipsos.com/sites/default/files/migrations/en-uk/files/Assets/Docs/Polls/ipsos-mori-veracity-index-2016-charts.pdf

55   Renwick, C. (2017) *Bread for All: The Origins of the Welfare State*, London, p 267.

56   Timmins, N. (2017) 'The "welfare state" should be something we're proud of. Not a term of abuse', 31 October, https://www.theguardian.com/commentisfree/2017/oct/31/time-bring-welfare-state-back-to-life-language-social-security

57   Attlee, C. (undated), quoted in Bew (2017) *op cit*, p 171.

58   MacAskill, E., Garside, J. and Pegg, D. (2017) 'Jeremy Corbyn leads criticism of Paradise Papers legal action: Labour leader among senior politicians alarmed by Appleby action against BBC and

Guardian over tax haven investigations', 19 December, https://
www.theguardian.com/world/2017/dec/19/jeremy-corbyn-
leads-criticism-of-paradise-papers-legal-action

59   Alvaredo, F., Chancel, L., Piketty, T., Saez, E. and Zucma, G.
(2018) *World Inequality Report 2018*, World Inequality Lab, http://
wir2018.wid.world/files/download/wir2018-summary-english.
pdf

60   Neate, R. (2017) 'World's richest 0.1% have boosted their wealth
by as much as poorest half: Inequality report also shows UK's
50,000 richest people have seen their share of the country's wealth
double since 1984', 14 December, https://www.theguardian.com/
inequality/2017/dec/14/world-richest-increased-wealth-same-
amount-as-poorest-half

Chapter Eleven

1   Aitken, J. (2013) *Margaret Thatcher: Power and Personality*, London,
Bloomsbury, p 302.

2   Thatcher, M. (1980) Speech to Conservative Party Conference, 10
October, https://www.margaretthatcher.org/document/104431

3   Parker, G. (2013) 'There is no alternative, says Cameron', 7
March, https://www.ft.com/content/3a39ea0e8723-11e2-bde6-
00144feabdc0

4   Thomas, D. (2018) 'Where did it go wrong for Carillion?', 15
January, www.bbc.co.uk/news/business42666275

5   Weale, S., Rawlinson, K. and Lynch, C. (2018) 'Fire services
ready to deliver school meals after Carillion collapse: Councils
prepare to protect vital services at schools, and doubts emerge
over construction projects', 15 January, https://www.theguardian.
com/business/2018/jan/15/fire-services-ready-to-deliver-school-
mealsafter-carillion-collapse

6   Carillion (2016) *Annual Report and Accounts 2016: Making Tomorrow
a Better Place*, http://annualreport2016.carillionplc.com/

7   Thomas (2018) *op cit*.

8   Quoted in S. Goodley (2018) 'Carillion's "highly inappropriate"
pay packets criticised: Stricken firm's bosses will still benefit
despite collapse', 15 January, https://www.theguardian.com/
business/2018/jan/15/carillion-highly-inappropriate-pay-
packets-criticised

9   Goodley (2018) *op cit*.

10   Edwards, J. (2018) 'KPMG believes it will be investigated over the collapse of Carillion: "We are standing by the work that we did"', 23 January, http://uk.businessinsider.com/kpmg-confirms-frc-investigation-over-collapse-of-carillion-2018-1

11   Williams, C. (2018) 'Carillion auditor KPMG faces scrutiny for approving books months before collapse', 15 January, www.telegraph.co.uk/business/2018/01/15/carillion-auditor-kpmg-faces-scrutiny-approving-books-months/

12   Curry, R. (2018) 'Carillion collapse could spark competition probe into accounting Big Four',30 January, www.telegraph.co.uk/business/2018/01/30/carillion-collapse-could-spark-competition-probe-accounting/

13   Chu, B. (2018) 'Why didn't anyone say it was going to fail?', 30 January, www.independent.co.uk/voices/carillion-kpmg-auditors-audit-hbos-financial-crisis-self-regulation-deloitte-a8185356.html

14   Lea, R. (2018) 'Carillion and KPMG face Financial Reporting Council's biggest-ever inquiry', 30 January, www.independent.co.uk/news/business/news/carillion-collapse-mps-accuse-big-four-accountancy-firms-operating-oligopoly-a8185921.html

15   Kollowe, J. (2018) 'KPMG to be investigated over Carillion auditing: Watchdog opens inquiry into accountancy firm's role in collapse of construction giant', 29 January, https://www.theguardian.com/business/2018/jan/29/kpmg-carillion-frc

16   Agerholm, H. (2018) 'Grenfell Tower inquiry hires KPMG despite firm earning millions from auditing council and contractors investigated over fire: Multinational consultancy company to be paid £200,000 over three months to provide "planning and programme management support"', 5 January, www.independent.co.uk/news/uk/home-news/grenfell-tower-fire-inquiry-kpmg-adviser-accountancy-firm-earning-millions-audit-council-contractors-a8143621.html

17   Alex, R. (2018) 'Advisers on Hinkley Point C nuclear power station had "cosy" ties to both sides: Apparent conflict of interest on Somerset project', 1 January, https://www.thetimes.co.uk/article/advisers-on-hinkleypoint-c-nuclear-power-station-had-cosy-ties-to-both-sides-xftxcl9sz

18   *Financial Times* (2018) 'PwC's multiple roles with Carillion come under scrutiny', 16 January, https://www.google.co.uk/search?ei=uBRyWr7COzWgAaQ5LqgDQ&q=https%3A%2F%2Fwww.

ft.com%2Fcontent%2Ffb913b2e-fac5-11e7-a4922c9be7f3120a+
&oq=https%3A%2F%2Fwww.ft.com%2Fcontent%2Ffb913b2e-
fac5-11e7-a4922c9be7f3120a+&gs_l=psy-ab.3...5196.7920.0.11
103.1.1.0.0.0.0.75.75.1.1.0....0...1c.1j2.64.psyab..0.0.0....0.ezqJ_
YN6bCY

19 BBC News (2018) 'Carillion collapse sparks break up call for "Big
    Four"', 30 January, www.bbc.co.uk/news/business-42870816

20 Sky News (2016) 'Construction "Blacklist" Settlement Reached',
    29 April, https://news.sky.com/story/construction-blacklist-
    settlement-reached-10262926

21 Smith, A. (2018) 'Carillion ruined my life by blacklisting me
    for raising health and safety concerns', 22 January, http://metro.
    co.uk/2018/01/22/carillion-ruined-my-life-by-blacklisting-me-
    for-raising-health-and-safety-concerns-7250856/

22 BBC (2013) 'Suffolk road crash: Wolverhampton firm fined
    £180,000', 8 November, www.bbc.co.uk/news/uk-england-
    suffolk-24863448

23 Martin, D. (2013) 'Failed firm's £53m from Labour NHS deal:
    Taxpayers foot huge bill after ministers terminated contract when
    GPs stopped referring patients to failing hospital unit', 2 August,
    www.dailymail.co.uk/news/article-2382926/Failed-firms-53m-
    Labour-NHS-deal-Taxpayers-foot-huge-ministers-terminated-
    contract-GPs-stopped-referring-patients-failing-hospital-unit.
    html

24 The Canadian Press (2015) 'Company fined $900k for not properly
    cleaning QEW in 2014', 6 October, www.cbc.ca/news/canada/
    hamilton/news/company-fined-900k-for-not-properly-cleaning-
    qew-in2014-1.3258973

25 Lintern, S. (2016) 'Trust seeks to terminate £200 million contract:
    Nottingham University Hospitals Trust will look to terminate a
    five year, £200m estates contract with Carillion amid concerns
    over poor standards', 28 November, https://www.hsj.co.uk/
    newsletter/hsj-local/providers/nottingham-university-hospitals-
    nhstrust/breaking-trust-seeks-to-terminate-major-200m-
    contract/7013653.article

26 BBC News (2018) *op cit*.

27 Jenkins, S. (2018) 'I'm not surprised by Carillion's failure –
    companies like this shouldn't exist', 15 January, https://www.

theguardian.com/commentisfree/2018/jan/15/carillion-failure-contracts-government-whitehall

28 Toynbee, P. (2018) 'It's not just Carillion. The whole privatisation myth has been exposed', 22 January, https://www.theguardian.com/commentisfree/2018/jan/22/carillion-privatisation-myth-councils-pfi-contracts

29 Hutton, W. (2018) 'Capitalism's new crisis: after Carillion, can the private sector ever be trusted?', 21 January, https://www.theguardian.com/politics/2018/jan/21/capitalism-new-crisis-can-private-sector-be-trusted-carillion-privatisation

30 Stewart, H. and Asthana, A. (2018) 'Corbyn on Carillion: We'll end outsourcing 'racket' in rule change: public sector would become first choice to provide government services, says Labour leader', 18 January, https://www.theguardian.com/politics/2018/jan/18/corbyn-on-carillion-well-end-outsourcing-racket-in-rule-change

31 Maidment, J. (2018) 'PMQs: Theresa May accuses Labour of being anti-business as Jeremy Corbyn attacks Government over collapse of Carillion', 17 January, www.telegraph.co.uk/politics/2018/01/17/pmqs-live-theresa-may-faces-grilling-governments-handling-carillion/

32 Jones, R. (2018) 'Ministers shake up contract bidding rules', 25 June, https://www.theguardian.com/business/2018/jun/25/ministers-shake-up-contract-bidding-rules

33 Pierce, A. (2018) 'George's sharp U-turn over Carillion crisis: Osborne backtracks over ailing construction firm after agreeing to boost its coffers while Chancellor', 22 January, http://www.dailymail.co.uk/news/article5295939/Osborne-backtracks-ailing-construction-firm-Carillion.html

34 *London Evening Standard* (2018) 'Who bails out Carillion?', 15 January, https://www.standard.co.uk/comment/comment/evening-standard-comment-the-last-straw-in-our-war-onneedless-plastic-a3740116.html

35 Yeatman, D. (2018) 'Carillion Gazillions', *Metro*, 16 January, p 16.

36 Davies, R.(2018) 'Carillion crisis: hedge funds rake in tens of millions: Short-sellers quietly targeted company as far back as 2015 with bets reaching peak before first profit warning in July 2017', 14 January, https://www.theguardian.com/business/2018/jan/14/carillion-crisis-hedge-funds-rake-in-tens-of-millions

37 BBC (2018) 'Carillion tried to "wriggle out" of pension contributions', 29 January, www.bbc.co.uk/news/business-42853895

38 Tovey, A. (2014) 'Serco issues profit warning and plans £550m rights issue: Serco shares plunge as the troubled outsourcer caught up in the tagging scandal warns on profits and announces plans for rights issue to shore up finances', 10 November, www.telegraph.co.uk/finance/newsbysector/supportservices/11220207/Serco-issues-profit-warning-and-plans-550m-rights-issue.html

39 *The Guardian* (2018) 'Editorial: The current outsourcing pattern is commercially unsustainable. It is time for a wider rebalancing of public and private provision of essential services', 31 January, https://www.theguardian.com/global/commentisfree/2018/jan/31/the-guardian-view-on-capitas-woes-another-warning-of-a-system-in-crisis

40 Toynbee (2018) *op cit.*

41 Chaplain, C. (2018) 'Businessman David Meller quits education post and as Mayor's Fund trustee amid Presidents Club Charity dinner "sexism" storm', 24 January, https://www.standard.co.uk/news/uk/businessman-david-meller-quits-e-a3748546.html

42 Marriage, M. (2018) 'Men Only: Inside the charity fundraiser where hostesses are put on show', https://www.ft.com/content/075d679e-0033-11e8-9650-9c0ad2d7c5b5

43 Puffett, N. (2018) 'Nadhim Zahawi to replace Robert Goodwill as children's minister', 11 January, https://www.cypnow.co.uk/cyp/news/2004744/nadhim-zahawi-to-replace-robert-goodwill-as-childrens-minister

44 Parliament UK (2018) 'Nadhim Zahawi', 1 February, https://www.parliament.uk/biographies/commons/nadhim-zahawi/4113

45 Adams, R. (2018) 'David Meller, the Tory donor "desperate to be part of establishment": Presidents Club groping scandal will deny wealthy Meller "his ultimate prize" of a peerage', 24 January, https://www.theguardian.com/uk-news/2018/jan/24/david-meller-presidents-club-groping-scandal-wealthy-tory-donor

46 *The Guardian* (2018) 'Presidents Club: who was invited to the all-male charity gala? The Guardian has obtained the full list of men allocated tables and seats at the event, though it is not confirmed they attended', 25 January, https://www.theguardian.

com/world/2018/jan/24/guest-list-presidents-club-all-male-charity-gala

47 Sparrow, A. and Walker, P. (2018) 'Corbyn to put May on spot by embracing EU customs union: Labour leader will pile pressure on PM before key vote, but avoid single market commitment', 26 February, https://www.theguardian.com/politics/2018/feb/26/jeremy-corbyn-to-confirm-labour-wants-a-customs-union-with-eu

48 *The Economist* (1998) 'The End of Privatisation?', 11 June, www.economist.com/node/134789

49 Gove, M. (2018) 'The failure of child protection and the need for a fresh start', 21 November, https://www.gov.uk/government/speeches/the-failure-of-child-protection-and-the-need-for-a-fresh-start

50 Jones, R. (2016) 'Six reasons to rethink moves to strip councils of children's services: The government's thrust towards trusts could do more harm than good to efforts to improve struggling services, argues Ray Jones', 5 September, www.communitycare.co.uk/2016/09/05/six-reasons-rethink-moves-strip-councils-childrens-services/

51 Hutton (2018) *op cit.*

52 Le Grand, J, 2016) 'Vision, Professional Social Work', 31 August, http://cdn.basw.co.uk/upload/basw_815343.pdf

53 Jones, R. (2016) 'I'm wary of Le Grand's brave new world of turmoil', *Professional Social Work*, September, p 11.

54 Eisenstadt, N. (2011) *Providing a Sure Start: How the Government Discovered Early Childhood*, Bristol, Policy Press.

55 Stevenson, L. (2018) 'Defining our social work practice: how a council is building on 12 years of stability: Why a council is taking the step to brand its existing social work practice, rather than import another model', 16 March, www.communitycare.co.uk/2018/03/16/defining-social-work-practice-council-building-12years-stability/

56 Sebba, J., Luke, N., McNeish, D., and Rees, A. (2017) 'Children's Social Care Innovation Programme Final evaluation report', November 2017, Rees Centre for Research in Fostering and Education, https://www.gov.uk/government/uploads/system/uploads/attachment_data/file/659110/Children_s_Social_C are_Innovation_Programme_-_Final_evaluation_report.pdf

57 Ofsted (2018) 'Bournemouth Inspection of children's social care services', July, https://files.api.beta.ofsted.gov.uk/v1/file/50015172

58 Donovan, T. (2018) 'Council gets "good" Ofsted rating after ending agency worker use', 24 August, https://www.cypnow.co.uk/cyp/news/2005681/council-gets-good-ofsted-rating-after-ending-agency-worker-use

59 Turner, A. (2018) 'Stability at heart of council's cross the board "outstanding" Ofsted grading', 6 August, https://www.communitycare.co.uk/2018/08/06/stability-north-yorkshire-council-outstanding-ofsted/

60 Lepper, J. (2018) 'Staff departures threaten progress at "inadequate" council, Ofsted warns', 31 August, https://www.cypnow.co.uk/cyp/news/2005734/staff-departures-threaten-progress-at-inadequate-council-ofsted-warns

61 *Community Care* (2018) 'Managers struggling to cover social worker sickness and leave at "inadequate" council', 6 August, https://www.communitycare.co.uk/2018/08/06/managers-struggling-cover-social-worker-sickness-leave-inadequate-council/

62 Hill, A. (2018) 'Courts for addicted parents work. So why are they being stripped of support?', 24 July, https://www.theguardian.com/society/2018/jul/24/courts-addicted-parents-funds-family-drug-and-alcohol-court-children-care

63 Goodman, S. and Trowler, I. (eds) (2011) *Social Work Reclaimed: Innovative Frameworks for Child and Family Social Work Practice*, London, Jessica Kingsley.

64 Goodman, S. (2017) Tweet, Morning Lane Associates, 14 October.

65 Bywaters, P., Bunting, L., Davidson, G., Hanratty, J., Mason, W., McCartan, C. and Steils, N. (2016) 'The relationship between poverty, child abuse and neglect: An evidence review', 3 March, https://www.jrf.org.uk/report/relationship-between-poverty-child-abuse-and-neglect-evidence-review

66 Hood, R., Goldacre, A., Grant, R. and Jones, R. (2016) 'Exploring demand and provision in English child protection services', June, https://academic.oup.com/bjsw/article-abstract/46/4/923/2472957

67 Bilson, A. and Martin, K. (2017) 'Referrals and child protection in England: one in five children referred to children's services and

one in nineteen investigated before the age of five', April, https://academic.oup.com/bjsw/article-abstract/47/3/793/2622314

68 Donovan, T. (2018) 'DfE "misguided and short sighted" on children's services spending', 21 June, https://www.cypnow.co.uk/cyp/news/2005436/dfe-misguided-and-shortsighted-on-childrens-services-spending

69 Ofsted (2012) 'Inspection of local authority arrangements for the protection of children: Isle of Wight', https://reports.ofsted.gov.uk/sites/default/files/documents/local_authority_reports/isle_of_wight/051_Inspection%20of%20local%20authority%20arrangements%20for%20the%20protection%20of%20children%20as%20pdf.pdf

70 Ofsted (2013) 'Inspection of local authority arrangements for the protection of children: Devon County Council', https://reports.ofsted.gov.uk/sites/default/files/documents/local_authority_reports/devon/051_Inspection%20of%20local%20authority%20arrangements%20for%20the%20protection%20of%20children%20as%20pdf.pdf

71 Jones, R. (2017a) *The Story of Baby P: Setting the Record Straight*, Bristol, Policy Press.

72 Jones, R. (2017b) 'Baby P death 10 years on: the case's lasting impact on child protection', 26 July, https://www.cypnow.co.uk/cyp/analysis/2003962/baby-p-death-10-years-on-the-case%E2%80%99s-lasting-impact-on-child-protection

73 Government UK (2018) 'Intellectual Property and Your Work', https://www.google.co.uk/search?q=Intellectual+property+and+your+work&rlz=1C1AKJH_enGB761GB761&o q=Intellectual+property+and+your+work&aqs=chrome..69i57j69i60&sourceid=chrome&ie=UTF-8

74 Munro, E. (2011) *Munro review of child protection: A child-centred system*, 10 May, https://www.gov.uk/government/publications/munro-review-of-child-protection-final-report-a-child-centred-system

75 Servelec Group (2018) 'Servelec Group', https://www.servelecgroup.com/about-us/

76 Servelec (2017) 'Making IT Work', https://www.servelechsc.com/media/2476/servelec-and-signs-of-safety-article-march-2017-final.pdf

77 Jones (2017a) *op cit.*

78   Ferguson, H. (2010) 'Walks, home visits and atmospheres: risk and the everyday practices and mobilities of social work and child protection', *The British Journal of Social Work*, 40(4), 1 June, pp 1100–1117, https://doi.org/10.1093/bjsw/bcq015

79   Stevenson, L. (2017) 'Hiring PAs for social workers cuts stress and saves money, finds study: Research into innovation-backed project shows successes of hiring administrative support for social workers', 21 March, www.communitycare.co.uk/2017/03/21/hiring-pas-social-workers-cuts-stress-saves-money-finds-study/

80   Stevenson, L. (2015) 'Council redesigns children's services to cut bureaucracy after innovation fund windfall: Hertfordshire council's head of family safeguarding tells Community Care how they plan to spend £4.86m from the innovation fund', 23 January, www.communitycare.co.uk/2015/01/23/council-redesigns-childrens-services-cut-bureaucracy-innovation-fund-windfall/

81   Burch, K., Green, C., Merrell, S., Taylor, V. and Wise, S. (2017) 'Social Care Innovations in Hampshire and the Isle of Wight Evaluation Report', The Institute of Public Care, Oxford Brookes University, https://www.gov.uk/government/uploads/system/uploads/attachment_data/file/600908/Hampshire_and_IOW_Evaluation_Report_March_2017.pdf

82   *Community Care* (2018) 'Private consultancies take share of £12 million for children's social care innovation implementation: Deloitte, Mutual Ventures and the Department for Education's Innovation Unit split the £12 million cost for implementing the innovation programme over the past four years', www.communitycare.co.uk/2018/08/30/private-consultancies-share-12-million-childrens-social-care-innovation-implementation/

83   LGA (2017) 'Bright Futures: We're calling for the services that change children's lives to be properly funded', https://www.local.gov.uk/sites/default/files/documents/LGA_Bright%20Futures%20key%20stats%20and%20summary_November%202017.pdf

84   Hayes, D. (2017) 'Goodwill: Children's leaders must make better use of existing resources', 13 October, https://www.cypnow.co.uk/cyp/news/2004351/goodwill-childrens-leaders-must-make-better-use-of-existing-resources

85   Puffett, N. (2018) 'DfE "examining children's services funding", Zahawi reveals', 14 March, https://www.cypnow.co.uk/cyp/

news/2005021/dfe-examining-childrens-services-funding-zahawi-reveals

86 Stevenson, L. (2018) 'ADCS rejects idea that too much money is spent on care placements: President of the ADCS tells ministers there is not enough money in the system "full stop"', www.communitycare.co.uk/2018/07/09/adcs-refutes-idea-much-money-spent-care-placements/

87 Stevenson (2018) *op cit.*

88 Stevenson (2018) *op cit.*

89 Hayes, D. (2018) 'DfE warns of uphill struggle to secure children's services funding', 9 July, https://www.cypnow.co.uk/cyp/news/2005524/dfe-warns-of-uphill-struggle-to-secure-childrens-services-funding

90 BBC (2018) 'Vulnerable children facing "catastrophe" over crisis-hit councils', 4 August, https://www.bbc.co.uk/news/uk-england-northamptonshire-45069057

91 LGA (2017) 'We're calling for services that change children's lives to be properly funded', November, https://www.local.gov.uk/sites/default/files/documents/LGA_Bright%20Futures%20key%20stats%20and%20summary_November%202017.pdf

92 All Party Parliamentary Group for Children (2018) Storing Up Trouble: A Postcode Lottery of Children's Services, July, https://www.ncb.org.uk/sites/default/files/field/attachment/NCB%20Storing%20Up%20Trouble%20%5BAugust%20Update%5D.pdf

93 Butler, P. (2018) 'Underfunding to blame for child protection "crisis", says report', 11 July, https://www.theguardian.com/society/2018/jul/11/underfunding-to-blame-for-child-protection-crisis-says-report

94 Jones, R., Matczak, A., Davis, K. and Byford, I. (2015) '"Troubled Families": a team around the family', in Davis, K. (ed) *Social Work with Troubled Families: A Critical Introduction*, London, Jessica Kingsley, pp 124–158.

95 Ofsted (2016) 'Royal Borough of Kensington and Chelsea Inspection of services for children in need of help and protection, children looked after and care leavers', 29 March, https://www.rbkc.gov.uk/sites/default/files/atoms/files/Single%20inspection%20of%20LA%20children%27s%20services%20and%20review%20of%20the%20LSCB.pdf

96   Ofsted (2015) 'Leeds City Council Inspection of services for children in need of help and protection, children looked after and care leavers', 27 March, https://reports.ofsted.gov.uk/sites/default/files/documents/local_authority_reports/leeds/051_Single%20inspection%20of%20LA%20children%27s%20services%20and%20review%20of%20the%20LSCB%20as%20pdf.pdf

97   Ofsted (2018) 'North Yorkshire County Council Inspection of children's social care services', July, https://reports.ofsted.gov.uk/sites/default/files/documents/local_authority_reports/north_yorkshire/070_%20North_Yorkshire_Inspection%20of%20local%20authority%20childrens%20services.pdf

98   Seebohm, F. (1968) *Report of the Committee on Local Authority and Allied Personal Services*, July, Cmnd. 3703, HMSO.

99   Featherstone, B., White, S. and Morris, K. (2014) *Re-imagining Child Protection: Towards Humane Social Work*, Bristol, Policy Press.

100 Featherstone, B., Gupta, A., Morris, K. and White, S. (2018) *Protecting Children: A Social Model*, Bristol, Policy Press.

101 Featherstone et al (2018) *op cit*, p 7.

102 Puffett, N. (2016) 'Government-ordered children's trust services rated "inadequate"by Ofsted', 17 February, https://www.cypnow.co.uk/cyp/news/1156006/government-ordered-childrens-trust-services-rated-inadequate-by-ofsted

103 Zahawi, N. (2018) Written Question 122430, 12 January, www.parliament.uk/business/publications/written-questions-answers-statements/writtenquestion/Commons/2018-01-12/122430/

104 Ofsted (2015) 'Doncaster Metropolitan Borough Council', 27 November, https://reports.ofsted.gov.uk/sites/default/files/documents/local_authority_reports/doncaster/054_Single%20inspection%20of%20LA%20children%27s%20services%20and%20review%20of%20the%20LSCB%20as%20pdf.pdf

105 Ofsted (2018) 'Doncaster Metropolitan Borough Council', 19 January, https://reports.ofsted.gov.uk/sites/default/files/documents/local_authority_reports/doncaster/059_Single%20inspection%20of%20LA%20children%27s%20services%20as%20pdf%20.pdf

106 Lepper, J. and Puffett, N. (2018) 'Children's trust boss steps down in wake of Ofsted report', 8 February, https://www.cypnow.co.uk/cyp/news/2004867/childrens-trust-boss-steps-down-in-wake-of-critical-ofstedreport?utm_content=&utm_campaign=080218_

DailyNews&utm_source=Children%20%26%20Young%20
People%20Now&utm_medium=adestra_email&utm_
term=https%3A%2F%2Fwww.cypnow.co.uk%2Fcyp%2Fnews%
2F2004867%2Fchildrens-trust-boss-steps-down-in-wake-of-
critical-ofsted-report

107 Kessen, D. (2018) 'Concern as Doncaster children's services
trust overspends by millions', 28 February, https://www.
doncasterfreepress.co.uk/news/concern-as-doncaster-children-
s-services-trust-overspends-bymillions-1-9040744

108 McNicoll, A. (2017) 'Virgin Care set to run social work service
in unprecedented deal: Bath and North East Somerset contract
would mark first time core adult social work services run by
for-profit firm', 9 November, http://www.communitycare.
co.uk/2016/11/09/virgin-care-set-run-social-work-service-
unprecedented-deal/

109 Miller, J. (2018) 'Doncaster's Direction', 6 February, https://www.
themj.co.uk/Doncasters-direction/210170

110 Dudman, J. (2016) 'Jo Miller: "Councils can't take more shocks
to an already shocked system"', 15 November, https://www.
theguardian.com/society/2016/nov/15/jo-miller-doncaster-
council-chief-executives-solace

111 Hayes, (2017) *op cit.*

112 Hood, R., Goldacre, A., Grant, R. and Jones, R. (2016) 'Exploring
demand and provision in English child protection services', *The
British Journal of Social Work*, 46(4), 1 June, pp 923–941, https://
doi.org/10.1093/bjsw/bcw044

113 Bywaters, P., Bunting, L., Davidson, G., Hanratty, J., Mason, W.,
McCartan, C. and Steils, N. (2016) 'The relationship between
poverty, child abuse and neglect: an evidence review', 3 March,
Joseph Rowntree Foundation, https://www.jrf.org.uk/report/
relationship-between-poverty-child-abuse-and-neglect-evidence-
review

114 Bilson, A. and Martin, K. (2016) 'Referrals and child protection
in england: one in five children referred to children's services and
one in nineteen investigated before the age of five', *The British
Journal of Social Work*, 47(3), 1 April, pp 793–811, https://doi.
org/10.1093/bjsw/bcw054

115 Stevenson, L, (2018) 'Council to invest £1.2 million to cover
overspend on children's social workers after "15% rise in work":

Social workers saw a "41% increase in monthly contacts" since local authority was rated 'inadequate' by Ofsted', 1 February, www.communitycare.co.uk/2018/02/01/council-invest-1-2-millioncover-overspend-childrens-social-workers-15-rise-work/

116 Puffett, N. (2015) 'Former Ofsted social care chief appointed DCS at Tower Hamlets', 16 July, https://www.cypnow.co.uk/cyp/news/1152656/former-ofsted-social-care-chief-appointed-dcs-at-tower-hamlets

117 Schooling, E. (2017) 'What social workers need to know about Ofsted's new inspection regime: Ofsted's national director for social care talks through the changes being made to social care inspection', 29 November, www.communitycare.co.uk/2017/11/29/social-workers-need-know-ofsteds-new-inspection-regime/

118 Hayes, D. (2016) 'LGA chief backs improvement role for councils', 2 February, https://www.cypnow.co.uk/cyp/news/1155794/in-the-new-edition-of-cyp-now-lga-chief-backs-improvementrole-for-councils

119 Michalska, A. (2018) 'DfE invest £17m in sector-led improvement', 15 March, http://adcs.org.uk/inspection/article/dfe-invest-17m-in-sector-led-improvement

120 BBC News (2015) 'Somerset children's services still "inadequate"', Ofsted says', 27 March, www.bbc.co.uk/news/uk-england-somerset-32085372 .

121 Stevenson, L. (2017) '"Inadequate" children's services praised by minister for improving social work practice: More manageable caseloads and a stable workforce were seen as key drivers of improvement in the authority rated "inadequate" by Ofsted twice', 19 January, www.communitycare.co.uk/2017/01/19/inadequate-childrens-services-praised-minister-improving-social-work-practice/

122 Ofsted (2014) 'Isle of Wight Council', 19 November, https://reports.ofsted.gov.uk/sites/default/files/documents/local_authority_reports/isle_of_wight/053_Single%20inspection%20of%20LA%20children%27s%20services%20and%20review%20of%20the%20LSCB%20as%20 pdf.pdf

123 Sharman, L. (2018) 'Plymouth agrees to manage Torbay's failing children's services: Plymouth City Council has agreed to take on full managerial responsibility for the 'inadequate' children's services

in Torbay', 31 January, https://www.localgov.co.uk/Plymouth-agrees-to-manage-Torbays-failing-childrens-services/44641

124 London Borough of Tower Hamlets (2017) 'Commissioners at Tower Hamlets: Role of Commissioners', https://www.towerhamlets.gov.uk/lgnl/council_and_democracy/Commissioners_at_Tower_Hamlets/Commissioners_at_Tower_Hamlets.aspx

125 BBC (2018) 'Northamptonshire County Council: Commissioners take over authority', 10 May, https://www.bbc.co.uk/news/uk-england-northamptonshire-44069130

Index

Note: Page numbers in *italics* refer to footnotes.

Numbers

A4e 221–2

A

Academies Enterprise Trust (AET)
181, *183*
academy schools
accountability 182
under Conservative governments
178–82
governing bodies 186
head teachers and teachers 186–7
looked-after children and 184
under New Labour 177–8
participation in LSCBs 183
accountability issues 22, 31, 33, 65,
141, 182, 281, 300
accountancy firms 160–2, 169
and conflicts of interest 267–70
see also KPMG
accreditation 82–90
government funding of 252–3
House of Commons Education
Select Committee concerns
over 87
KPMG awarded contract to
develop 69, 82–3, 86, 93
opposition to 83–6
pilots 86–7
power of Secretary of State for
Education to set standards 88
and relevance to privatisation
journey 89
Achieving for Children 32–3, 103
Action for Children 187, 188, 189

ADCS (Association of Directors of
Children's Services) 84–6, 96, 97,
290–1
The Adolescent and Children's Trust
(TACT) 46–7
adoption 41–2, 47, 100
adult social care
agency social workers 248
concept of choice in 134
direct (cash) payments 134–5
in Northamptonshire 38–9, 249
private companies replacing public
sector organisations 243–5
purchaser–provider separation
118–21, *122*
rigging the market 121–7
AET (Academies Enterprise Trust)
181, *183*
agency workers 247–52
AILC (Association of Independent
LSCB Chairs) 63, 66, 67
Aitken, Jonathan 130
All Party Parliamentary Group for
Children (APPG Children) 289,
293, 294
All Wales Strategy on Mental
Handicap 125
Angel Solutions 181
APPG Children (All Party
Parliamentary Group for
Children) 289, 293, 294
Archer, Graham 291–2
arrest, powers of 204–5

Association of Directors of
Children's Services (ADCS)
84–6, 96, 97, 290–1
Association of Independent LSCB
Chairs (AILC) 63, 66, 67
Atos 222, 223–4
Attlee, Clement 175, 259
austerity, policy of 8, 39–40, 42–3,
101, 154–7, 171–2, 263–4

B
'Baby P' 3, 35, 37, 42, 286, 287
Baginsky, M. 183
banking crisis 2007-8 7, 150–3, 162
Darling on coalition government's
actions after 154–5
Jones on 155
Barker, Roger 266–7
Barnardo's 47, 100, 125, 126
Bath and North East Somerset
Council 243–4
BBC reports 181–2, 184, 201,
206–7, 215–16, 217, 219, 236,
264–5, 270
'Best Value' requirements 138–9
Beveridge Report 109–10
adding two new 'giants' to 174
'five giants' of 173–4
Bew, John 257
billionaires 170–1
Birmingham, children's services in
24, 28
Birmingham Prison 215
Blackrock 274
Blair, Tony 137, 138–40, 149
Brazil, Eleanor 102
Brexit 158
British Association of Social
Workers (BASW) 83–4, 111
Brook House 217, 218, 219
Brown, Gordon 141, 150
Butler, Patrick 11–12, 16, 25, 30,
45–6, 50–1

C
Cambridgeshire community health
services 198–9
Cameron, David 36, 38, 42, 43–4,
45–6, 47, 125, 159, 169, 171–2,
263–4
Campbell, Jane 135

Capita Business Services Ltd. 200,
222, 224, 256, 275
Cardy, Simon 3
care homes 232–9
financial collapse of private 233–4
Four Seasons 237–8
local authorities and payments to
private 233, 238–9
rigging the market 121–2
right-to-buy policy and impact
on 122–3
social security subsidies 121
Southern Cross 234–7
care management 119
care to tackle neglect 174, 231
for children 239–43
for older people 232–9
private companies replacing public
sector organisations 243–7
Carillion 264–8, 269–71, 271–4,
275
case management 119
Cavendish, Camilla 42
charities
expanding into family and
community services 125–6
grants available to voluntary
organisations and 125, 188–9
and involvement in outsourced
children's services 48–9
senior management of children's
47, 100
Chief Social Worker for Children
and Families 58–9, 71–2, 80, 81,
91–4, 95–6, 291
see also Trowler, Isabelle
child abuse, 'mandatory reporting'
of 78–9
child poverty 8
Child Safeguarding Practice Review
Panel 66, 67
Children Act 1989 51, 55, 293
Children Act 2004 63, 121, 281
Children and Social Work Bill
52–90
accreditation 69, 82–90
aim of increasing political control
of children's services 67–8
Child Safeguarding Practice
Review Panel 66, 67
'exemption clauses' 54–61

Knowledge and Skills Statement (KSS) 81–2
Labour response to 50–1
lack of consultation prior to 53
Local Safeguarding Children Boards 61–4, 65
Lord Watson commenting on 58–9
regulation of social workers 70–3
serious case reviews 64–7
social work education 74–80
children's centres 187–90
Children's Commissioner for England 104, 252, 292
children's homes, privatisation of 239–43
children's public health services 49, 245
Children's Services Improvement Boards 35, 57
children's social work and child protection services
  agency social workers 248
  alternative framework for future 294–9
  consultation on contracting out services to private companies 11–15
  DfE and meetings with private companies 23–9
  DfE-commissioned report on developing market 28–9, 99–100
  foundations of privatisation in place 132
  funding 37, 290–2
  funding gap, concerns over 292–4
  inherent weaknesses in contracting out process 278–9
  local authorities coerced into contracting services to independent trusts 33–4, 98, 102–3
  momentum to move services out from local authorities 29–34
  narrative of privatisation shaped by Cameron and Gove 39–51
  new providers for 45–6, 49–50
  Ofsted used to drive removal from local authorities' control 34–9
  partnerships between councils for improvement 303–4
  performance indicators 302
  poor performance, responding to 299–304
  promotion of sector-led improvements 302–3
  rethinking government strategy on trusts 279–81, 299–300
  separation from adult services 121
  six stages to privatising child protection 8–9
  statutory regulation changes, 2014, in move towards privatisation of 11–23
  under Thatcherism 131
  thresholds for accessing 293–4
  timeline 2013–15 10
  turnover of children's social workers 252
choice
  as an argument for creating markets 132–4
  direct (cash) payments and 134–5
  integral to 'third way' 146–7
  for patients 191–2
  'Tenants Choice' 225
Circle Holdings 56–7, 195–7
Clark, Alan 112
Climbié, Victoria 63, 281
Clinicenta 270
Coalition government 7–8
  2014 changes in statutory regulations 11–23
  austerity policy 8, 39–40, 42–3, 101, 154–7, 171–2, 263–4
  DfE and meetings with private companies 23–9
  pushing ahead with privatisation 157–63, 263–4
Cockburn, Jim 242–3
College of Social Work 69–70, 82–3, 93, 94
Community Care 49–50, 69, 73, 243–4, 252, 279
Community Care: An Agenda for Action 118–20
Community Care (Direct Payments) Act 1996 134, 135, 190
community health services, contracting out of 197–9
community safety and criminal justice 174

police 201–8
prisons 212–20
probation 208–12
compulsory competitive tendering (CCT) 127–30, 208
Conservative-led governments post 2010 7–8
2014 changes in statutory regulations 11–23
austerity policy 8, 39–40, 42–3, 101, 154–7, 171–2, 263–4
battles over funding under 289–94
DfE and meetings with private companies 23–9
improvement and innovation 283–9
momentum to move services out from local authorities 29–34
narrative of privatisation shaped by Cameron and Gove 39–51
pushing ahead with privatisation 157–63, 263–4
schools policy 178–81
using Ofsted to drive removal of children's services from local authorities 34–9
see also Children and Social Work Bill
consultancy firms 45
see also accountancy firms
contracts
A4e and issues with 221, 222
accreditation process 69, 82–3, 86, 93, 253
business competence concerns of private companies running 275–6
challenging award of 245–6
collapse of Carillion 264–71, 274
concerns over Atos and Capita 222–4
concerns over G4S running of 61–2, 206–7, 215–20
issues in management of 61–2, 256–7, 271
letting, public service 167–8
local authorities held to account over external 20–1, 27, 28
need for greater diversity in companies bidding for 273

performance of prisons under private 213, 214
probation service 206, 208–12
termination of 168, 179, 196, 197, 198, 199, 206, 212, 234, 271
track record on NHS 192–200
Virgin Care winning 243–7
Corbyn, Jeremy 257, 272, 277
corporations, power of 170
Coughlan, John 37
Crewe, Ivor 128, 128–9
criminal justice and community safety see community safety and criminal justice
Croisdale-Appleby, David 79, 101
Cusick, James 180

D
Daily Mail 204–5, 222, 242, 273–4
Daily Telegraph 38, 43, 195
Darling, Alistair 154–5, 156
Delivery Unit, public sector change 139
deregulation 115, 150, 229
Deregulation Bill, children's social services in 26–8
direct (cash) payments 134–5
disability benefit assessments 222–4
Donaghy, Baroness 26–8
Doncaster Children's Trust 30, 31, 32, 299, 300–1
Doncaster Council 29–32, 102, 300
Drakeford, Mark 143–4
Durham University 77

E
Edwards, Steve 287
electronic-tagging 202, 206–7, 209
Elvin, Andy 46–8, 56–7, 241–2
employment
agencies 248, 250–1
getting benefit claimants into 221–2
and recruitment of social workers 247–52
social security and 220–4
equalities helpline 220
Evans, Kathy 3–4
Evening Standard 237, 274
'exemption clauses,' Children and Social Work Bill 54–61

F

facilities management and
maintenance contracts 142–3,
271
family courts 207
fast-track work-based training
programmes 9, 41, 75–7, 78,
79–80
Featherstone, Brid 74, 298–9
Financial Times 208–9, 211, 236–7,
263–4
Firstline 95
Under Fives Initiative 125
foreign ownership of previously
public-owned resources 168–9
Forensic Science Service 207–8
foster care 101–2, 241–3
Foster Care Associates 242–3
Four Seasons 237–8
Fowler, Norman 124, 125
free schools 185–6
Frontline 44, 75–7, 78, 79, 80, 94, 99
and Josh Macalister 94–5
restrictions in Scotland and
Northern Ireland 79–80
see also Cavendish, Camilla
funding, battle over 289–94

G

G4S 203, 215–20, 219
2012 London Olympics contract
206
electronic tagging of offenders
202, 206–7, *209*
examination suites, sexual assault
247
failings in running prisons 215–16
government's equalities helpline
220
immigration removal centres
(IRCs) 217–18
policing involvement 202, 205
Secure Training Centres for young
people 61–2, 215–16, 218–19
Gallimore, Stuart 290–1
Garrett, Paul Michael 3
General Social Care Council
(GSCC) 71
Gibb, Moira 30, 104
Giddens, Anthony 144–5
Gilbert, Christine 181

Gilmour, Ian 116
Goodman, Steve 62, 95–6, 97
Goodwill, Robert 289–90
Gove, Michael 24, 29, 30, 39–43, 79,
180, 278
grants available to charities and
voluntary organisations 125,
188–9
Greening, Justine 59, 61, *68*, 88–9,
187, 188, 189
Grenfell Tower 227–30
Fire Inquiry 268–9
Griffiths, Roy 117–20, 134
The Guardian 8–9, 11–12, 16–17, 20,
25, 30–1, 38–9, 44–5, 51, 141–2,
156, 192–3, 202–3, 205–6, 212,
214–15, 218–19, 238, 239–40,
244, 247, 272–3
Gupta, Anna 298–9

H

Hackney Council 285
Haringey Council 35, 37
Harrison, Emma 221
Health and Care Professions
Council (HCPC) 70, 71
Heath, Edward 112, 113
Hennessy, Peter 110, 175–6
Hewitt, Patricia *162*
Hibbert-Biles, Hilary 184
Hillier, Meg 199
Hinchingbrooke Hospital 56–7,
195–7
Hinkley Point 269
Hodge, Margaret 194–5, 197
Holman, Bob 131
homelessness 224, 226, 229
House of Commons Home Affairs
Select Committee 217–18
House of Commons Justice Select
Committee 209–10
House of Commons Library
Briefing Paper 232
House of Commons Public
Accounts Committee 185–6,
193–4, 197, 199–200, 213, 256–7
housing
Grenfell Tower 227–30
history of council 224–6
New Labour policy 226
Thatcher's policy 122–3, 225–6

Westminster City Council scandal
226–7
Housing Act 1980 225
Hudson, Annie 30–1
Hutton, Will 272, 281–2

I
immigration removal centres (IRCs)
217–18, 219
The Independent 180, 210–11,
211–12, 245, 268–9
Independent Children's Homes
Association (ICHA) 241
innovation and improvement 283–9
Reclaiming Social Work model
83, 96, 97, 284–6
Signs of Safety model 287–8
Innovation Fund 95, 96, 97, 284,
288–9
internal markets, creation of 117–21
International Monetary Fund (IMF)
crisis 113–14
investment banks 115, 142–3
Isle of Wight 67, 286, 288, 304

J
Jackson, Mary 95
Jenkins, Simon 137, 271
Jones, Owen 155
Jordan, Bill 147–8
Jordan, Charlie 147–8

K
Kensington and Chelsea Council
227–30
children's services 296–7
key players 91–102
lack of professional experience in
social work 103–4
marginalisation of other relevant
organisations 104–5
networks of 104
taking statutory children's social
work out of local authorities
102–3
Kingston and Richmond Council
32
Klein, Naomi 157–8
Knapp, M. 132–3
Knowledge and Skills Statement
(KSS) 81–2

KPMG
accreditation process development
69, 82–3, 86, 93
Carillion and 267–8
Grenfell Fire Inquiry 268–9
Sedgemoor administrator 240
Kynaston, David 175, 224–5

L
Labour
commits to reversing privatisation
trend 257, 272, 277
manifesto 2017 78, 257
response to Children and Social
Work Bill 50–1
response to revised statutory
regulation proposals 19–21, 26
see also New Labour
Labour-controlled councils, forced
into contracting out children's
services 33–4, 38
LaingBuisson 29, 99, 233, 305
Lancashire County Council 245–6
Lansley, Andrew 191, 192
Le Grand, Julian 28, 29, 30, 98–100,
146–7, 163
Leeds children's services 297–8
Letwin, Oliver *123*
Lewell-Buck, Emma 21, 53, 59, 88
Lewisham Council 249–50
Liquid Personnel Ltd, 250–1
Local Authority Social Services Act
1970 111
Local Government Association
(LGA) 35, 56, 57, 72–3, 289, 292
Local Safeguarding Children Boards
(LSCBs) 61–4, 65, 183
London Olympics 2012 206
looked-after children and schools
184
Loughton, Tim 60–1, 69, 293–4
LSCBs (Local Safeguarding
Children Boards) 61–4, 65, 183
Luyendijk, Joris 151

M
Macalister, Josh 94–5, 104
Major, John 130, 140
managerialism 117–18
mandatory reporting 78–9

May, Theresa 7, 52, 67, *89*, 156, 272–3
McCabe, Steve 19
McCarthy, Mike 124
McNicoll, Andy 69
media attacks on social workers 42
Medway Secure Training Centre (STC) 215–16
Meek, James 168
Meller, David 276
Mendoza, Kerry-Anne 170, 171–2
Metro 270, 274
Michalska, Alison 291, 303
Milburn, Alan 161–2, 190
Miller, Jo 31, 300–1
Milne, Seamus 156
Mitchell, Andrew 259
Morgan, Nicky 41, 49, 82
Morning Lane Associates (MLA) 82, 93, 95–6, 97, 284, 285
Morris, Kate 298–9
Mott Macdonald 84, 253
MTCnovo 216–17
Munn, Meg 19–21
Munro, Eileen 60, 78, 287

N
Narey, Martin 41, 79, 80, 98, 100–2, 104, 163, 213–14, *216*
Nash, Lord 53, 68
National Audit Office (NAO) 95–6, 140, 199, 211–12
National Health Service (NHS) 190–201
  Carillion contracts 270, 271
  concerns over privatising of services 200–1
  continuing costs of PFI to 141–2
  contracting out of community health services 198–9
  Foundation Trusts 190–1
  Hinchingbrooke Hospital 56–7, 195–7
  out-of-hours GP services contract 192–5
  outsourcing to Capita 200
  profits taken out by private sector 192
  purchaser–provider separation 118
  spending on agency staff 248
  Virgin Care contracts 244, 245–7

Warner on 24
National Intermediate Treatment Fund 125
National Offender Management Service (NOMS) 213
National Society for the Prevention of Cruelty to Children (NSPCC) 15, 65, *126*
neglect, care to tackle 174, 231
  for children 239–43
  for older people 232–9
  private companies replacing public sector organisations 243–7
New Labour 137–53, 253
  assessments of 147–50
  banking crisis 2007-8 150–3
  'Best Value' requirements 138–9
  a continuum of Thatcherism 137–8, 148, 149
  housing policy 226
  NHS Foundation Trusts 190–1
  opening up public services to private sector 139–40, 143
  prisons policy 213
  public–private finance initiatives (PFI) 140–3
  public sector change Delivery Unit 139
  schools policy 177–8
  third way 140–50
  welfare system 220–1
Newsam, Malcolm 102
NHS and Community Care Act 1990 120, 121, 134, 190
North Yorkshire children's services 298
Northamptonshire County Council 38–9, 248–9, 304
Nottingham University Hospitals NHS Trust 271
nursing services, children's 49, 245

O
Ofsted
  actions after 'inadequate' judgements of children's social services 98, 103, 286, 299–304
  changed inspection process 301–2
  on children's homes 241
  findings on stability and continuity in leadership and workforce 284

'good' and 'outstanding' children's
    services 296–8
impact of 'inadequate' ratings on
    local authorities 36–8, 301
inspections of multi-academy trust
    chains 179
outsourced service inspections 28
school inspections 180, 181
Spielman appointed chief
    inspector 66–7
statistics on 'inadequate' children's
    services 46
used to drive removal of children's
    services from local authorities
    34–9
Oliver, Michael 135
Open Public Services White Paper
    2011 159
Opportunities for Volunteering
    grants 125
Osborne, George 156–7, 172, 273–4
out-of-hours GP services 192–5
outsourcing
    changing attitudes to 255–6
    companies moving beyond core
        competencies 275–6
    concerns over 167–8, 201, 256–7
    DfE meeting with large
        companies to explore, children's
        services 23–9
    to increase consumer choice
        132–4
    inherent weaknesses in 278–9
    momentum to move children's
        services out from local
        authorities 29–34
    Northamptonshire County
        Council 38–9, 248–9, 304
    political bias and skew in forcing
        of 33–4, 38
    track record with private
        companies and NHS 192–200
    undermining public trust in 256
ownership of previously public-
    owned resources, foreign 168–9
Oxfordshire County Council 184

P
partnerships between councils
    303–4

pay and bonuses 120, 142, 171,
    229–30, *242*, 251, 266, 274
Pemberton, Max 195–6
performance
    addressing poor 299–304
    indicators 302
Perry, Roy 36, 303
Persimmon 229–30
personal independence payments
    (PIP) 222–4
personal social services and social
    work, future of
    alternative framework 294–9
    a new agenda 278–83
Peston, Robert 151–2, 170
PFI *see* public–private finance
    initiatives (PFI)
police 201–8
poor
    discourse of 'welfare' and 258–9
    and politics of austerity 8, 39–40,
        42–3, 101
    under Thatcher 127
Poor Law 110
Porter, Shirley 226–7
Poyner, Chris 214–15
Pratley, Nils 238
Presidents Club 276–7
Prison Reform Trust 213, 214
prisons 212–20
private equity 45, 152–3, 235, 238,
    239, 287
private security firms 202–3, 204
    see also G4S
privatisation
    accountancy firms' role in
        promoting and pursuing 160–2
    an alternative agenda to 278–83
    banks as main beneficiaries of 143
    of care homes for older people
        121–2, 232–9
    Carillion collapse and possible
        turn against 264–71, 271–4,
        277–8
    challenges in changing narrative
        on 257–9
    Coalition pushing ahead with
        157–63, 263–4
    companies moving beyond core
        competencies 275–6
    concerns over 167–72

Corbyn commits to reversing
  trend 257, 272, 277
foreign ownership and 168–9
of health services and hospitals
  190–201
of housing 224–30
May seeks a more diverse market
  place 272–3
morality and behaviour concerns
  of private company leaders
  276–7
moves under New Labour
  139–40, 143
of police 201–8
policy of austerity used to push
  for greater 154–7
priorities of owners and
  shareholder 109
of prisons 212–20
of probation 208–12
prospects for an end to moves
  towards 277–8
Public Accounts Committee
  comments on 256–7
public opinion on 255
reflections on 253–60
of schools and children's centres
  177–90
of social care services 243–7
of social security and employment
  220–4
of social work workforce 247–53
of youth custody training services
  61–2, 216–17, 218–19
privatisation moves under
  Thatcherism
alleged improvements often not
  delivered 129–30
'choice' as an argument for
  creating markets 132–4
compulsory competitive tendering
  (CCT) 127–30
direct (cash) payments 134–5
purchaser–provider separation
  117–21, 122
rigging the market 121–7
selling policies to electorate 129
privatisation of children's social
  services and child protection
  services
children's care 239–43

concerns that 'exemption clauses' a
  gateway to 56–7, 59
consultation on contracting out
  services to private companies
  11–15
deregulation proposals and House
  of Lords debate 26–8
DfE and meetings with private
  companies 23–9
DfE-commissioned report on
  developing market 28–9, 99–100
government-controlled
  accreditation and 89
momentum to move services out
  from local authorities 29–34
narrative shaped by Cameron and
  Gove 39–51
new providers for 49–50
Ofsted used to drive 34–9
six stages to 8–9
statutory regulation changes in
  move towards 11–23
probation services 208–12
Professional Capabilities Framework
  (PCF) 81, 83, 93
public opinion on privatisation of
  public services 255
public–private finance initiatives
  (PFI) 140–3, 192
making profits out of facilities
  management and maintenance
  contracts 142–3
purchaser–provider separation
  117–21, 122, 190
PwC 160, 161, 269

R

Rainsbrook Secure Training Centre
  216–17, 218–19
Randox Testing 207
Rawnsley, Andrew 149
Reading Council 34
Reclaiming Social Work model 83,
  96, 97, 284–6
recruitment and employment of
  social workers 247–52
Rees, Janet 242–3
regulation
  of public services 133–4
  of social workers 70–3, 150
Renwick, C. 258

Ridley, Nicholas 123–4, 126–7
rigging the market 121–7
right-to-buy policy 122–3, 225
Rogowski, Steve 4
Rotherham 300–1

S

Sampson, Anthony 140–1, 142–3, 160–1
Sanctuary Personnel 251
Sandbrook, Dominic 113–14
Schooling, Eleanor 301–2
schools 177–87
  free 185–6
  local authorities and 178, 179, 182, *183*, 185
  looked-after children and 184
  making profits from 179–80, 180–1
  marketisation and competition 183–4, 185
  under New Labour 177–8
  see also academy schools
Scourfield, Peter 234–5
Secure Training Centres for young people 61–2, 215–17, 218–19
security firms, private 202–3, 204
  see also G4S
Sedgemoor children's homes 239–40
Serco 205–7, *209*, 220, 247, 275
  out-of-hours GP services contract 192–5
serious case reviews (SCRs) 64–7
  'national panel of independent experts' 65, 66
Serwotka, Mark 220
seven 'I's of being 287–8
Shaxson, Nicholas 169
Signs of Safety model 287–8
six Ts in rethinking government strategy on children's social work services 279–81
Sky News 217
Slough Children's Services Trust 300
social security and employment 220–4
social work and personal social services, future of
  alternative framework 294–9

  a new agenda 278–83
social work education 74–80
  costs of different programmes 80
  Department of Health commissioned report 101
  fast-track work-based training programme 9, 41, 75–7, 78, 79–80
  Gove critical of 39–40
  Narey's commissioned report 41, 79, 81, 101
  universities, social work degree programmes 77–8
  see also Croisdale-Appleby, David; Frontline
social workers
  accreditation process *see* accreditation
  Gove critical of 39–40, 41
  Knowledge and Skills Statement (KSS) 81–2
  media attacks on 42
  privatisation of recruitment and employment of 247–52
  regulation of 70–3, *150*
  and shift in perception of public servants 146–7
Society of Local Authority Chief Executives (SOLACE) 35
Sodexo 209, 210–11
Southern Cross 234–7
Spielman. Amanda 66–7
Stevenson, Luke 49–50
subsidies, social security 121
The Sun 42
The Sunday Times 202, 204
Sunderland Council 34, 103, 300
Sure Start children's centres 187–9, 190, 283
Surrey Council 250
Sutton Trust 181–2, 189

T

tax havens 169, 259
Tett, Gillian 150–1
Thatcher, Margaret 114–16, 263
  housing policy 225–6
  out of step with electorate on tax cuts 128
  privatisation a part of philosophy of 130

puzzle of re-election of 128–9
on welfare state 110–11
Thatcherism
'choice' as an argument for
creating markets 132–4
Coalition government and
enhanced 158–60
compulsory competitive tendering
(CCT) 127–30
direct (cash) payments 134–5
Giddens on 144
Holman on impact of 131
New Labour a continuum of
137–8, 148, 149
purchaser–provider separation
117–21, 122
push to privatise and minimise
welfare state 114–16
rigging the market 121–7
third way 140–50
assessments of 147–50
Giddens on 145
Le Grand on shift in perception of
public servants 146–7
public–private finance initiatives
(PFI) 140–3
social work and 147–8
Thoburn, J. 74
The Times 42, 269
Timmins, Nicholas 112–13, 225,
258–9
Timpson, Edward 17, 28, 29, 41, 49,
56, 60, 65, 67, 100
Tower Hamlets 301, 304
Toynbee, Polly 142, 149–50, 152–3,
159, 160, 162–3, 172, 226, 271–2
trade mark protection 287
transparency issues 33, 48, 275–6,
279, 281, 300
Trowler, Isabelle 28, 29, 56, 62, 72,
80, 82–3, 87, 91–4, 97, 98, 99,
291
potential conflict of interest with
MLA 95–6
see also Chief Social Worker for
Children
trust, public 256, 257
Turnell, Andrew 287

U
Unison 84
UnitingCare Partnership LLP 198–9
universities, social work degree
programmes 77–8

V
Virgin Care 243–7

W
Wakefield City Academies Trust
178–9
Walker, David 129, 149–50, 152–3,
159, 160, 162–3, 172, 226, 229
Warner, Norman 23–5
Watson, Lord 53, 58–9
wealth, ownership and distribution
of 170–1, 259
welfare state
changing attitudes and language
258–9
period of consensus 109–11
rolling back 173–6
Thatcherism and push to
minimise 114–16
wearing away of consensus
112–14
Westminster City Council scandal
226–7
White, Alan 167
White, Sue 298–9
Whitfield, Nick 32, 33, 34, 102–3
Willow, Carolyne 4, 51, 55
Wilshaw, Michael 37, 182
Wiltshire Council 122, 135, 138
Windsor and Maidenhead Council
32–3
Wood, Alan 28, 29, 30, 61–2, 62–3,
64, 66, 97–8, 304
Wood, Zoe 239–40
Worcestershire County Council 34

Y
YouGov 255
Young, Hugo 127–8

Z
Zahawi, Nadhim 37, 276, 289, 290